ACHIEVING ACCESS

A volume in the series
The Culture and Politics of Health Care Work
Edited by Suzanne Gordon and Sioban Nelson

A list of titles in this series is available at
www.cornellpress.cornell.edu

Achieving Access

Professional Movements and the
Politics of Health Universalism

Joseph Harris

ILR PRESS
AN IMPRINT OF
CORNELL UNIVERSITY PRESS
ITHACA AND LONDON

First published 2017 by Cornell University Press

Printed in the United States of America

Library of Congress Cataloging-in-Publication Data

Names: Harris, Joseph, 1976 August 23– author.
Title: Achieving access : professional movements and the politics of health
    universalism / Joseph Harris.
Description: Ithaca : ILR Press, an imprint of Cornell University Press, 2017. |
    Series: The culture and politics of health care work | Includes bibliographical
    references and index.
Identifiers: LCCN 2017009676 (print) | LCCN 2017010235 (ebook) | ISBN
    9781501709968 (cloth : alk. paper) | ISBN 9781501709975 (pbk. : alk. paper) |
    ISBN 9781501714740 (epub/mobi) | ISBN 9781501714832 (pdf)
Subjects: LCSH: Health services accessibility—Thailand. | Health services
    accessibility—Brazil. | Health services accessibility—South Africa. | AIDS
    (Disease)—Treatment—Government policy—Thailand. | AIDS (Disease)—
    Treatment—Government policy—Brazil. | AIDS (Disease)—Treatment—
    Government policy—South Africa. | Medical policy—Thailand. | Medical
    policy—Brazil. | Medical policy—South Africa.
Classification: LCC RA395.T5 H37 2017 (print) | LCC RA395.T5 (ebook) |
    DDC 362.1—dc23
LC record available at https://lccn.loc.gov/2017009676

Cornell University Press strives to use environmentally responsible suppliers and materials to the fullest extent possible in the publishing of its books. Such materials include vegetable-based, low-VOC inks and acid-free papers that are recycled, totally chlorine-free, or partly composed of nonwood fibers. For further information, visit our website at cornellpress.cornell.edu.

Contents

Acknowledgments

When I first set out to study a sweeping new health care program in Thailand that was being praised by the rural poor and pilloried by the rich, I never could have imagined the monumental nature of the journey I was about to undertake, the remarkable stories I would have the privilege to hear, or the incredible debts that I would owe to so many extraordinary people who showed me endless generosity along the way.

While many scholars had written book-length works about HIV/AIDS in the developing world, comparative study of universal health coverage in the industrializing world had yet to find many takers. This is perhaps because the idea of resource-constrained countries making such commitments has until recently seemed preposterous. So the notion of a wave of countries making such expansive commitments to both universal health care *and* life-saving AIDS medication at the same time seemed completely implausible.

And so it was that for the first few years that I studied this wave of expansive commitments by nations in the industrializing world, I would sometimes wonder if what I had stumbled upon was real or all in my head. The process of sense-making (and polishing) has been a long one that began in graduate school and has extended right up to the publication of this book. In the process, concern with universal access to antiretroviral therapy and "universal coverage" has become regular features of the broader development landscape, most recently embodied in the Sustainable Development Goals. A book about a previously unidentified phenomenon now has an audience. That this manuscript is a book at all is due to the countless people who have helped and supported me along the way.

The largest debt I owe is to Gay Seidman, who encouraged me to look outside Thailand to see if other countries were adopting similar policies as Thailand's Universal Coverage program. When I found that they were, she encouraged me to make my work comparative and provided the assistance and contacts that would play an important role in making my case studies on Brazil and South Africa successful. While this book has taken a shape of its own since those early days, Gay's vision, tireless support, and incisive feedback are enormous reasons why this book exists today.

Chad Goldberg, Christina Ewig, Sida Liu, and Mara Loveman have each contributed powerfully to the development of this book. Chad Goldberg was responsible for turning me on to the welfare state literature, and his advice, suggestions, and encouragement played a key role in the development of my thinking. Christina Ewig deepened my appreciation for that literature as it had been applied to the developing world, and was very generous in acquainting me with the field of health politics, while also serving as a bridge to political science. Sida Liu's encyclopedic knowledge of the professions literature provided me with an important foundation in a field many had lost an appreciation for but would prove crucial in helping me to develop my idea of "professional movements." Mara Loveman's incisive criticism improved my work immensely, and her expertise on ethnoracial politics would help me to produce a related article on those issues. Mustafa Emirbayer, Myra Marx Ferree, Erik Olin Wright, Katherine Bowie, Thongchai Winichakul, Kannikar Elbow, Michael Cullinane, and Larry Ashman also deserve acknowledgement for their support of my work. The Center for Southeast Asian Studies at the University of Wisconsin-Madison and the U.S. Department of Education played an important role in supporting my graduate work through fellowships from the Foreign Language and Area Studies Fellowship Program. Marie Villemin, Alison Porri, and the World Health Organization deserve thanks for their assistance.

Since graduate school, my ideas have perhaps been even more thoroughly shaped by friends and peers, among them Tod van Gunten, Shiri Noy, Brent Kaup, Amy Quark, Adam Slez, Matt Desmond, John Gerring, Jim McGuire, Sanyu Mojola, Laura Heideman, Oriol Mirosa, Mytoan Nguyen, Carly Schall, Bob Seifert, Steve Kemble, and Philip Verhoef. Harel Shapira deserves special recognition for his thoughtful criticism, support, and encouragement. Michael Reich generously offered a round of comments on the final version of the manuscript.

Many who visit Thailand regard the Land of Smiles as an easy place to live. This is certainly true. However, the language and cultural differences can make it a hard place to know well. While I am fortunate to have developed strong language and cultural capacities over nearly two decades, many people helped make study and comprehension of these issues easier, among them Thitinan Pongsudhirak and the staff at the Institute of Security and International Studies at Chulalongkorn University, Viroj NaRanong and the Thailand Development Research Institute, Chayan Vaddhanaphuti and the Regional Center for Sustainable Development at Chiang Mai University, Viroj Tangcharoensathien, Wirun Limsawart, Suwat Chariyalertsak, Aphaluck Bhatiasevi, Mukdawan Sakboon, Wisit Wangwinyoo, Nuttarote Wangwinyoo, Peter Cox, Michael Nelson, Peter Shearman, Nalinee Tantuvanit, Chanetwallop Khumthong, Scott Stonington, and Felicity Aulino. Nathchar Naowarojna, Oraphan Tatha, and Uravadee Chanchamsang served as able research assistants. I would also like to thank Dr. Kijja Jearwattanakanok, Dr. Worawut Phowatcharakul, and Dr. Prajin Laothiang and the many other wonderful people who helped deepen my knowledge of the Thai health care system at Nakorn Ping, San Sai, and Om Koi Hospitals. My research in Thailand was funded through the generous financial support of a Fulbright-Hays Doctoral Dissertation Award with assistance from the National Research Council of Thailand.

Suriya Wongkongkathep of Thailand's Ministry of Public Health deserves more thanks than I could possibly give. Much of my understanding of the intricacies of Thailand's health care system and its politics has been shaped by the many conversations we have had and the countless doors he opened for me to a variety of important voices. To say his generosity has been immense would be an understatement.

Comprehension of South Africa's complicated political history (and health care system) would never have been possible without the assistance of many kind and generous South Africans who provided assistance in a myriad of ways, among them Cathi Albertyn and the Centre for Applied Legal Studies, Mark Heywood and Section 27 (formerly the AIDS Law Project), Heinz Klug, Neva Makgetla, Shula Marks, Shireen Ally, Alex van den Heever, Sue le Roux, Catherine van de Ruit, David Fowkes, and Sara Compion. Nicole Lyn and Michael Chau served as research assistants on South Africa. A Scott Kloeck-Jenson award and a departmental fellowship provided financial support for my work in South Africa, and the South African Historical Archives served as an indispensable resource for materials of use to the project.

Understanding the intricacies of Brazil's approach to providing access to health care and medicine was an equally tall order. However, Kurt Weyland, John Stephens, Amy Nunn, Tulia Falleti, Matthew Flynn, Gabriela Costa Chaves, Sandi Chapman, Elize Massard da Fonseca, Carlos Ocké-Reis, Fabio de Sa e Silva, Carlos Siqueira, and Alecia McGregor helped make that task immensely more manageable. Juliana de Mello Libardi Maia deserves special recognition for her research assistance on the history of Brazil's health system and AIDS policies, along with Adel Faitaninho, Paula Sanchez, and Samantha Rick.

I have had the incredible fortune to be surrounded by the most amiable and supportive colleagues one could ever ask for at Boston University's Department of Sociology. It has been a blessing to see this project through to fruition there as a member of the faculty. At BU, the project has benefited from feedback at numerous forums, including the Society, Politics, and Culture Workshop run by Julian Go; the Center for Global Health and Development Scientific Meeting; and the Tertulia Junior Faculty Forum. Especially warm thanks are reserved for Alya Guseva, Pat Rieker, Sigrun Olafsdottir (the department's health team). Current chair Nazli Kibria and immediate past chair Nancy Ammerman have been incredible sources of support.

The project also benefited from substantial feedback and criticism outside BU. Here, the generous insights, feedback, and criticism I received following presentations at six forums are particularly worth noting: the Sampran Forum maintained by the founding members of Thailand's Rural Doctors' Society; the Southeast Asia Research Group, run by Allen Hicken, Eddy Malesky, Tom Pepinsky, and Dan Slater (who is owed special thanks); a graduate seminar at the Harvard School of Public Health hosted by Tom Bossert and Kevin Croke; the Revisiting Remaking Modernity Miniconference Session on the Professions hosted by Ming-Cheng Lo; a symposium on Professions and Professionals in the Developing World at Brown University hosted by Nitsan Chorev and Andrew Schrank; and a session of the American Political Science Association meetings organized by Erik Kuhonta.

Earlier presentations of this work were made at the Thailand Development Research Institute and the Chiang Mai Regional Center for Sustainable Development in Thailand; the American Sociological Association Annual meetings; the Association for Asian Studies; the Joint Meeting of the Midwest/North Central Sociological Association; and the Sociology of Economic Change and Development brownbag, the Politics, Culture, and Society brownbag, and the Center for Southeast Asian Studies Friday Forum at the University of Wisconsin-Madison.

I am also grateful to the College of Arts and Sciences Dean's Office and the Department of Sociology at BU for their generous subvention that has helped make this project a reality. The Department's Morris Fund helped defray the cost of formatting, indexing, proofreading, and editing, to which Rebecca Farber contributed much.

Portions of chapter 2 (including table 2.1 and figure 2.1) have been published previously as "Who Governs? Autonomous Political Networks as a Challenge to Power in Thailand" in *Journal of Contemporary Asia* (2015), copyright © Journal of Contemporary Asia, reprinted by permission of Taylor & Francis Ltd, www.tandfonline.com on behalf of Journal of Contemporary Asia.

An earlier version of this material appeared in *The Journal of Health Politics, Policy, and Law* under the title "'Developmental Capture' of the State: Explaining Thailand's Universal Coverage Policy" (2015).

There truly could not have been a better team of people to work with than the editors and staff at Cornell University Press. Frances Benson immediately saw the promise of this project when we first met. Both she and series editor Suzanne Gordon have helped to sharpen the argument and broaden the appeal of the book. They have been a real pleasure to work with. I am also grateful to the assistance of Emily Powers, Susan Barnett, Karen Laun, Martin Schneider, and the input and feedback of the editorial committee and of the anonymous reviewers.

My wife, Stefanie Shull, and our two children, Christoph and Dominick, have been the most wonderful, patient, and tolerant fellow travelers on this journey that one could ask for. Special thanks are reserved for Stefanie, who forsook two job offers in Washington, D.C., to move to Wisconsin with me on the promise that my graduate school career would go somewhere. She has been my companion from the project's beginning, through all its ups and downs. I could not have done it without her.

While the kind assistance of these people and institutions has no doubt improved my manuscript immeasurably, any errors or mistakes are my own responsibility.

This book is dedicated to people engaged in the struggle to expand access to health care and medicine around the world. A portion of the proceeds from the sale of this book will go toward supporting their efforts.

Abbreviations

ABRASCO	Brazilian Post-Graduate Association for Public Health
AIDS	Acquired Immune Deficiency Syndrome
ALP	AIDS Law Project
ANC	African National Congress
ARENA	National Renewal Alliance
ARV	antiretroviral medication
AZT	zidovudine
CALS	Centre for Applied Legal Studies
CEBES	Center for Brazilian Health Studies
CL	compulsory licensing
COSATU	Congress of South African Trade Unions
CPMF	Provisional Contribution on Financial Contributions Tax
DSG	Drug Study Group
GEMS	Government Employee Medical Scheme
GEAR	Growth, Employment, and Redistribution Program
GPO	Government Pharmaceutical Office
GTPI/REBRIP	Working Group on Intellectual Property of the Brazilian Network for the Integration of Peoples
HIV	Human Immunodeficiency Virus
ILO	International Labor Organization
IMF	International Monetary Fund
INAMPS	Instituto Nacional Assistência Médica Previdência Social
MASA	Medical Association of South Africa
MSF	Médecins Sans Frontières (Doctors without Borders)
NACOSA	National AIDS Committee of South Africa
NAMDA	National Medical and Dental Association
NAPWA	National Association of People with AIDS

NEHAWU	National Education Health and Allied Workers Union
NGO	nongovernmental organization
NHI	National Health Insurance
NPPHCN	National Progressive Primary Health Care Network
PEPFAR	President's Emergency Plan For AIDS Relief
PMDB	Brazilian Democratic Movement Party
PSF	Family Health Program
PT	Workers' Party
RDP	Reconstruction and Development Programme
SACP	South African Communist Party
SAHSSO	South African Health and Social Services Organisation
SAHWCO	South African Health Workers Congress
SAMA	South African Medical Association
SUDS	Unified and Decentralized Health System
SUS	Unified Health System
TAC	Treatment Action Campaign
TNCA	Thai NGO Coalition on AIDS
TRIPS	WTO Agreement on Trade-Related Aspects of Intellectual Property
UNDP	United Nations Development Programme
WHO	World Health Organization
WTO	World Trade Organization

ACHIEVING ACCESS

Introduction

This book is about explaining historical change: how parts of the developing world transitioned from a moment characterized by what I call "aristocratic health care" to an altogether different moment characterized by "health universalism." Prior to the 1990s, access to health care and life-saving drugs in the developing world was largely a matter of privilege. In the era of "aristocratic health care," only the privileged (and politically active) few—the rich, civil servants, and employees of large businesses—enjoyed the benefits of modern medicine. Very generally, the aristocracy paid for care themselves or received it through membership in elite state or private health insurance schemes. The vast majority—many of whom were poor and living in rural areas—relied on state programs that were narrow and limited, the individual charity of doctors, and the unpredictable effects of "traditional medicine." In the 1990s, however, these exclusionary health care regimes began to give way to a more inspiring but largely unexpected new mode of health universalism. Standing far apart from the kinds of health care programs that existed before them, these programs were "anti-elitist" by nature and, in line with their European counterparts in the Global North, aspired to make increasingly comprehensive access to health care and medicine available to all.

The broadening of state obligations to health care and medicine was especially puzzling because it took place at a time when a variety of factors would seem to have predisposed governments to rein in government spending rather than expand government programs. During the tenures of Ronald Reagan in the United States and Margaret Thatcher in Great Britain, a neoliberal logic had achieved hegemonic status in the 1980s. This policy program emphasized the privatization of government services, the weakening of social entitlements, and the liberalization of government regulation. At the same time, the emergence of the HIV/AIDS epidemic—an epidemic that disproportionately affected the developing world—had decimated populations and left governments and international organizations scrambling over how to respond. Yet the expansion of access to health care and treatment for AIDS occurred in countries that experts had generally deemed too poor and resource-constrained to support such programs. Moreover, they took place at a time when health care costs were exploding and medical expertise was scarce.

While the broadening of state obligations to health care and medicine unfolded unevenly throughout the world, by the 2000s their growing significance and clout could increasingly be seen in bold new transnational institutions. In January 2012, Thailand hosted an awards conference for scholars and practitioners in public health, with the theme "Moving towards Universal Health Coverage." At the conference, representatives from some sixty countries agreed to the Bangkok Statement on Universal Health Coverage. The statement made reference to the World Health Organization's *World Health Report* of 2010 and the World Health Assembly's Resolution 64.9 of May 2011, both of which drew attention to the issue of universal health coverage. Just three months later, delegates from twenty-one countries (including the United States) met in Mexico and signed the Mexico City Political Declaration on Universal Coverage. However, the surprising shift in support of universal coverage was perhaps embodied nowhere more forcefully than at the United Nations, where on December 12, 2012, the UN General Assembly passed a resolution in support of universal coverage with some ninety co-sponsors. WHO Director General Margaret Chan has since called universal coverage the "single most important concept that public health has to offer" (Chan 2012), and in recent years, more than one hundred countries have sought WHO technical assistance to achieve universal coverage (Chan 2016, 5).

Illustrating the extent of the shift, even conservative international organizations, which had previously promoted policies eroding health care coverage, embraced the movement toward universal health care. David de Ferranti, former vice president of the World Bank, and Julio Frenk, former minister of health for Mexico and dean of the Harvard School of Public Health, penned an op-ed in the *New York Times* in 2012 titled "Towards Universal Health Coverage" that drew attention to efforts to institutionalize universal health care programs in such places as Brazil, China, Colombia, Ghana, India, Mexico, the Philippines, Rwanda, South Africa, Thailand, and Vietnam (de Ferranti and Frenk 2012). The op-ed was particularly symbolic given that de Ferranti, while an executive at the World Bank, had coauthored the 1987 flagship report *Financing Health*

Services for Developing Countries: An Agenda for Reform. The report expressly called on government to *get out of* the business of health care and to dismantle measures intended to make access to health care easier. The World Bank itself would subsequently embark on not one but two major projects that aimed to support national efforts to implement universal coverage.

However, as remarkable and sweeping as this shift was at the international level, even more remarkable were the dynamics driving policy change inside many countries. Often, the countries making radical new commitments to universal coverage were newly emerging democracies. And in some of these countries, reform efforts were being led *not* by those most in need but rather by movements of doctors who had seen the devastating effects of exclusion under dictatorship and had sought to expand access to health care *on behalf of* those in need following democratization. In countries like Thailand, progressive doctors working as state bureaucrats convinced an innovative new political party to put universal health care on their campaign platform. They then ensured that the party fulfilled its promise by implementing the policy as a national pilot project before it became law. In Brazil, a similar movement of medical professionals concerned with public health embedded principles of universalism, equity, and participation in the country's new constitution. They then played key roles drafting legislation in the Health Ministry and promoting programs to bring health care to the masses and to hold the state accountable.

At the same time that this movement to expand access to health care was gaining steam, a separate but related movement to expand access to medicine for victims of HIV/AIDS was also forming. While scientists had discovered that AZT (zidovudine) could slow the progress of the AIDS virus in the mid-1980s, in 1996 scientists at the International AIDS Conference announced that a combination of these antiretroviral (ARV) drugs had the power to stop the progression of AIDS in its tracks and turn a once-fatal illness into a chronic disease. By 2015, some 17 million AIDS patients around the world would have access to this life-saving cocktail of medication (UNAIDS 2016). The international community would play an important role helping to finance national efforts to expand access to the cocktail through new global health institutions—like the Global Fund to Fight AIDS, Tuberculosis, and Malaria—as well as the U.S. government's President's Emergency Plan for AIDS Relief (PEPFAR). Collectively, these organizations would funnel billions into efforts to provide ARV treatment in countries devastated by AIDS. Yet the uneven expansion of access to this new "essential medicine" in different countries would underscore the critical role of *national* politics in the life-and-death stakes of emerging treatment for AIDS.

Unlike the movements to expand access to health care, the movements to expand access to life-saving medicine were by and large not being driven by doctors. A vocal AIDS movement played an important role in advocating for treatment through traditional social movement activities that included street protests and demonstrations. While physicians were frequent participants, even more important was the role of lawyers and other activist medical professionals with legal training. In countries like South Africa and Thailand, these movements were embodied in organizations like the AIDS Law Project and the Drug Study Group, social movement organizations in which use of the law was not merely a tactic to expand access to medicine but was inscribed much more fundamentally into the organizations' identity.

This book examines efforts to expand access to health care and AIDS medicine in Thailand, Brazil, and South Africa. Although these countries are geographically far apart, they share many similarities as newly industrializing countries engaged in processes of democratic opening. Scholars have often suggested that expansionary social policy is the product of left-wing parties and labor unions or bottom-up people's movements. From a strictly rational perspective, that these groups would be at the forefront of such change makes perfect sense. After all, expanding access to health care and medicine would seem to be in their interest, and they would appear to have a lot to gain.

While this book recognizes the role they often play, it focuses on a different, more puzzling set of actors whose actions are sometimes even more decisive in expanding access to health care and medicine: elites from esteemed professions who, rationally speaking, aren't in need of health care or medicine themselves and who would otherwise seem to have little to gain from such policies. This group includes doctors like Sanguan Nitayarumphong and Paulo Teixeira, whose work with the poor and needy informed their advocacy for universal health care in Thailand and Brazil while also putting them into conflict with the medical profession of which they were a part. How is it that these people would play such an important and active role in making change happen?

In the countries I examine, efforts to expand access to health care and AIDS medication have been led by a certain kind of elite. While specialists and other doctors working in large urban (and often private) hospitals often hold conservative ideological positions, oppose major reforms, and seek to uphold a status quo that serves their interests, my work draws attention to "professional movements" of progressive doctors, and lawyers, and other medical professionals with access to state resources and training in the law. Doctors and lawyers in these movements often began their careers as activists championing the interests of marginalized populations. Although their knowledge, networks, and privileged positions in the state set them apart from ordinary citizens, they frequently occupy a status on the periphery of the profession. How these relatively marginal professional subdivisions manage to triumph over the opposition of the broader profession is therefore an important issue taken up in this book.

This focus on professional movements is not to suggest that the traditional social movement activism of HIV-positive AIDS activists played no role in some of the dramatic changes that swept the globe related to access to AIDS treatment. After all, important accounts have illustrated how lay citizens have "forced science to be open to nonscientific frames of reference based on human rights" (Chan 2015, 7) and, in South Africa, turned "a dry legal contest into a matter about human lives" (Heywood 2001, 147). Yet, I argue that popular narratives that stress traditional social movement activism leave underappreciated the role that elite professionals with specialized knowledge in the law have played in the expansion of access to AIDS medicine. They also leave untouched the processes by which those in need have had to become experts in the law—often vis-à-vis the efforts of elite professionals who derive relatively limited benefits from these new policies themselves.

At a time when international trade accords increasingly compel countries to protect the patents of brand-name pharmaceuticals under the World Trade Organization's 1995 Trade Related Intellectual Property Rights (TRIPS) accord, expertise in the law plays an especially important role in enabling countries to take advantage of flexibilities that allow them to maintain affordable access to pharmaceuticals. The professional movements I study have dedicated themselves to expanding access to health care and medicine over opposition from the medical profession, pharmaceutical companies, private industry, and conservative international organizations. In making sense of this broad puzzle, this book both offers an account of how changes happened in the fields of health care and medicine and makes a larger contribution toward understanding the role of progressive elites in politics.

The positive role of elites and, more particularly, of members of esteemed professions who would otherwise seem to have little to gain (and potentially much to lose) by upsetting the status quo, has been widely acknowledged but woefully under-theorized. The stories related here are significant because scholars have frequently conceived of elites as self-interested and incapable of delivering for society the promise of a better future. Professions likewise have all too often stood on the "wrong side" of reforms that challenge the status quo, serving as obstacles to policies that would benefit the masses but hurt their own interests. Although conventional wisdom has emphasized the way in which democratization empowers the masses, this book draws out an underappreciated dynamic: the extent to which *democratization empowers elites*, who in turn can have a progressive impact on politics. As I show, these newly empowered (and public-minded) elites, in turn, often work on behalf of the poor and needy to institute important new social rights.

Grounded in the cases of Thailand, Brazil, and South Africa, this book asks: What explains the difference between the laggard response to expanding access to health care and HIV/AIDS medicine in South Africa and the pioneering responses of Thailand and Brazil? Thailand and Brazil are two countries whose approaches to universal health care and AIDS treatment would lead them to be praised internationally as models for the developing world. However, of the three countries, South Africa would seem to have been most predisposed to the adoption of such sweeping new programs, given the need for improved access to health care and medicine following the transition from apartheid, the unrivaled majorities of the African National Congress, the close ties between the ANC and the South African Communist Party, and plans for a universal health care program by professionals that predated the transition to democracy. And yet, these three countries took remarkably different paths, with Thailand and Brazil enjoying relative success in both domains and South Africa making only incremental gains; in South Africa the government actively obstructed efforts by professional movements seeking more transformative reform.

While important contributions have already been made that have focused on transnational relationships, struggles, and change (Chan 2015; Kapstein and Busby 2013), this book aims to give more fine-grained attention to the domestic politics at play in these national contexts, which I would suggest is sorely needed given that state policy outcomes are the book's ultimate concern.[1]

Health Care through the State, Medicine through the Law

The politics of expanding access to HIV/AIDS medicine and the politics of expanding access to health care would, on its face, appear to be related, given their similar goals and underpinnings in human rights, access, and equity concerns. However, the professions that dominate the politics of each of these fields are different. The politics of health care access operates primarily within the domain of doctors, who control entry into the medical profession; who oversee health care facilities and supervise legions of nurses, midwives, and other public health officials; and whose medical associations mobilize to protect the interests of physicians when their sovereignty and autonomy are challenged.

The politics of access to medicine operates differently. In a world governed by international trade rules that center on the protection of patents, knowledge of intellectual property law is increasingly understood as critical to effective advocacy for human rights. Success often hinges on the skills and expertise of professionals trained in the law who interpret and build national and international laws; who negotiate with and bring challenges against the pharmaceutical industry; and who hold the state accountable for obligations written into national law and represent the needs of ordinary citizens in court. While lawyers with formal training often lead these efforts, they frequently work hand in hand with other professionals—pharmacists, doctors, and health economists—whose knowledge and expertise in the law comes through professional experiences working on issues related to pharmaceutical access.

Transformative health care reform that makes access to comprehensive care a right of citizenship typically relies on the cooperation and interest of political parties who must pass laws in Parliament. In the face of competing policy priorities and tight government budgets, movements seeking to enact major new reforms must look for resources that enable them to have influence on the policy process. The case studies illustrate how access to state offices and legal expertise provides professional movements not only with the type of agenda-setting power frequently associated with "epistemic communities" but also with more wide-ranging influence on the policy process.[2] While their power is not complete in matters of public policy, I show that their influence is much more sweeping than currently accounted for in the literature.

In the domain of universal health care, the cases draw out the way in which the occupation of the state bureaucracy (a phenomenon I have in other work called "developmental capture"[3]) provide professional movements with access to resources that allow them to outmaneuver larger entrenched professional associations who oppose reform. These resources include but are not limited to the ability to set principles, mandates, and guidelines for state responsibilities for health care in new constitutions; to implement national pilot projects of health care programs before statutory laws that give such programs legal standing are even in place; to draw on the support of international organizations to advance reform in Parliament and stem the influence of opposition; and to put in place mechanisms that give citizens an active role in ensuring new policies operate as they should. Operating from these privileged positions in the state, professional movements push policy outcomes by affecting agenda-setting, policy formulation and adoption, and implementation as well as mechanisms that hold the state accountable for the policy once it is in place.

In the field of AIDS treatment, the case studies suggest that state occupation can be useful for the expansion of access to pharmaceuticals. However, this book points to an even more important, if overlooked, insight that bears centrally on the domain of pharmaceutical access: When authoritarian governments relinquish absolute control over the "rules of the game" following democratic transition, this frequently has the effect of dramatically empowering progressive elites with legal training, who become free to pursue social change through legal avenues that were closed to them under dictatorship. And they are likewise afforded greater opportunities to forge alliances with other technically savvy organizations abroad. These resources set them apart from ordinary citizens and allow them to hold the state accountable for rights outlined in newly created constitutions and to design effective strategies for countering pressure from pharmaceutical companies and industrialized nations. Drawing on these resources, legal movements act on behalf of patients in need of medication through litigation in court and hold the state accountable for living up to the promises embedded in a country's laws; challenge efforts by foreign governments and pharmaceutical companies to restrict access to medicine cheaply; and create new transnational institutions aimed at building an international environment that is more conducive to affordable access to generic medication.

The argument developed in this book points to the role that heightened political competition in the wake of democratic transition plays in providing openings for well-organized professional movements to influence the policymaking process. As the successful cases of Thailand and Brazil illustrate, environments in which political competition is fierce and no one party dominates predispose parties to being receptive to policy innovations proffered by professional movements who use the state to advance health care reforms and the law to widen access to treatment. However, the case of South Africa demonstrates that heightened political competition does not always result from democratic transition. In such cases where an ascendant party's dominance is essentially guaranteed and the ruling party enjoys the luxury of unrivaled power, entreaties for transformative reform from even the most well-organized professional movement may be ignored or taken up in piecemeal fashion.

Where legal cases demanding that the state expand access to medicine have strong grounds, governments may eventually be compelled to act, even in contexts where political competition does not flourish. However, initial government intransigence and the long and drawn-out process of legal mobilization (which sometimes includes appeals to higher courts) helps explain why we often see delayed action by governments in this area rather than no action at all. But this delay can have disastrous consequences for citizens' health in countries where a party's electoral success is a foregone conclusion versus those in which it is not.

In drawing together disparate threads of theory related to the importance of professionals in health care policymaking and fashioning a broader theory of the importance of professional movements in the expansion of social policy during periods of democratic transition, this work has implications for broader theories of the professions, political transitions in emerging nations, the welfare state, and democracy. In pointing to the important role played by professional movements in policy reform in these cases, this work draws attention to some counterintuitive findings, chief among them that democratization empowers elites; that those most responsible for advancing major social policies are frequently those least in need; and that professional movements achieve reform by virtue of privileged positions in the state, knowledge, and networks that are largely inaccessible to the common man.

The Cases

Enormous complexity characterizes different countries' health care systems, which are themselves shaped by social, economic, and demographic factors; unique individual political histories and struggles; and past policy decisions. These factors ensure that no two countries' health care systems will ever be exactly the same. Of course, this does not mean that the reform experiences of different countries should never be compared. Rather, it means that the complex differences between them have to be acknowledged, since countries frequently operate from different starting points, hold different values, and have different constellations of interest groups and political dynamics. These differences frequently make reforms easier or harder. In writing such complex comparative history, one must therefore strive to make these differences clear and explicit while observing scope conditions that make comparison reasonable.

As emerging economies engaged in processes of democratization, study of Thailand, Brazil, and South Africa gives us purchase for understanding how commitments to universal health care are shaped in countries grappling with high levels of inequality, limited resources, and competing policy priorities. All three countries emerged from authoritarian political arrangements and experienced an opening of the democratic sphere. In this new environment, the optimism associated with democracy in the wake of a repressive past left the countries ripe for more inclusionary social policies. Thailand experienced a shift from authoritarian rule (before 1992) to competitive democracy under a new constitution (1997–2006). Brazil saw the end of rule by the military and a competitive democracy emerge (beginning in 1985), and South Africa experienced the fall of apartheid and the transition to a democratic era marked by rule of the ANC (after 1994).

However, the selection of Thailand, Brazil, and South Africa for study is also beneficial for another reason: with 35 million deaths around the world since the epidemic began, HIV/AIDS is *the* major epidemic our time (UNAIDS 2016). As countries that all confronted the HIV/AIDS epidemic at the same time that discussions around health care reform occurred, examination of these countries offers a window into the ways in which the dynamics of AIDS policymaking related to HIV/AIDS compares with the dynamics of policymaking related to universal health care.

Given their status as similar public goods, one might expect the politics of expansive health care reform and AIDS treatment to be the same. And yet the comparison highlights the tensions that characterize the relationship between the two policy domains, offering some insight that helps explain why we cannot lump them together: Apart from the different professions that dominate the domains of health care and essential medicine, universal health care and AIDS treatment are each very costly endeavors. The former program serves a very broad population, while the latter serves a much narrower (and frequently marginalized and stigmatized) one. Frequently, funding support for AIDS treatment can be found abroad, while the financing of universal health care remains predominantly an entirely domestic enterprise. These dynamics sometimes lead advocates of these policies alternately into partnership and conflict with one another. In comparing reform dynamics in these two areas, this study aims to elucidate how and why professional movements succeed in some contexts and fail in others in two separate but related policy domains.

While providing openings for progressive change, decisive moments of democratic transition do not by themselves determine the content or the type of social policies to be enacted. The content of policy in these critical moments was of course shaped in part by past policies and current socioeconomic realities but above all by *agents* of social change who acted strategically to put policy innovations on the political agenda in cooperation with receptive political parties who held power in this new era. The study therefore explores the interaction between democratic transition and major social reforms, an area that other scholars have noted is in its infancy (Wong 2004).

In my study, Thailand—a country that has received scant attention from sociologists and political scientists—is my primary case, and Brazil and South Africa are secondary cases. The selection of these cases helps to extend literature on the welfare state beyond its traditional focus on Europe and North America. Recent work on social policy in Latin America (Ewig 2010; Huber and Stephens 2012; Kaufman and Segura-Ubiergo 2001; Nelson and Kaufman 2004; Weyland 2007), Eastern Europe (Nelson 2001), and Asia (Kasza 2006; Kwon 2011; Wong 2005) has sought to expand focus to the developing world. However, while attention to broad patterns that have occurred across regions is growing (Gough and Wood 2004; Haggard and Kaufman 2008; Sandbrook et al. 2007), rigorous comparative historical study of universal health care and AIDS treatment policy in the industrializing world remains remarkably thin. While the few comparative studies that do exist on universal health care (Wong 2004) and AIDS treatment (Lieberman

2009) are of great quality, they have principally taken aim at comparing the historical experiences of two countries. This book is therefore one of the first to explore the politics of health policy in three major industrializing countries. It is also the first to compare the politics of advocacy in both the domains of universal health care and AIDS treatment.

Thailand

Thailand took a gradualist approach to expanding state obligations toward health care under predominantly authoritarian governments in the 1970s and 1980s. However, in 2001 it made a decisive break with the past by instituting a tax-funded program that expanded health care access to the 30 percent of the population who lacked it. The proportion of the population without coverage was approximately double that lacking coverage in the United States at the time of the signing of the Patient Protection and Affordable Care Act in 2010. And yet, while the ACA did not expand coverage to everyone, Thailand's Universal Coverage program expanded coverage nationwide in less than a year, with expansion beginning just four months after a new political party came to power. This new program made access to health care a right of citizenship and sat alongside two existing state programs for workers in the formal sector and civil servants and their families. Thailand's reform also brought with it important improvements, ranging from new financing arrangements that sought to introduce greater accountability and control costs to a new health information system which aimed to provide policymakers with better data on which to base decisions. Shortly after the country's program was implemented nationwide, on the anniversary of World AIDS Day in 2001, the nation's health minister made a commitment to expand access to antiretroviral medications for AIDS patients. And in the years that followed, Thailand's leadership on the issue of HIV/AIDS access would become even more celebrated on the world stage after its health minister in 2007 became the first to declare a "compulsory license" on the "second-line" AIDS drug, Kaletra, and Plavix, a heart disease medication. This announcement followed an earlier compulsory licensing declaration on a first-line AIDS drug, efavirenz, in 2006.[4] And in 2008 the ministry would issue additional compulsory licenses on four other cancer drugs. The international notoriety Thailand gained on the issue of HIV/AIDS treatment built on the country's earlier fame as a leader on HIV/AIDS prevention and its well-known condom campaigns.

Brazil

Beginning with passage of a universal health care law in 1990—a mere five years removed from military rule—Brazil's health care reform took place in a similar context of democratization. Prior to reform, the distribution of medical services in Brazil was highly skewed toward developed urban areas, particularly in the south and southeast, and the government's main social insurance program excluded or otherwise provided minimal benefits to some 52 percent of the population (Weyland 1996, 97, 132). Although the military regime extended a thin measure of social insurance to the rural, unemployed, and self-employed, largely to coopt rural pressures for change (Falleti 2010, 40), in practice it provided the rural poor with minimal protection while leaving urban informal workers excluded from coverage entirely (Weyland 1996, 91–92). The country's 1990 Unified Health System (SUS) law sought to correct this by creating a British-style National Health Service that provided equal access to health care for all through the public system and contracting private providers. One of the leading strategies for implementation of the SUS legislation was the Family Health Program, which brought health care to the masses via teams of health care providers working in communities. The SUS also opened up important new avenues for citizen participation in health care decision-making and governance through city, state, and national health councils.

An announcement that the government would provide AIDS medication designed to slow the progression of the virus to sufferers of the disease followed the SUS legislation in 1991. Following discovery that combination antiretroviral therapy could stop the AIDS virus in its tracks, the country passed a law in 1996, making it the first industrializing country in the world to make access to combination ARVs free and universal to its citizens. The country's pioneering negotiations with drug companies would help drive down the cost of ARVs and would lead its response to HIV/AIDS to be hailed as a model for the developing world. Professionals from Brazil with knowledge of intellectual property law would play an active role in institutionalizing new norms related to access to AIDS medication at the WHO, the World Trade Organization, the UN Commission on Human Rights, and the UN General Assembly Special Session on AIDS. The country's impressive achievements, however, are even more remarkable when weighed against the political and economic context of the time: Politics in Brazil had been defined by clientelism. The country had the world's largest foreign debt (Biehl 2007, 54) and between 1980 and 1991 undertook seven structural adjustment packages from the World Bank and IMF (Parker 2003, 180). While the country's new universal health care and antiretroviral therapy programs have taken time to realize their potential, the expansion that occurred did so in improbable fashion, against a backdrop of debt, hyperinflation, and austerity that saw actual per person federal spending on health plunge from $83 in 1989 to $37 in 1993 (Biehl 2007, 59).

South Africa

If Thailand and Brazil's achievements in the provision of health care and AIDS medicine might be regarded as successes, then South Africa's experience in both domains stands in sharp contrast. Christian Barnard performed the world's first successful heart transplant in South Africa in 1967. But under apartheid, the real benefits of the country's health care system were unequally distributed, enjoyed primarily by the country's white minority. However, in the last years before apartheid's end in 1994, reformers sought to change this situation and laid the groundwork for a new universal health care program. The program aimed to overcome the deep divide between the country's top-rated private health care system, which largely served the country's white minority, and the crumbling means-tested public health care system, which served the black African majority.[5] Proposals discussed at the time included plans for both a British-style National Health Service, in which the government both pays for and provides health care for everyone, and a Canadian-style National Health Insurance system, which offered the promise of access to the country's system of private hospitals and clinics by providing everyone with insurance-based health care coverage. Yet the African National Congress has initiated only smaller reforms that aimed to pro-vide free comprehensive health care for children under six and pregnant women through the public system in 1994 and free basic "primary health care" for every-one in 1996, again through the already overburdened public sector.[6] In a politi-cal context that is completely uncompetitive, more transformative health care reforms have languished for more than twenty years. Caught between ideological desires and practical realities, the government has convened task force after task force to explore transformative reform but has so far avoided major changes, choosing instead to embrace national health insurance in name only.

However, if progress on transformative health care reform in post-apartheid South Africa might be described as glacially slow, then government policy toward expanding access to AIDS medication in post-apartheid South Africa might be described as moving in the wrong direction altogether. According to data from UNAIDS, in the year before Mandela's transition to the presidency in 1993, HIV prevalence rates in South Africa among adults aged 15 to 49 stood at 2 percent. Having inherited a weak institutional apparatus from the outgoing apartheid gov-ernment and failing to put into place an effective preventative response, that num-ber climbed significantly under the tenure of South Africa's first two presidents after apartheid, Nelson Mandela and Thabo Mbeki. And while it is also important to acknowledge not only colonial institutions but also the distinct epidemiological profile of HIV/AIDS in South Africa as major factors contributing to the growth of the disease,[7] under President Mbeki the government embarked on its disastrous policy of AIDS denialism, suggesting that HIV does not cause AIDS, asserting that ARVs are dangerous, and proffering charlatan advice on AIDS treatment that emphasized the use of garlic, olive oil, and beetroot. In taking these steps, the administration aligned itself with the views of radical scientific dissidents and actively took steps to prevent the rollout of national programs aimed at preventing the transmission of the AIDS virus from mothers to children. By 2003, when the government finally changed course and agreed to commit itself to a national plan to roll out treatment for pregnant mothers, HIV prevalence rates in South Africa had climbed to nearly 18 percent (UNAIDS 2015). South Africa would have the largest population of HIV-infected people in the world, and scholars would estimate that some 330,000 lives had been lost because a more general ARV treatment program for people infected with AIDS had not been implemented sooner (Chigwedere et al. 2008).

Research Strategy

In the area of social policy, comparative and historical work has been used to explain the creation of major new social programs, as well as differences in state commitments to social programs—and in doing so, this approach has arguably made larger theoretical contributions in the area of social policy than those in other areas (Amenta 2003, 92–103). This work builds on and complements other important quantitative scholarship on globalization and the welfare state (Garrett and Mitchell 2001; Huber and Stephens 2001; Rodrik 1998; Rudra 2002; Rudra and Haggard 2005) and emerging research on the politics of health policy in the developing world (Lieberman 2009; Selway 2015; Wong 2004).

My research utilizes comparative and historical methods as a way to gain analytical leverage on three cases of professional movement-led efforts to expand access to health care and medicine in the industrializing world. As a methodological approach, comparative and historical methods have helped to spur the development of middle-range theory, including efforts to explain empirical anomalies. Building on foundational work in comparative and historical analysis (Moore 1966; Skocpol 1979; Skocpol and Somers 1980), this book takes an inductive approach that aims to build theory through comparative analysis of the cases. In so doing, it follows a well-established path taken by other scholars of health politics who have used comparison to develop arguments and generate hypotheses (Lieberman 2009; Wong 2004). Here, I suggest that the comparison of Thailand and Brazil with South Africa is particularly instructive. While the broad dynamics of political transition in these two countries were marked by important differences, elections in the years that followed were marked by pronounced political competition. In both cases, professional movements (the Rural Doctors' Movement in Thailand and the *sanitaristas* in Brazil) drew on the power of the bureaucracy to institute universal health care reforms. And in both cases, newly empowered movements of legally minded medical professionals (led by the Drug Study Group in Thailand and *sanitaristas* and lawyers within the AIDS movement in Brazil) drew on legal knowledge and institutions to make their countries the envy of the world in terms of AIDS treatment policy.

Whereas Brazil serves as a kind of ally to the claims I make about the sources of social change in Thailand, in South Africa I find something different altogether. Here, too, vigorous professional movements attempted to play an active role in the expansion of health care and medicine, led by a progressive health movement in the field of health care and the Treatment Action Campaign and AIDS Law Project in the field of AIDS treatment. However, professional movements in South Africa did not achieve the same level of success for reasons I suggest have to do with the lack of political competition in the wake of democratic opening. In the 1994 election, the African National Congress won nearly 63 percent of the vote, and in the election that would follow in 1999, it increased its share to almost 66 percent of the vote with no serious challengers (the Democratic Party finished a distant second, reaping only 9.6% of the vote). Even though the second national election under the new constitution in Thailand in 2005 would bring the first elected majority (rather than coalition) government to power in the country's history, the lopsided political dynamics in South Africa would have no rival with either the cases of Thailand or South Africa—and indeed, few democratic countries ever in the world.

These dynamics, which have essentially brought a one-party government that has no true rivals into power in the years that followed, have created serious and fundamental differences in political interests and incentives that I argue help explain why South Africa's policy outcomes on the issues of health care and medicine differ so radically from those found in Thailand and Brazil. In the absence of serious political competition—and in spite of being the only country of the three whose people have embraced a party with a commitment to communist ideology and that had also already laid the groundwork for transformative health reform at the time of transition—the South African government had the luxury of being able to ignore the entreaties of a well-organized professional movement, to function as an echo chamber and entertain its own flights of fancy, and ultimately to embrace incremental reforms that were easier and less risky than more radical transformative reforms. As prominent scholars have written, the situation has only gotten worse over time, as the ANC has hollowed out structures of participatory governance and extended hegemony over mass politics, largely sidelining civil society from politics (Evans and Heller 2015).[8] The case therefore exists as a kind of contrary example that highlights the way in which the character of political competition interacts with professional movement advocacy.

As an understudied country whose health policies in both the areas of universal health care and AIDS treatment have garnered attention internationally, Thailand serves as my primary case. While there has been some analysis of the development of the Universal Coverage policy in Thailand, it has generally emphasized the importance of incentives embedded in new constitutional and electoral rules (Hicken 2006; Kuhonta 2008; Selway 2011, 2015) or the importance of a populist political party (McCargo and Pathmanand 2005; Phongpaichit and Baker 2004) and has not explored the role of professional movements in the policy development and implementation. While important work on Thailand's HIV/AIDS policy has drawn out the role that social movements have played (Ford et al. 2004; Ford et al. 2009; Kijtiwatchakul 2007, Suwanphattana et al. 2008; Tantivess and Walt 2008), this public health literature has generally left the legal roots of change underexplored and ignored the broader theoretical implications. My research builds on and complements these studies by drawing out the role that movements of medical and legal professionals have played in expanding access to health care and AIDS treatment. The main source of data in this study comes from primary and secondary materials collected at various archives[9] and in-depth interviews with over 120 key informants in both Thai and English.[10] This research took place over one year (January 2009 to December 2009) with typical interviews lasting between a half hour and two hours, under the auspices of a Fulbright-Hays Doctoral Dissertation Fellowship.

South Africa serves as an important secondary case that puts the findings from Thailand in broader perspective. There is a well-developed literature in the health policy field that emphasizes the roles of various committee deliberations over national health insurance in South Africa (McIntyre and van den Heever 2007; Thomas and Gilson 2004), but this literature generally takes 1994 as its entry point and does not consider the earlier role that professional movements played in putting health care reform on the political agenda. Similarly, there has been an abundance of work on the politics of HIV/AIDS in South Africa (Decoteau 2013; Fassin 2007; Friedman and Mottiar 2005; Gauri and Lieberman 2006; Gevisser 2009a; Lieberman 2009; Nattrass 2004). This work has generated critical insights but has not seriously considered the events in relation to broader processes of democratization and has left the professional character of the movement to expand access to antiretroviral therapy relatively unexplored. My research on South Africa employed the consultation of primary and secondary data,[11] attendance at several local conferences, and interviews with twenty-five key informants in South Africa.[12] This research took place in Johannesburg, Durban, and Cape Town over approximately three months from September to December 2008, with interviews typically lasting between a half hour and two hours. It was supported through a University of Wisconsin-Madison departmental research grant and a Scott Kloeck-Jenson Award.

Brazil serves as another secondary case that helps broaden the comparison further. Of the three countries, Brazil has enjoyed the greatest scholarly attention to date. A robust literature has developed that considers both the development of the 1990 Unified Health System reform (Buss and Gadelha 1996; Cornwall and Shankland 2008; Elias and Cohn 2003; Falleti 2010; Huber and Stephens 2012; Weyland 1995) and of the country's HIV/AIDS programs (Biehl 2004; Daniel and Parker 1993; Flynn 2013, 2014; Gauri and Lieberman 2006; Lieberman 2009; Nunn 2009; Parker 2003). Because of the abundant work that has already been done, I rely exclusively on secondary sources on Brazil and the helpful advice and assistance of seasoned scholars of Brazil.

Aside from this fieldwork, my knowledge of what has become known as "universal coverage" in health care and AIDS treatment was further informed through my attendance at the 35th Annual Conference on Global Health in 2008 and the 17th and 19th International AIDS Conferences (the theme for the first of which was, appropriately, "*universal* action now") in 2008 and 2012. Since that time, I have become further enmeshed in the practical problems faced by countries seeking to achieve universal health coverage in the developing world through consulting projects. While I do not draw on that knowledge in the telling of the stories that are related here, that experience has been informative in its own right.

The Plan for the Book

The book is organized in the following manner. Chapter 1 explores the literature related to health, welfare, and democracy, providing an account of the major theoretical issues that motivate the study. In this chapter, I lay out how this book builds on previous work and investigates the relationship between well-organized movements made up of elites with professional training and the character of political competition in the wake of democratic transition. Drawing on literature from social movements and the professions, I fashion the concept of "professional movements" and explain why elite professional movements, whose membership is narrower than mass movements, at times exercise such sweeping influence in times of democratic transition.

The first half of the book explores the politics of universal health care in Thailand, Brazil, and South Africa. Chapter 2 looks at the politics of universal health care in Thailand in the wake of transition to democracy. It illustrates the critical role played by a professional movement made up of doctors who put universal coverage on the political agenda and drew on their privileged positions in the state, their knowledge, and their social networks to institutionalize the policy over opposition from the World Bank and the broader medical profession. Chapter 3 explores these same dynamics in the case of democratizing Brazil, drawing out surprising parallels with Thailand and acknowledging important differences between the two countries. In Brazil, we find a movement of public health professionals (the *sanitaristas*) that is remarkably similar to Thailand's Rural Doctors' Movement, which also drew on the offices of the state, albeit in different ways, to institutionalize universal health care at the most unlikeliest of times. Chapter 4 explores the failure of transformative health care reform in South Africa, where a longstanding movement of medical professionals confronted political dynamics markedly different from the other two countries. Here I show how these dynamics predisposed the ruling African National Congress to commit to only incremental reform and embrace more transformative health care reform (national health insurance) in name only.

The second half of the book examines the politics of antiretroviral access in the three countries. Chapter 5 examines the politics of antiretroviral access in Thailand, drawing out how a movement of pharmacists and medical professionals with training in the law helped make Thailand a global model for AIDS treatment. Chapter 6 highlights the underappreciated legal dimensions of Brazil's well-known AIDS treatment story, which contributed not only to Brazil becoming the first industrializing country to make combination antiretroviral therapy available to all free of charge but also to international efforts to make antiretroviral access more accessible. Chapter 7 explores the reasons for failure of the AIDS treatment policy in South Africa, where ANC executives moved slowly in addressing the AIDS epidemic and adopted a charlatan AIDS policy in an electoral context that allowed them the luxury to do so. While a legal movement eventually succeeded in forcing the hand of the government, these different political dynamics eventually led to the deaths of more than three hundred thousand people. Finally, in chapter 8, I offer some concluding observations, briefly discuss how the current political situation has affected the continued prospects for professional movements and health universalism in those countries, and explore the relevance of professional movements to social change in other policy domains and parts of the world.

DEMOCRATIZATION, ELITES, AND THE EXPANSION OF ACCESS TO HEALTH CARE AND MEDICINE

"We trust our health to the physician, our fortune, and sometimes our life and reputation, to the lawyer and attorney. Such confidence could not safely be reposed in people of a very mean or low condition."

—Adam Smith, *The Wealth of Nations*

"Organizations of teachers, doctors, and lawyers are still apt to look out, first of all, for 'number one.' "

—Abraham Flexner, "Is Social Work a Profession?"

What accounts for the emergence of health rights in new democracies, and why should progressive members of elite professions—who frequently receive no benefit themselves—play such an important role in their expansion? In sociology, the power of elites has often been viewed with a mixture of contempt and suspicion. From C. Wright Mills's *The Power Elite* to William Domhoff's *Who Rules America?*, the discipline has rarely thought of elites as figures capable of delivering for society the promise of a better future. More frequently, they have been imagined as shadowy figures bent on pursuing ways to increase their own power, standing, and capital at the expense of broader society.

Classic work within sociology and political science has more frequently pointed to the role of labor unions and left-wing parties who serve as champions of the masses and advance egalitarian social policy. T. H. Marshall's theory of citizenship (1950), now taken as a foundational work in sociology, pointed to the gradual expansion of civil, political, and social rights in Great Britain over three centuries. Although the state ultimately served as the vehicle for the expansion of what Marshall termed "citizenship," social struggle—and the role of labor unions and other actors in society—was at times explicit in his accounts. More recent work by scholars working in the "power resources" school (Korpi 1983; Stephens 1979) has emphasized the importance of working-class power and in particular the role of labor unions and left-wing political parties in the expansion of social policies. The generous social democratic welfare regimes advanced by left-wing parties and labor unions have frequently been set against less generous arrangements in liberal and corporatist welfare regimes (Esping-Andersen 1990). While the influence of left-party power on the expansion of social policy in Europe has long been acknowledged, its importance in developing countries has only recently received attention (Heller 1999; Huber and Stephens 2012; Sandbrook et al. 2007).

By contrast, Amartya Sen's (1999) theory of development as freedom has spawned an abundance of work that has emphasized the importance of direct citizen participation in human development. From accounts of participatory governance (Fung and Wright 2003) to the role of ordinary (even illiterate) citizen participation in processes of participatory budgeting in Brazil (Baiocchi 2005) to innovative institutional mechanisms of public involvement in Brazil (Cornwall and Shankland 2008), India (Gibson 2012), and twenty-first century developmental states more broadly (Evans and Heller 2015), scholars have convincingly shown that direct citizen participation plays a vital role in human development.[1,2]

While a consensus that democracy enhances human development has been longstanding (Boix 2001; Dreze and Sen 1989; Lenski 1966; Lipset 1959), recent work has interrogated the relationship between democracy and health more specifically. These studies have found mixed evidence on the relationship between regime type and health (Gauri and Khaleghian 2002; Gerring, Thacker, and Alfaro 2012; Gómez and Harris 2015; Ross 2006; Shandra et al. 2004). While some research has found "little evidence that the rise of democracy contributed to the fall in infant and child mortality rates" (Ross 2006, 872), these findings have been called into question (Gerring, Thacker, and Alfaro 2012; Martel-García 2014). Besley and Kudamatsu (2006) find a strong relationship between democracy and life expectancy. James McGuire (2010) suggests that it is not a country's wealth (or spending) that determines its citizens' health but rather a government's commitment to well-financed social services, in particular primary health care. In this context, democratic elections encourage politicians to attend to these needs. Wigley and Akkoyunlu-Wigley (2011) find that democracy has a positive effect on life expectancy independent of its effect on redistributive policies. Following Sen (1999), they theorize that this pro-health effect is due to the fact that democracy enables active citizen participation in decision-making processes and because of the protection democracy affords individual civil and political rights. While Gerring, Thacker, and Alfaro (2012) find only a weak relationship between level of democracy in a given year and health, they report substantially stronger support for the relationship between a country's total stock of democracy over the previous century and infant mortality. McGuire (2013) reports lower infant mortality rates among democracies than authoritarian regimes and likewise finds support for the idea that long-run democratic experience contributes to health.

Within this literature, the relationship between democratization and health is a related issue that has recently been taken up by scholars. In a survey of twenty-eight countries in sub-Saharan Africa, Kudamatsu (2012) finds that infant mortality falls by nearly two percentage points after democratization. Wong (2004, 13, 26, 28) contends that the transition from authoritarian to democratic politics provides policymakers with new incentives to consider universal, rather than selective and piecemeal, health care reforms. The emergence of new actors in civil society broadens existing policy networks and forces new ideas to be taken into account. Frenk, Gómez-Dantés, and Knaul (2009) and Carbone (2011) have likewise pointed to the importance of new political opportunities that emerged in Mexico and Ghana which helped to facilitate the adoption of national health reform.

This book builds on this emerging literature and complicates existing theories in three ways. First, whereas scholarship has emphasized the way in which democratization empowers the masses, this book turns that conventional wisdom on its head by suggesting that democratization empowers elites. Second, it calls attention to the role that newly empowered (and public-minded) professionals play in expanding access to health care and medicine *on behalf of* the poor and those in need. Third, it highlights the importance of differences in the character of political competition in the wake of democratic transition in conditioning the possibilities for well-organized professional movements to institute such changes.

In light of the literature that has emphasized the critical role played by left-wing political parties and broad-based mass movements in expanding human freedom and broadening notions of citizenship, this book points to the need to revise and refine our understanding of the sources of major policy change in industrializing societies. In the developing world, some of the institutions that have typically been relied on for progressive change in the Global North, like labor unions, often represent only the needs of those in the formal sector, leaving out the needs of vast majority—and sometimes even entrenching inequality when new health care programs are enacted that serve only comparatively well-off civil servants and workers in the formal sector.

This book therefore refocuses our attention away from these typical explanations for social policy expansion and points to the important role played by actors from a narrower stratum of society than existing theories suggest. It draws attention to the importance of movements comprised of medical and legal experts who advocate for health care rights on behalf of the poor and disenfranchised in the face of well-established professional and corporate interests. While classic scholarship within the Marxist tradition (including work by Gramsci and Lenin) has also theorized that intellectuals have a role to play in revolution and that the primary beneficiaries of social change do not always have to be the drivers, my work shows how the knowledge, networks, and positions of elites from esteemed professions play a particularly important role in concrete policy domains characterized by technical complexity.

An Elite-Centered Theory of Welfare State Expansion

Doctors have long been central to health care reform. However, nearly all of the prominent scholarship from sociology and political science suggests that they have been on the "wrong side" of reform, posing as obstacles to efforts to extend access to health care to members of the population who do not have it (Hacker 1998, 2002; Quadagno 2004, 2005; Skocpol 1997; Starr 1982). Classic scholarship in the professions has emphasized the unique professional autonomy extended to the medical profession (and other professions) by the state and efforts by the profession to preserve professional autonomy, authority, and jurisdiction and to protect professional interests in the face of change (Abbott 1988; Freidson 1970; Larson 1977; Starr 1982). This work has explored the historical basis of power, dominance, and authority of the medical profession, its reliance on knowledge and competence for this power, and the degree to which doctors' power sometimes "spills over its clinical boundaries into arenas of moral and political action for which medical judgment is only partially relevant" (Starr 1982, 4–5). This scholarship has suggested that "over the politics, policies, and programs that govern the system, the profession's interests have also tended to prevail" (Starr 1982, 5).

While the influence of professional associations may vary by national context (Immergut 1992), the interests and power of the professions is something that scholars have generally taken for granted. Medical associations have played a key role in mobilizing against efforts to extend coverage to citizens when presidential administrations have led efforts to enact health care reform (Quadagno 2004, 2005; Skocpol 1997). Hacker, for example, has suggested that "[i]n no country has the medical profession wholeheartedly embraced national health insurance" (1998, 66) and has pointed to the enduring consequences of early instances of professional resistance to health reform in shaping the character of health care systems today (2002). The historical success enjoyed by the medical profession in resisting threats to its professional autonomy has led Paul Starr to suggest that the United States is perhaps the paradigmatic case in this respect: "Hardly anywhere have doctors been as successful as American physicians in resisting national insurance and maintaining a predominantly private and voluntary financing system" (1982, 6). While important work has since enumerated challenges to the dominance of the medical profession—the corporatization of health care, the growing influence of the pharmaceutical industry, new health care purchasing arrangements, and large new federal programs—and pointed to evidence of the decline of its autonomy in important respects (Conrad 2008; Light 2010; Timmermans and Oh 2010), few if any are willing to go so far as to suggest that the influence of organized medicine is dead; it is taken for granted as a potent force in politics today in the United States and abroad.

Scholars have pointed to the need to go beyond these traditional ways of understanding the professions and to question the assumptions that have led us to conceptualize professionals as "unproblematic agents of professions" (Lo 2005, 390–91). Although there have been calls for sociologists to investigate the multiple and even ambiguous identities of professionals for some time (Balzer 1996; Hafferty and McKinlay 1993; Lo 2005), with few exceptions (Bucher and Strauss 1961; Bucher 1962; Hoffman 1989; Wolfson 2001) professional subdivisions—and more specifically, their relationships with social movements—have not been a central focus of this literature. While I acknowledge the tendency of medical associations to oppose health care reform efforts, to suggest that the attitude of a profession toward health care reform is always uniformly negative would also be an overstatement. Within the United States, groups such as Physicians for a National Health Program have provided an important alternative to the once-dominant American Medical Association by advocating for national health insurance for almost forty years. In other words, while national associations have traditionally sought to represent the interests of professions as a whole, research has long acknowledged that professions may contain opposing factions, splinter groups, and subdivisions (Abbott 1988, 247; Freidson 1986, 195–96)—even if it has generally been a footnote within the broader literature.

Only recently has work in medical sociology turned its attention to social movements working in the health domain and formalized the study of "health social movements" (Brown et al. 2004; Brown and Zavestoski 2005). While valuable, this scholarship has generally encouraged us to think about social movements in relation to health, rather than in relation to the broader organizational category of the professions, of which movement advocates are a part. And until recently (O'Brien and Li 2006; Steinhoff 2014), study of the interface between law and social movements has likewise been limited, with social movement researchers generally demonstrating little interest in law and legal scholars not taking up social movements (McCann 2006). While growing attention has been given to "cause lawyering" within the scholarship on law and society (Sarat and

Schiengold 2006), the literature on medical sociology has more frequently treated litigation and engagement in legal action as tactics that health social movements might use rather than as professional identities around which to construct new social movements (for example, Brown and Zavestoski 2005, 13; Wolfson 2001, 38–39).

Scholarship has more frequently shown how their different needs, goals, and methods have put scientists and laypeople into conflict in battles over the science related to illness and health (Brown 1992; Epstein 1996; Hess 2005; Joffey, Weitz, and Stacey 2005). Steven Epstein (1996), for example, has documented the struggle over access to experimental drugs before the advent of combination antiretroviral therapy by AIDS activists in the United States. By documenting processes of knowledge-building and the "expertification" of lay citizens, Epstein's work has illuminated the ways in which activists have themselves worked to become knowledgeable about the science of AIDS in order to be able to challenge scientists and advocate more forcefully for improved access to experimental medicines. This work can be read as existing within a broader scholarship that has taken "embodied health movements" as its concern (Brown et al. 2004).

While the work of Epstein and others has drawn attention to efforts by activists to become experts in science in an era in which access to pharmaceuticals could prolong life, but not extend it indefinitely, scientific advances have since changed the game, with new technologies turning previously fatal illnesses into chronic ones. However, the price of these new medicines has not always come cheap, and the need for life-saving medicines has at times come into conflict with their affordability. This conflict has in turn bred both cooperation and contestation among state bureaucrats responsible for public health, activists representing those in need of pharmaceuticals, and pharmaceutical companies tasked with making innovative new medicines. Given the centrality of both intellectual property and human rights to what has come to be known as "essential medicine," the battles between these actors have frequently taken place in a jurisdiction well beyond the established clinical setting of the doctor. Courts have played important roles in distributional conflicts related to expanding access to medicine, leading both activists and doctors to venture outside of their core jurisdictions, to undergo training in the law, and to engage in contentious struggles that rely on expertise. By showing how lawyers and activist medical professionals have engaged the law, I extend this line of research and highlight the way in which treatment advocates have both relied on lawyers and themselves sometimes undergone processes of "expertification," not just in important issues related to science but also in the law. And by pointing to the professional character of these movements, this work interfaces with recent debates within Science and Technology Studies on the democratization of science and the relative contributions of lay people and elites to problems that are both scientific and social (Benjamin 2013; Brown 2009; Shim 2014).

Professional Movements: Political Actors Who Occupy an In-Between Space

I advance the notion of "professional movements" to describe a category of collective action that occupies an in-between space among the broader categories of the professions and social movements, referring to social movements that operate within and sometimes against broader professions. While others have used the idea of professional movements as an entry point for exploring intra-professional conflict over ideas—particularly in the transnational economic field (van Gunten 2015, 29, 8; also Hirschman and Berman 2014)—this work has not generally taken national policymaking processes as its central focus, exploring instead contests that have taken place in the realm of ideas rather than examining overt strategic political action by professional movements to make policy concrete in national environments. This book examines professional movements as political actors who frequently operate outside the academy, acting purposefully and strategically—drawing on privileged positions within the state and legal institutions—to put policy ideas on the political agenda, to institutionalize new policy innovations, and to hold the state accountable for robust implementation.

In the domains of health care and medicine, professional movements—comprised of medical professionals—engage in strategies and actions that take place *outside* their normal professional jurisdiction. For example, these professional movements include doctors who leave work in clinical practice to take up positions in the state bureaucracy and advance health reform and pharmacists who leave the hospital dispensary to accrue legal expertise on intellectual property issues, which they then deploy on policy issues related to pharmaceutical access. But such movements are not necessarily limited to the domains of health and medicine: In the domains of business and finance, for example, professionals may leave high-paying industry jobs to work to improve consumer protection or advocate for regulation that benefits the marginalized.

Professional movements are distinct from scientific and intellectual movements in that scientific and intellectual movements involve "collective efforts to pursue *research* programs or projects for thought in the face of resistance from others in the scientific or intellectual community" (Frickell and Gross 2005, 206, emphasis added). Professional movements are also distinct from "identity movements within professions," which aim to critique the existing orthodoxy within a profession and promote cultural change through the reshaping of institutional logics and the redefinition of role identities within the profession (Rao, Monin, and Durand 2003). While the actions of professional movements may impact the institutional logics of a profession, cultural change within the profession is not their primary objective or interest. Rather, they seek to advance *policy changes* that stand to affect broader society in the face of professional resistance.

Whereas identity movements within professions occupy professional societies to promote new institutional logics *within* the profession (Rao, Monin, and Durand 2003, 835), professional movements that aim to promote broader policy reforms must look elsewhere to do so. Professional movements frequently step outside the confines of their own professional jurisdictions to have a broader impact on society (and on their own professions) when the hierarchies and power structures within their own professional jurisdiction limit opportunities for far-reaching reform. While the reforms they promote may seem radical and revolutionary to those who would be affected by them, the socialization processes involved in becoming experts in their fields and their engagement with the law, state institutions, and policymaking processes exert some natural constraints on their agendas. On the revolutionary/reform spectrum, relative to truly radical social movements that operate untethered from such institutions, professional movements fall squarely on the reform side of the spectrum in terms of aims and goals, favoring engagement with the state and policy advocacy over actions aimed at toppling or smashing the state. This does not mean that the agenda of professional movements cannot be transformative. Indeed, professional movements like to use the infrastructure and resources of the state and legal and policy levers cleverly to advance their agenda, to undermine entrenched professional interests, and to build the world they want.

The case studies show that the influence of professional movements goes well beyond that implied by existing work on scientists and professionals who engage the policymaking process through their roles as experts. This work, exemplified by the "epistemic communities" approach, has generally circumscribed their influence to agenda-setting and defining state interests (Haas 1992). In line with other recent work that is beginning to recognize the role of technical experts (Dargent 2014), the cases also challenge scholarship that has suggested that experts rarely take strategic actions to advance the development of policy, either because they don't have interests or because their influence is peripheral and is most often limited to obscure technical issues (Brint 1994, 363, 366; Freidson 1986, 192; also Dobbin, Simmons, and Garrett 2007; Gutiérrez 2010, 81; Krücken and Drori 2009, 191; Scott 2008). However, it also points to the moral foundations that motivate participants in professional movements as opposed to members of *epistemic communities* who, "[i]f confronted with anomalies that undermined their causal beliefs, would withdraw from the policy debate" (Haas 1992, 18). Value-driven members of professional movements, elite and knowledgeable experts though they may be, are not like that; a commitment to science, though important, does not come at the expense of commitment to cause. As with members of other social movements—and transnational advocacy networks (Keck and Sikkink 1998)—shared normative commitments are at the heart of what motivates their actions. They are motivated primarily by longstanding shared normative beliefs, rooted in concerns related to social justice and human rights, rather than narrower career interests and incentives that scholarship has emphasized in explaining the behavior of state officials (Geddes 1994; Evans 1995).

In pointing to the way in which professional movements use the infrastructure and resources of the state to advance policy, this work brings together two related but distinctive lines of research: one that has noted that in health and other social policy reforms key players "tend not to be presidents or political parties, but rather experts embedded in national bureaucracies" (Ewig 2010, 63; also Dargent 2014; Haggard and Kaufman 2008, 197; Kaufman and Nelson 2004; Weyland 2007; on bureaucrats' influence in international organizations, Chorev 2012a) and a second that has pointed to the increasingly blurred lines between state and society and has drawn out efforts by activists to take over parts of the state to advance their agenda (Eisenstein 1996; Falleti 2010; Gilbert and Howe 1991; Harris 2015; Keck and Sikkink 1998; Mitchell 1991; Rich 2013; Santoro and McGuire 1997; Weyland 1995; Wolfson 2001). This scholarship can be read against classical Marxist scholarship that has more frequently envisioned the state to be an instrument of another elite group whose purposes are typically much narrower, the upper class.

In this vein, important scholarship has outlined both the strategic value of the state for activists (Gamson 1990) as well as offered ideas about the durability that professional movements occupying different parts of the state might expect. This work has shown that high-ranking political appointees can enable networks of activists to wield particular influence on state policy (Keck and Sikkink 1998, 103). Likewise, Haas has suggested that the influence and ability of experts is a function of "the extent to which an epistemic community consolidates bureaucratic power within national administrations and international secretariats" (1992, 30). Whereas political appointees suffer from frequent turnover and do not have a window into the details of particular programs, meso-level bureaucrats, such as bureau and division chiefs, "are sufficiently elevated to observe differences across offices but low enough to know the necessary details about programs" (Carpenter 2001, 22). In addition, few are better positioned "to know both political elites and the grass-roots constituency of an agency's programs (potential and actual)" (Carpenter 2001, 21–22). In those rare cases where a reputation for competence and expert knowledge links up with the support of external actors outside the bureaucracy—in such places as political parties, civil society, and international organizations—state, or bureaucratic, autonomy can be achieved, granting members of professional movements in the meso level of the bureaucracy sweeping influence on the policy process.

While one reading of this work might suggest the value of taking a "state-centered" approach (Evans et al. 1985; Skocpol 1979) to the examination of social policy expansion, the approach I follow here implores us to recognize the value of state resources while at the same time recognizing the underlying movement identities of the actors involved in pursuit and use of those resources. While capture of state offices does, arguably, fall outside the range of normal channels of social movement influence, it does not suggest a disdain for institutions (though in some cases the relationship with the bureaucracy is complex). More broadly, these accounts call to question both Weberian and political science conceptions of the state that emphasize its rational character (Geddes 1994; Weber 1978). They also challenge the general focus of the literature on health care reform, which has firmly revolved around interests, including those of business, which some have interpreted as consistently opposing welfare state development (Esping-Andersen 1990; Stephens 1979) and others as supporting it (Mares 2003; Swenson 2002); those of professional associations, insurance companies and, employer groups (Quadagno 2004); and those expressed by political actors at all important veto points in the policy process (Immergut 1992).

The contrast I draw between elite professional movements and mass movements (comprised of laypeople) focuses attention on the bases of social movements and puts into sharp relief the different kinds of resources (in the health care domain, knowledge, networks, and powers derived from state office) that different kinds of social movements have access to, and in turn, the different transformative possibilities open to them. My approach also points to the need to recognize the multiple identities of state bureaucrats, particularly their role as "moral agents," and to give greater emphasis to the moral and ideological facets of the state. By pointing to the underlying networks of relations that motivate actors working within the state to use state resources to advance policy, we both distinguish them from other bureaucrats and also highlight the important powers professional movements can access vis-à-vis privileged positions in the state. This willingness to operate within the state may constrain more radical revolutionary agendas. However, as the cases show, drawing on the infrastructure of the state also enables quite a lot of far-reaching change. In this way, it offers an important intervention in the debate over the political consequences of social movements (Baumgartner and Mahoney 2005; Burstein and Sausner 2005; Piven 2006; Skocpol 2003) and responds to calls to consider movement influences beyond the agenda-setting stage in comparative historical perspective (Amenta et al. 2010).

Structuring the Possibilities for Professional Movement Influence: Heightened Political Competition in the Wake of Democratic Transition

"Transitions are highly interactive moments. The bargaining context is defined, and issues are placed on the agenda concurrently or sequentially, as a result of the relations among the actors involved and the historical sequence that informs their evaluation of the situation."

—Margaret Keck, *The Workers' Party and Democratization in Brazil*

Recent work has taken aim at specifying the conditions that lead to policy change in countries transitioning from authoritarianism and engaged in processes of democratization. Amid the broader context of democratic breakthrough, Wong, for example, suggests that authoritarian governments in Taiwan and South Korea that are no longer insulated from political pressures in society needed to compete for votes and preemptively initiated programs to make access to health care universal (2004, 15). While many commonalties marked the political contexts of Taiwan and South Korea, the case studies I consider in this book lend themselves to an altogether different kind of analysis. Specifically, I explore the way in which important *differences* in political contexts following democratic transition lead to different kinds of interactions between states and professional movements and, ultimately, different policy outcomes.

The central contention of this book is that, even when outgoing authoritarian governments do not preemptively initiate universalistic programs, democratic transition creates new political opportunities for the expansion of important new social rights—opportunities that professional movements are uniquely predisposed to take advantage of. These opportunities come about because heightened political competition creates incentives for new political parties to be receptive to innovative policy ideas that can help them capture important segments of the electorate. Although such incentives would not, on their face, appear to advantage professional movements any more than labor unions, left-wing political parties, or vocal mass movements, I suggest that professional movements are particularly empowered because of their occupation of privileged positions in the state and their knowledge of the law.

When authoritarian governments relinquish absolute control over the "rules of the game" following democratic transition, professionals holding legal training and occupying privileged positions in the state stand newly empowered to pursue major social change through legal and other avenues previously closed to them under dictatorship. This book therefore draws out the role that "professional movements" play in the expansion of health policy in two different policy domains (universal health care and HIV/AIDS treatment) in three major industrializing countries engaged in processes of democratic transition (Thailand, Brazil, and South Africa).

Heightened Political Competition

Sociologists and political scientists have pointed to the importance of changes in "political opportunity structures," "windows of opportunity," and "critical junctures" to social and policy change (Capoccia and Kelemen 2007; Kingdon 1984; Kitschelt 1986; McAdam, McCarthy and Zald 1996; Tarrow 1996). More generally, this work dovetails with other scholarship that has charted the importance of critical moments of flux in which politics and policy become more fluid and enable the possibility of change (Gourevitch 1986) and related work that has emphasized the possibility of rapid institutional change during crisis, followed by consolidation and long periods of stasis (Krasner et al. 1984). While some variation exists among these accounts, very generally they suggest that major change can come from within society or exogenous pressures from outside.[3] Recent scholarship on social policy in the industrializing world has built on this work by concretely emphasizing the importance of transitions to democracy and "critical realignments" in opening possibilities for expansive social reforms (Haggard and Kaufman 2008; Huber and Stephens 2012; Wong 2004).

I build on this work by advancing the term "heightened political competition" to refer to specific moments in the process of democratic transition when the status quo shifts and it becomes advantageous for parties or governing executives to consider innovative policy initiatives that may help them to either maintain or capture political power. Most commonly, I theorize that heightened political competition may take place when authoritarian governments introduce and compete in national elections for the first time (as in South Korea or Taiwan in the late 1980s and early 1990s); when corruption and electoral fraud become so endemic and associated with a dominant political party that political parties that had been shut out of the process are afforded opportunities to win votes (Mexico in the late 1990s and early 2000s); and when new "rules of the game" (North 1990), defined typically by the introduction of new constitutions or similar overhauls in the electoral rules change the usual political calculations of political parties (Colombia in the early 1990s). While this is not intended to be an exhaustive list of such moments of heightened political competition, it does illustrate a range of possible situations. Broadly speaking, the conditions that produce heightened political competition usually involve some marked change that substantively alters the dynamics of political competition. However, the factors that create these new dynamics—whatever they may be—must lead to relative parity among political parties (relatively greater competition than before) or, at the very least, not result in immediate electoral dominance after their introduction. Some have emphasized the vote share by the largest party to be a meaningful measure of competitiveness (Gerring, Thacker, and Alfaro 2012, 10); I point instead to the difference between the first and second vote-getters, since these dynamics—rather than the overall vote share of the largest party—seem to bear most on the openness of leading political parties to change and, in turn, the potential influence of professional movements.

This concept bears similarities to Grzymala-Busse's notion of "robust competition" (2007). However, whereas Grzymala-Busse explores how the threat of replacement by another party prompts ruling parties to adopt formal institutions that constrain state behavior, my work explores a different phenomenon altogether: how democratic transition creates new channels for the expansion of state social policy through mechanisms that are both legal and organizational. Rather than focusing on party transformation as an independent causal variable, I explore how the introduction of political competition has sociological consequences, specifically how it provides an opening for professional movements. And in contrast to other recent work that has explored cases in which outgoing authoritarian governments preemptively institute universalistic reforms in order to maintain power in new democratic political environments (Wong 2004), my work explores cases in which the authoritarian incumbent no longer expects to compete seriously on the national political stage.

The important point I am making here is that we cannot take the quality or character of processes of democratic transition for granted. The political interests and incentives of incumbents are not always the same in all cases, nor are the dynamics limited to mass organizations in civil society. This is to say that even among cases in which the authoritarian incumbent no longer seeks to have a sustained future on the national political stage, greater attention is needed to understand the way in which the dynamics of democratic transition affect policy choice differently in different cases. Comparison of the political dynamics within these cases of emerging economies engaged in the politics of democratic transition is therefore useful for drawing out differences that have been neglected by theory. In the cases of Thailand and Brazil, immersed in a political context of heightened political competition, parties competed savagely for opportunities to represent constituents. In South Africa, however, transition led to an electoral outcome that most regarded as a foregone conclusion. However, most unexpectedly, rule by a party that would seem to have had more of a mandate than the governments in the other two countries led to mostly unfulfilled dreams of expanded social rights in the areas of health care and medicine.

It is important to note that I am not suggesting that the crucial difference that delineates the cases of Thailand and Brazil from South Africa—heightened political competition—necessarily secures or guarantees policy innovation by itself. Rather, as the literature before me suggests, it creates opportunities for policy innovations to take root. In order to understand who put the health care and medicine issues on the political agenda and drove them through the political process in countries where heightened political competition provides such opportunities, exploration of the strategic actions of health care reformers is required to understand where specific reform ideas come from and how and why an expensive policy reform, such as health care expansion, makes its way through the political agenda amid possible alternatives. In this way, it answers calls to deepen analyses of the role of politics in explaining health policy outcomes (Reich 1994; Schneider 2002), while complementing quantitative research that has explored the relationship between democracy and health (Bor 2007; McGuire 2010; Ross 2006; Shandra et al. 2004).

Part I

ACCESS TO HEALTH CARE

2

THAILAND: CHASING THE DREAM OF FREE MEDICAL CARE FOR THE SICK

"Access to health care should be viewed as a right and not charity."

—Dr. Sanguan Nitayarumphong

Thailand's dramatic adoption of universal health care in 2001 garnered worldwide attention. The program was put into place just four years after a landmark constitution took effect amid a broader backdrop of democratic opening. The reform made major improvements to the health care system and extended access to health care to millions of citizens who had previously been without it in the unlikeliest of moments: just four years after the Asian financial crisis had led the country's currency to collapse and the government to assume major debt obligations from the IMF. Thailand's program has since been heralded by health care analysts as a model for the developing world and spurred other industrializing countries to take an interest in universal health coverage (Damrongplasit and Melnick 2009; Somkotra and Lagrada 2008; WHO 2010). While existing scholarship has emphasized the importance of electoral rule changes (Hicken 2006; Selway 2011) and a populist political party (McCargo and Pathmanand 2005; Phongpaichit and Baker 2004) in bringing about the policy, these accounts neglect the critical role played by a longstanding movement of elite medical professionals in the policy's institutionalization. This chapter highlights the important role played by progressive physicians in Thailand's Rural Doctors' Movement who drew on their knowledge, social networks, and privileged positions to institutionalize universal health care over powerful opposition forces. In the absence of the strategic actions of this network, there is little evidence to suggest that Thailand's universal coverage policy would ever have been a major issue in the 2001 election, much less a policy that would have been implemented and gone on to receive international acclaim.

Progressive physicians in Thailand's Rural Doctors' Movement forged bonds working to advance the cause of health equity in Thailand's poorest rural areas when the country was under a military dictatorship in the 1970s. At a time when other doctors were leaving the public service to take more lucrative positions abroad or in private urban hospitals in Bangkok, doctors in this movement actually sought positions in community hospitals in the country's poor regions in the north and northeast, founding an organization called the Rural Doctors' Society.

Following democratization in the 1990s, founding members of the Rural Doctors' Society moved up the ranks within the Ministry of Public Health and acted strategically to make changes that would pave the way for the country's landmark universal health care reform in the absence of mass demand. Playing leading roles in a movement for constitutional reform, they helped prompt changes that altered the character of political competition, leading political parties to compete on the basis of policy proposals, as opposed to personality, while introducing changes that would lead to greater citizen participation in political affairs. In this new political environment, the doctors then drew on their knowledge, networks, and positions in the state to make universal coverage an issue in the 2001 election, convening a panel of experts to provide support and legitimacy to proposals for universal coverage; drawing on funding from international organizations to finance and mobilize a grassroots petition campaign for universal health care; embedding the policy in the campaign platform of an innovative new political party named Thai Rak Thai; implementing the policy as a national pilot project before politicians could go back on their word or the medical profession could mobilize against it; and co-opting attempts by conservative international organizations to implement neoliberal policy and retrench Thailand's fledgling universal coverage reform.

The Thailand that has become known today as a global destination for health care is hardly recognizable from the Thailand of the 1970s. In the 1970s, men, on average, did not live to 60. Infants died at five times the rate they do today, and children died at more than six times today's rate (UN Department of Economic and Social Affairs 2015). State programs that aimed to provide access to health care for citizens were in their infancy, focused mainly on providing care to relatively well-off urban civil servants and their families. Where public health care infrastructure did exist, it was often more concentrated in urban areas and provided care to only a fraction of the country's citizenry. Although this description hints at the broad challenges the country faced related to health and development at the time, it does little to capture the stark differences between the lives of people in Thailand's moneyed urban areas and those of the vast majority of the poor living in rural areas.

In the mid-1970s, 84 percent of the country's poor lived in rural villages—nearly two-thirds of those in the impoverished north and northeast—while just over 8 percent lived in Bangkok and the country's municipal areas (National Statistical Office 1979). At the end of the decade, per capita income in Bangkok was six times that of people in the country's rural northeast (AusAid 1983, 1); by 1981, urban incomes would be ten times higher than those in rural areas (World Bank report in Bunpanya 1982, 5). With few exceptions, physicians were drawn almost exclusively from the elite (urban) classes (Maxwell 1975, 483). And very broadly, the medical profession held few allegiances to the problems of the rural areas: Between 1965 and 1966, 90 of the 93 doctors graduating from Chiang Mai University went abroad to work immediately after graduation (Cohen 1989, 162), and over the course of the decade, as many as one thousand Thai doctors left to work in the United States permanently (Pongsuphap 2007, 37–39). Use of medical facilities, not surprisingly, was therefore principally an urban phenomenon: Even though the vast majority of people living in the country lived in rural areas in the 1970s, by 1977 visits to urban provincial hospitals accounted for nearly half of all outpatient doctors' visits (Wibulpolprasert and Pengpaibon 2003, 8).

The Activist Origins of a Professional Movement to Expand Access to Health Care

Set against the backdrop of the Vietnam War, the plight of the country's rural poor appeared even dimmer amid the political repression of military rule. A series of harsh military dictators with ties to the United States would rule Thailand for much of the 1950s through the 1980s, and the country would enjoy only a brief window of democracy from 1973 to 1976. It was not until around this time that the government would begin to address the problem of rural health inequity in a serious, albeit limited, way. During this democratic period, socialist ideas that had been banned for some time would begin to circulate (Lertsuridej interview 2009), and grassroots social movements in Thailand began to flourish, particularly among students and farmers. The Peasants' Federation of Thailand, founded in 1974, was "the most broad-based, well-organized association of poor, rural villagers in Thailand," while the National Student Center of Thailand became an influential center of activism after 1969 and became a home to Marxist activists beginning in 1974 (Missingham 2003, 23, 25–26). Amid this wave of activism, a small group of activist doctors and medical students began to nurture a commitment to addressing the problems faced by the rural masses and to play an active role in the political awakening that was occurring.

One such medical student—Sanguan Nitayarumphong—served as editor of the school newspaper and head of the Mahidol University Student Union (Pongpisut interview 2009; Ungpakorn interview 2009). After a means-tested government program that sought to provide health care to the poor was implemented in 1975, Sanguan began to publish articles in the school newspaper on health security, enlisting medical professors to write for the paper, including Dr. Prasan Tengjai, the co-founder of a new Buddhist socialist political party called Palang

Mai (Nitayarumphong 2006, 21). Jon Ungpakorn, a physics professor at Mahidol and son of Puey Ungpakorn, the well-known rector of Thammasat University, began working with student activists on another student newspaper at the time, called the *Voice of Mahidol* (Ungpakorn interview 2009). Collectively, these venues provided student activists with opportunities to give voice to social justice concerns and to establish ties with aspiring like-minded professionals with whom they would work more closely later.

These doctors-in-training envisioned themselves as having a role to play in the process of social development in the countryside. As early as 1974, students and professors at Mahidol University collaborated to create a seminar to revise the existing curriculum and to encourage young doctors to go to the countryside to volunteer in order "to acquaint themselves with rural health problems" (Drug Study Group 1984, 5). Many of the young medical students became involved in the broader political movement of the time. Some also used their skills to address the issues through a technical organization they set up called the Equality Action Group, which provided education and awareness programs at the secondary school level on population issues, such as venereal disease and contraceptives (Wibulpolprasert interview 2009). Over four thousand student volunteers joined what became known as the Return to the Countryside Campaign to spend a month in rural villages, getting acquainted with and trying to understand local problems. This event coincided with the Public Health for the Masses campaign, another major effort designed to bring attention to the problems faced by the rural poor (Cohen 2007, 110).

The progressive work of these medical activists took place at a time when the idea of "primary health care," which emphasized the importance of basic health promotion and disease prevention activities, the use of volunteers, and community participation in health care, was just beginning to be popularized around the globe. While public health professionals generally recognize the WHO-UNICEF Conference on Primary Health Care in Alma Ata in 1978 as a watershed moment in the diffusion of ideas related to primary health care, Thailand's experimentation with primary health care dated back to the 1960s and early 1970s when community health volunteers were used in the control of malaria and other aspects of health services in two different pilot projects.[1]

Working with senior doctors in the Ministry of Public Health, a group of medical activists would form an organization called the Rural Doctors' Federation in 1976. The Federation would meet and produce a journal aimed at sharing doctors' experiences in the countryside; collectively, they set a goal of traveling to communist China to learn firsthand about the work of the "barefoot doctors" there (Wibulpolprasert interview 2009). A few medical activists at this time openly described their radical views as socialist (Tangcharoensathien interview

2009), while some tried to cast their views more moderately as concerned student activists interested in the welfare of rural people. Others refused such labels altogether and emphasized instead the public health benefits of "primary health care." Sanguan himself expressed an interest in visiting Sweden as a student because of its universal health care system and suggested that the social democratic aims of countries like Denmark, Sweden, and West Germany meshed well with his own ideology (Nitayarumphong 2006, 22–23). Concern with plight of the rural poor animated them all.

The founding of the federation took place, however, at an inauspicious moment. A U.S.-backed military junta mounted a coup and then took power in October of 1976. A wave of repression by the new military government was accompanied by the rise of conservative paramilitary forces, an increase in violence against the left, and broader efforts to stanch the spread of communism in Southeast Asia following the fall of Vietnam. Despite growing global concern with the social and economic development of rural communities, progressive efforts to empower villagers by the Rural Doctors' Federation left them open to charges of being communist agents. Amid growing violence and disappearances by military and paramilitary forces, such activism stood to have very real consequences on their lives.[2]

The period following the military coup was a particularly dangerous time for Sanguan, who as president of the Mahidol Student Union had attained quite a high profile as a student activist and had been charged with being a communist (Lertsuridej interview 2009). Sanguan went into hiding and consulted with the professors he most trusted—Dr. Ari Valyasevi, the dean of Mahidol's Ramathibodi Medical School, and Dr. Prawase Wasi and Dr. Sem Pringpaungaew, two luminaries connected to the Ministry of Public Health—to discuss his options (Lertsuridej interview 2009; Nitayarumphong 2008). Amid the conservative backlash, protection was not an easy task, since even the university's vice rector was reported to be a member of one of the right-wing movements (Ungpakorn interview 2009). In time, though, with the support of his professors Sanguan took gradual steps back into public view to test the police and military's interest in him and eventually continued his studies free of harassment. Some of Sanguan's friends, however, were not so lucky, including two young medical activists who had been high-achieving students at the country's top medical school: Surapong Suebwonglee, who later served as editor of the *Rural Doctors' Bulletin*, and Prommin Lertsuridej, a close friend of Sanguan who was secretary-general of the radical student organization, the Mahidol Front. Along with several thousand others, Surapong and Prommin were forced to go into hiding with communist insurgents in the forest.[3]

While the 1976 coup halted the activities of the Rural Doctors' Federation, in 1978 the group was reconstituted with a less inflammatory name, the Rural

Doctors' Society, as the word *federation* brought to mind radical labor and farmers' organizations that had been targeted by right-wing militant groups (Trirat 2000, 15). The "society" brought together medical professionals who were similarly concerned about the harsh social and economic inequalities in the country, the lack of access to health care, and the plight of the country's rural poor. Rather than leave the public service for more lucrative careers, doctors who joined the Rural Doctors' Society sought to work in the country's poorest rural areas, especially in the country's north and northeast. The motivations that animated the work of the Rural Doctors are perhaps best summed up in the words of a senior member of the Rural Doctors' movement, Dr. Wichai Chokewiwat: "When I was a rural doctor, I saw many people taken ill and becoming almost penniless. They had to sell their farmland or even their daughter to get enough money to pay for their medical treatment. It was such a painful and bitter experience that we dreamt of providing free medical care to the sick" (quoted in Kijtiwatchakul 2007, 17).

Together the Rural Doctors' Society sought to improve the lives of the rural poor and build morale among physicians serving in rural areas by starting management training programs; developing handbooks, activities, newsletters, journals, and awards; and organizing visits by senior doctors to support their work (Wibulpolprasert and Pengpaibon 2003, 13). They imagined their work extending far beyond the walls of the hospital, connecting with what we now popularly call the "social determinants of health," working with villagers to develop community gardening projects, revolving funds, village banks, and drug cooperatives[4] with the goal of improving the broader inputs into people's health.[5] Some of the first projects promoted socioeconomic development (Quinn 1997, 94).

Aware of their power to heal and their high university status, uneducated villagers frequently thought of doctors as gods.[6] Even today, ordinary citizens still hold doctors in esteem above cabinet members, ambassadors, generals, governors, and professors (Ockey 2004, 159). However, the Rural Doctors' work with villagers challenged some of the traditional hierarchies between doctors and patients and led some conservative members of the medical profession to perceive such medical activism as a threat to physicians' elite professional status (Bamber 1997, 233). So the social justice commitments of the Rural Doctors fostered something of a chasm between conservative doctors who were more interested in maintaining a strict relationship between doctors and patients and those seeking to use their revered status to mobilize action to improve the health status of the masses, particularly in rural areas (Bunpanya 1982, 5).

While in the rural areas, Rural Doctors began to develop stronger ties both with one another and with other progressives working to improve the plight of the poor. These ties would later prove important in efforts to expand access to health care and medicine. Dr. Mongkol na Songkhla, who would go on to play a critical role in the implementation of both universal health care and antiretroviral access in Thailand, served as the director of a hospital and chief provincial medical officer in the northeastern province of Korat at the same time that the young Dr. Sanguan became director of another hospital in the same province. Rural Doctors also developed ties with Jon Ungpakorn, an activist university professor who in 1980 had started the Thai Volunteer Service (TVS), a Peace Corps–style program that built on his father Puey's Graduate Volunteer Project and the Thailand Rural Reconstruction Movement.[7] One of the first TVS volunteers to work with the Rural Doctors was based in Korat with Dr. Sanguan. Jon had met Sanguan when Sanguan was a medical student at Ramathibodi Medical School in Bangkok but really got to know him during this period (Ungpakorn interview 2009). To these young doctors, Jon served as a "respected mentor" (Tangcharoensathien interview 2009).

While these progressive doctors stood in the minority within their profession, they also enjoyed the support of senior administrators in universities and in government. In particular, Dr. Prawase Wasi, a respected physician at Mahidol University who served as adviser to the deputy minister of health, provided the young doctors with a much-needed patron to stand behind them and legitimize their activities.[8] And although a loyalist in matters related to the Thai monarchy, Prawase did not mince words in identifying what he saw as impediments to social progress. At a Primary Health Care conference organized by some members of the Rural Doctors' Society in 1986, he singled out "the state, the religious establishment, colonialism, and the economic and educational systems as the '*oppressive social structures*' that people must '*liberate themselves from*' in the course of attaining good health" (quoted in Lohmann 1986, 8; emphasis in original). The doctors' commitments to the broad-based participatory development of rural communities and their common bonds were therefore shaped by Dr. Prawase in the ideas he laid out in his book *Public Health for the People* in 1976 (Wibulpolprasert interview 2009) as well as the principle of "Health for All" articulated at Alma Ata in 1978.

Gradual political opening in the 1980s, including an order of amnesty for insurgents hiding in the forest, allowed some of the doctors who had been in hiding to resume their studies, including Dr. Surapong and Dr. Prommin. Taking advantage of this opening, the Rural Doctors deepened their engagement in the countryside by founding nongovernmental organizations (NGOs) dedicated to community development. Dr. Sanguan chaired the Primary Health Care (PHC) Group while also holding the position of director of the Buayai District Hospital; in time, the PHC Group grew from a two-person operation to include a credit union and activities involving handicapped children and malnutrition

(*Thai Development Newsletter* 1986a, 31). A diverse set of progressive professional organizations working with Jon Ungpakorn's Thai Volunteer Service helped form the Thai Development Support Committee (TDSC) in 1982 to bring international attention and funds to support Thailand's development. In 1983, the doctors had a hand in creating the Primary Health Care Coordinating Network, chaired by Dr. Prawase Wasi, with other interested organizations (Cohen 1989, 168; Drug Study Group 1984, 5–6, 17). And in 1990, working with Dr. Prawase, Sanguan formed another NGO called the Local Development Institute (LDI).[9]

Entering the National Bureaucracy

Because of their dedication to the countryside and their connections to elites in the ministry, Rural Doctors found opportunities for advancement when they left hospital service and joined the national Ministry of Public Health, including as liaison to the World Health Organization and as director-in-waiting in the ministry's Office of Primary Health Care (on early work, Chunharas interview 2009). As bureaucrats in the ministry, the doctors in the movement would gain experience managing the development of some of the country's nascent state health insurance programs, including the program that aimed to provide care to low-income people started in 1975 (Nitayarumphong 2006, 58); a subsidized government program for low- and middle-income Thais started in 1983 (Supachutikul and Sirinirund 1993); and a social health insurance program for workers in the formal sector started in 1990 (Burns interview 2009).

As they rose up the ranks, the Rural Doctors' shared interest in advancing the cause of health equity led them to create an informal network in 1986 called the Sampran Forum that united the energy and spirit of the younger generation with some respected figures from the older generation that had supported them.[10] While one history of the organization suggests that its founding evolved out of debates among group members over technical issues (Nitayarumphong 2006, 48), an alternative account provided by an informant suggests that the forum was actually originally conceived after a contentious row erupted among people in the movement over who would be most appropriate to lead the Ministry of Public Health. In other words, the subject matter around which the forum originally cohered was inherently political, rather than technical.

The group's mentor, Prawase Wasi, observed that "it might be difficult for the group to resolve [its differences], and that structured attempts to do so might only stimulate additional conflicts, especially given the level of ego among the participants" (Nitayarumphong 2006, 48). He therefore instead suggested that it serve as "a mechanism to share experiences and lessons on a range of issues, and allow each participant to take from it what they could, without trying to force consensus on any issue" (Nitayarumphong 2006, 48). Rather than serve as "an intellectual boxing ring," the forum became a kind of informal think tank or, in the words of the late Dr. Sanguan, a "continuous means to improve our intellectual capabilities" (Nitayarumphong 2006, 49). The forum would become a monthly opportunity to nurture their own ideas related to health equity and would include talks by senators, doctors working in rural areas, and occasionally even foreign medical experts.

After a social security program that included health care benefits for workers in the formal sector was passed in 1990, the Sampran Forum "immediately took action to initiate extensive research on the policy" (Nitayarumphong 2006, 49). One of the forum's members, Dr. Viroj Tangcharoensathien, a medical doctor and economist-in-training, gave presentations with Sanguan on the potential impacts of the law and began work with the Department of Labor to ensure that the program would be designed and implemented effectively to avoid pitfalls that had led to the fragmentation of health systems in other countries (Nitayarumphong 2006, 49–50). The doctors played an important role in the program's development by convincing the Department of Labor that it did not need to build its own hospitals to serve the program. Doing so would not only help control costs but also derail new avenues for clientelism and make possible integration with other state programs easier in the future. Second, several of the doctors played leading roles in a costing study that provided a basis for the program's reimbursement rate for participating hospitals (Tangcharoensathien interview 2009; Wallee-ittikul interview 2009; Wibulpolprasert interview 2009). The study led to more extensive collaboration with international consultants on issues related to health financing and economics and built on earlier experiences that members of the movement had had with health economics in the 1980s through workshops sponsored by international organizations like the WHO and via on-the-job training gained while managing some of the country's pilot state health insurance programs.

While most in the Sampran Forum got to know each other as students at Mahidol University's Ramathibodi Medical School during Thailand's turbulent 1970s, some met during their time working in rural areas after graduating medical school. Others met in graduate school at Antwerp's Royal Institute of Public Health, which some the doctors attended. Some were identified by Prawase Wasi or other members of the forum and invited to participate. But some common causes were advancing health equity, standing against professional interests that put profit over the needs of the community, and serving as a stalwart voice of people's concerns. The forum would become a natural venue for doctors in the movement to nurture their concerns related to rural health and development and maintain strong ties as they rose up the ranks of the Ministry of Public Health.

By the early 1990s, the power of the Rural Doctors within the broader medical profession in Thailand was growing. Between 1987 and 1993, the Rural Doctors enjoyed clear majorities on the board of the Medical Council, which was charged with setting the country's ethical standards, investigating complaints, and representing the interests of doctors (Wibulpolprasert 2003, 122). The Rural Doctors' interest in controlling the council was aimed at ensuring that the council "protected the interests of the public more than the profession" (Wibulpolprasert interview 2009).

While control of that organization was earned on the basis of elections by members of the profession (at a time when the profession did not perceive the movement as a threat to its interests), core members of the movement also sought to increase their power by creating new autonomous parastatal organizations that were affiliated with the Ministry of Public Health but without being subject to the same bureaucratic rules and procedures.[11] In some cases, the parastatal organizations founded and controlled by the movement would come to enjoy significant funding and exercise considerable influence in the country's political affairs. The Thai Health Promotion Foundation, for example, had a budget of $45 million in 2001 (Vathesatogkit 2005, 17, 24) and entertained multi-million-dollar proposals aiming to encourage grassroots political participation by contentious political factions (*Fah Diaw Kan* 2009). And the National Health Assembly—a nationally representative body modeled after the World Health Organization's governing body in Geneva that aims to get citizens more involved in health care decision-making and governance—has cultivated a new crop of activist leaders friendly to the doctors' causes. The semiautonomous nature of some of these organizations not only reduced the level of political interference in their operations but also gave executives more independence and authority to direct them, while providing them with the ability to draw on expertise from outside the bureaucracy (Chunharas personal communication 2013).

One project in which doctors in the movement exercised their growing autonomy to experiment with new models of health care provision was the Ayudhya Project. Started in 1989 in partnership with two professors with whom they had studied at the Antwerp Royal Institute of Hygiene and Tropical Medicine, the project posted a doctor who lived and worked in the community in a family medicine practice. In providing care to community members for 70 baht per visit—a rate that had been carefully negotiated with community members—the project served as a demonstration project, offering a model of how a universal health care program working at the local level might work at the national level (Nitayarumphong 2006, 39–43).

While experimental programs like Ayudhya and the state health insurance programs that the doctors played a role in developing helped to extend health care access to growing segments of the population, the expansion of health care access in Thailand's brief window of democracy and longer periods of authoritarian rule took place in fits and starts, and access to health care was still far from universal. However, the political environment would begin to change in 1989, followed by a more serious process of democratization beginning in 1992. The doctors themselves would not only play a significant role in these changes, they would also take advantage of some of the new opportunities inherent in the new political environment they had a hand in creating.

Thailand's Slow Road to Democratization: The Central Role of the Rural Doctors

Whereas a military dictatorship ruled Brazil for twenty consecutive years (1964–1985) and apartheid lasted for nearly fifty years in South Africa (1948–1994), the contemporary history of authoritarianism in Thailand was marked by greater discontinuity. Following the country's brief period of democracy from 1973 to 1976, Thailand did not see another civilian prime minister elected until 1989.[12] However, even this government would be short-lived, as it was interrupted by another coup in 1991. Citizens could not protest openly during this time (Encarnacion-Tadem 2001, 49), although there was evidence that political parties and Parliament were gaining power over time, with politicians gradually coming to pose a challenge to soldiers and bureaucrats (McCargo 2001, 92). While political factions did exist during the period dominated by the military (1976–1992), more generally self-interest, a contempt for electoral politics, and a desire to limit mass political participation animated the concerns of those in power (McCargo 1997, 19–24). Political participation was generally confined to the upper class (Hewison 1997; McCargo 2002).

After the restoration of democracy in 1992 following the death of civilians at the hands of the military, the country embarked on a slower and more deliberate process of democratization that culminated in a new constitution in 1997 (McCargo 2003, 135). Efforts to create a new constitution were largely the result of pressure from progressive elites, most notably Dr. Prawase Wasi, the patriarch of the Rural Doctors' movement (McCargo 2005, 511). Prawase had been centrally involved with efforts to promote democracy at the time of transition. Just one month before the September 1992 elections, he worked with the doctors in the Rural Doctors' movement to form the Health Assembly for Democracy, which sought to involve the medical profession in the institutionalization of democracy (Bamber 1997, 242). The public stance for democracy and against military repression was particularly meaningful to Rural Doctors like Surapong

Suebwonglee, who had experienced repression firsthand in the 1970s and sought to ensure that violence at the hands of the military did not happen again (Sakboon 1992). Aside from promoting democracy and encouraging the masses to vote, the doctors also played a prominent role in the creation of the democracy watchdog organization PollWatch (Bamber 1997, 242).

Even more important, Prawase wrote a letter to Anand Panyarachun, the caretaker prime minister in 1992, asking him to amend the constitution and create a better political system (Wasi 2002, 22). Following transition to the country's first elected government under the old constitution, Prawase was named chairman of the Democracy Development Committee (DDC) by the new government in 1994; the Prawase-led DDC recommended that a new constitution be drafted to promote real political reform (Wasi 2002, 22–23).

Activists at the time had disagreed with Prawase's decision to become chair of the committee, believing that the Democrat Party in power was not sincere about embarking on political reform (Chokewiwat interview 2009). Prawase too felt that the Democrat Party was trying to use the deliberations of the committee to avoid doing any real work on the problem (McCargo 2001, 94). Wary that politicians would reject attempts to institute checks on their political power, Prawase therefore drew on the expertise of one of Thailand's most recognized specialists in public law who had written a book on constitutionalism; as a doctor, and not a lawyer or politician, Prawase reportedly brought the book everywhere and read it between ten and twenty times, seeking to gain a strong understanding of constitutionalism (Chokewiwat interview 2009). With this expertise in hand, he then sought to involve the masses in the constitution's formation to ensure that the process of reform would continue (Wasi 2002, 22–23).

While Prawase would describe his efforts to create a reform movement as involving a combination of personal lobbying, media outreach, and public involvement (Wasi 2002, 22–24), some of his concerns were also animated by a desire to institutionalize a stable political order that would mitigate against the potential chaos and violence that royal succession caused by the death of an aging king might eventually stir (McCargo 2005, 511). In one reading, his desire to replace corrupt politicians who occupied ministerial positions with "morally-upright technocrats" was connected to a desire to ensure that the monarchy would be preserved (McCargo 2001, 95, 98). Although the constitutional drafting process was dominated by elites, the "People's Constitution," as it would come to be known, was more than at any point in the past also informed by input from the people and aimed to correct some of the problems of Thailand's political past—among them, poor (and frequently corrupt) leadership and the influence of money in politics. This would be achieved through a system of checks and balances that would ensure greater institutional responsiveness, accountability, and capacity (Hewison 2010, 121; McCargo 2003, 130; Winichakul 2008, 19).

The drafters aimed to professionalize politics and create a stronger executive and political party system that would widen politicians' commitment to the national interest, reduce patronage, and increase popular participation (McCargo 2003, 141). The constitution sought to address these problems in three ways. First, the constitution instituted electoral reform that involved replacement of the appointed Senate with a two-hundred-person elected upper house and the creation of a five-hundred-person lower house, while making political parties stronger and more coherent by reducing the incentives for politicians to switch parties. Second, the constitution created new watchdog agencies, including the Electoral Commission, the National Human Rights Commission, and the National Counter-Corruption Commission. Finally, the constitution contained new provisions that outlined the rights of the people and included new articles that gave citizens the power to challenge elected officials in new ways (McCargo 2003, 135). After collecting a petition with the required fifty thousand signatures, citizens gained the power to prompt Parliament to consider legislation (Zurcher 2005) and to petition a new anti-corruption body to investigate corrupt politicians or even to have politicians impeached (Thabchumpon 2002, 320).

These provisions, combined with the broad rhetoric of popular empowerment that had framed the constitution's development, emboldened citizens to make their voices heard and led to the growth of popular protests around a wide variety of issues (McCargo 2003, 139, 148). While these interventions by no means completely solved the problems that led the constitution to be created, they did have important effects on the quality and character of democracy in Thailand. Amid rampant allegations of vote-buying and fraud, the new Electoral Commission, for example, invalidated the election victories of nearly half of the members of the new Senate in the country's 2000 senatorial elections, which led to six election reruns, and also required three election reruns in the 2001 general elections (McCargo 2003, 138). Even more importantly, the reforms provided incentives for political parties to reject solely provincially focused strategies that centered on delivering benefits to their home constituencies and to create more nationally oriented policies and more coherent party platforms (Hicken 2006; Hicken and Selway 2012; Kuhonta 2008; Selway 2011; Selway 2015).

The stamp of the Rural Doctors' movement on the constitution—in particular their effort to create a more stable political system and institute a system of checks and balances—led some Rural Doctors involved in the process to dub Prawase Wasi, the patriarch of the Rural Doctors' movement, as a "mastermind of the constitution" (Chokewiwat interview 2009).[13] Had he and those working closely with him not acted strategically to create the conditions for a substantive political reform process, it is unclear what other sources would have prompted Thailand to usher in such a new and different era of political competition in the years that followed.[14]

Incremental Progress in the Early Years of Democratic Transition

In the early years of Thailand's democratic transition, prior to the creation of the new constitution in 1997, the Rural Doctors would make important, albeit limited, progress toward universal health care, and access to health care would remain a major problem in the country. In 1993, just half of the population in Thailand enjoyed access to health care through one of the state's health insurance programs (Pitayarangsarit 2004, 22). A workshop on health care financing in 1993, co-sponsored by the Ministry of Public Health, the National Economic and Social Development Board, and the World Bank, provided a somewhat unlikely opportunity for doctors in the movement to put forward a plan for universal coverage.

Just six years earlier, the World Bank had released a landmark report, *Financing Healthcare Services for Developing Countries,* that emphasized the importance of cost recovery for state health care programs through the charging of user fees and the expansion of private health insurance as a way of alleviating burden on the state. And in 1993, the *World Development Report* (whose theme was "Investing in Health") continued to advocate for neoliberal principles but in a slightly more circumscribed manner (Ewig 2010, 70). In spite of these broader developments, which had been spearheaded by the Bank, the Rural Doctors used the event to advance their cause: "The agenda was set by us . . . most economists at the time . . . they think about efficiency more than equity, so universal coverage which provides equal access . . . will be against their ideology" (Pannarunothai interview 2009). There they circulated for the first time a very primitive roadmap on how to achieve universal coverage, which "marked the beginning of the national health insurance movement in Thailand" (Nitayarumphong 2006, 59). Given its recent history of policies that had the effect of reducing access to health care services, the World Bank sponsoring a conference that unveiled a plan to expand access to services amounted to a surprising outcome. That it did so underscored the cunning way in which doctors in the movement used their positions, networks, and knowledge to set the political agenda in a most unlikely venue.

Further opportunities for the doctors to put universal health care more sub-stantively on the political agenda emerged when Sanguan became adviser to the Committee on Public Health in the House of Representatives. In that role, San-guan immediately began advocating for a national health insurance law and suc-ceeded in getting a bill drafted in 1995; however, in the context of an electoral system marked by weak political parties that had not yet been touched by consti-tutional reform, momentum for the bill died following the demise of a govern-ment and a reshuffle in the ministry (Nitayarumphong 2006, 65–66).

The laissez faire–minded Democrat Party had for some time resisted calls by the Rural Doctors' movement for universal health care. However, the Asian financial crisis of 1997 provided politically expedient reasons for them to expand coverage incrementally without having to make more substantial and transfor-mative health care commitments that would be in conflict with the party's ide-ology. During the tenure of Prime Minister Chuan Leekpai (1997–2001), the Democrats expanded the budget for two of the state's health insurance programs for poor and middle-income people, leading to sizable increases in the number of people with access to health care between 1996 and 2001 (Selway 2011, 177, 180).

The sudden growth in coverage by the state's health insurance programs under the Democrats, however, should be read as a temporary reaction to economic crisis and not a demonstration of the party's ideological commitment to universal health care. At the same time that it expanded state welfare programs to cushion the people against the effects of the growing economic crisis, the country was coming to grips with a $17 billion structural adjustment program by the IMF and a $500 million loan from the Asian Development Bank that aimed to stabi-lize the country's currency in the wake of the Asian financial crisis. Just as larger IMF loans had often done, the ADB loan included conditions that required the country to reform its health, education, and labor sectors. Fearing what would happen if the ADB went about reform on their own, the doctors sought to influ-ence the process by bidding to become the external team that would advise the ministry on the reforms. Since the external advising team could not be an offi-cial government agency, the movement assembled a winning bid using the Rural Doctor–controlled semiautonomous Health Systems Research Institute as the external team. Through these efforts, those involved resisted a corporatization agenda promoted by the World Bank and the ADB (Chunharas interview 2009). While not expanding access to coverage, the professional movement's actions avoided institutionalization of a policy that would ultimately have served as an impediment to efforts to make coverage universal. As the financial crisis abated and the effects of the constitutional reform began to be felt, the movement would take advantage of new opportunities to advance the cause of universal health care.

Drawing on the Unique Powers of the State to Institutionalize the Policy

Financing and Mobilizing the Grassroots Petition Campaign for Universal Coverage

By the late 1990s, the Rural Doctors' movement had come to exercise significant control over the Ministry of Public Health, holding leadership positions in the ministry and its affiliated institutions as well as executive positions in international organizations and civil society (table 2.1 and figure 2.1). The new

TABLE 2.1   List of prominent members of the Sampran Forum and positions held

NAME	POSITIONS HELD
Prawase Wasi	Chairman of the 2010 Assembly for Reform, Chairman of Democracy Development Committee, Founder of *Village Doctor* and *Folk Doctor* magazines, Folk Doctor Society, Local Development Institute, New Consciousness Network, prolific author, revered social critic
Sanguan Nitayarumphong (deceased)	Architect and first Secretary-General of the National Health Security Office, Former Deputy Permanent Secretary MoPH, Founder (with Prawase) of Local Development Institute, Past Member of the Medical Council of Thailand
Amphon Jindawattana	Architect and first Secretary-General of the National Health Assembly, Past Member of the Medical Council of Thailand
Wichai Chokewiwat	Chairman of the Government Pharmaceutical Organization, Former Food and Drug Administration Chief, Past Member of the Medical Council of Thailand
Suwit Wibulpolprasert	Former Vice-Chair of the Global Fund, Thai Representative to the WHO, Chair of the Program Coordinating Board of UNAIDS, Former Deputy Permanent-Secretary MoPH and Senior Adviser to MoPH with involvement in a wide range of projects from Compulsory Licensing to representation at the World Health Assembly, Past Member of the Medical Council of Thailand
Somsak Chunharas	Secretary-General of the National Health Foundation and first Director of the Health Sciences Research Institute, on many boards, Past Member of the Medical Council of Thailand
Supakorn Buasai	CEO, Health Promotion Foundation
Pongpisut Jongudomsuk	Director, Health Sciences Research Institute
Supattra Srivanichakorn	Dean of the ASEAN Institute of Health Development at Mahidol-Salaya, Former Director of Office of Primary Health Care research, First female President of the Medical Council of Thailand
Komatra Chuengsatiansup	Director, Society and Health Institute
Viroj Tangcharoensathien	Director, International Health Policy Program

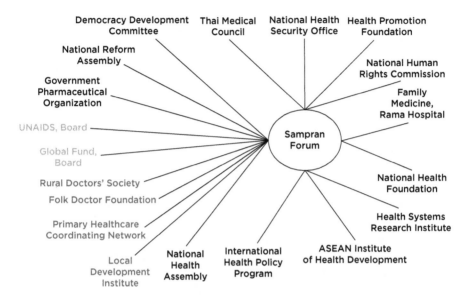

FIGURE 2.1   Historical bases of power of members of the Sampran Forum

Source: Courtesy of the *Journal of Contemporary Asia*.

environment created by the elite-led "People's Constitution" provided citizens with new ways of getting involved in politics and prompted civil society organizations to become more engaged. Doctors in the professional movement used this opportunity to mobilize civil society organizations with whom they had ties dating back to the 1970s to advocate more forcefully for universal health care. The doctors drew, in particular, on ties to two organizations that shared an interest in transforming the health care system.

The Foundation for Consumers (FFC)—led by Saree Ongsomwang, a former nurse who had worked with the Rural Doctors in the 1980s—was an organization that grew out of the work of the Primary Health Care Coordinating Network (Ongsomwang interview 2009). In 1999, health care access became an issue of particular concern to FFC, which released a report that highlighted the problem of unequal access to health care services using a series of fifteen case studies (Foundation for Consumers 2004). The Rural Doctors' movement also reconnected with Jon Ungpakorn, who had, since his time working with the Rural Doctors in the 1970s and 1980s, founded the AIDS Access Foundation in 1991, one of the country's leading HIV/AIDS organizations. Working with these organizations and a broader network of civil society organizations, the doctors sought to take advantage of the provision in the 1997 constitution that would force Parliament to consider legislation when petitions containing fifty thousand signatures had been collected.

In a meeting at the Richmond Hotel in Bangkok, Sanguan shared the results of public opinion polls that pointed to public interest in universal health care; however, Sanguan wanted to frame the campaign for universal health care not as an initiative of government but as "an initiative coming from civil society," with his team acting "technical supporters" (Ungpakorn interview 2009). Aside from giving a common vision and sense of purpose to an otherwise diverse set of civic groups that included labor and youth organizations, the Rural Doctors' movement provided direct financial support in the form of a million baht from the EU-funded Ayudhya Project to help defray the administrative costs of the petition campaign and to pay for technical assistance in drafting a bill for universal coverage (Jongudomsuk interview 2009; Leechanavanichaphan interview 2009). Beginning in March 2000, the AIDS movement—led by Jon Ungpakorn, who had just been elected a senator in the first elections under the new constitution—began to collaborate with ten other grassroots NGO networks to promote universal health care. A campaign to collect signatures in support of the initiative in local communities across the nation kicked off on October 11, 2000—the anniversary of the 1997 "People's Constitution" (Sirisinsuk interview 2009; Ungpakorn interview 2009). The campaign promoted a model of universal health care that involved providing access to all people, regardless of socioeconomic status or nationality, and that included free comprehensive benefits, such as combination antiretroviral medication that could stop the progression of AIDS (Campaign for Universal Health Care brochure 2000).

The inclusion of antiretroviral medication in the benefits package promoted by the campaigners underscored the degree to which the AIDS movement saw universal health care as a ticket to the life-saving medicine so desperately needed by victims of HIV/AIDS. Although eleven different networks were involved in the drive to collect the fifty thousand signatures, the vast majority of the signatures (37,000) were collected by the AIDS movement, which demonstrates that no one understood more keenly than AIDS activists the life-and-death consequences of a government commitment to universal health care (Leechanavanichaphan interview 2009; Suwanphattana et al. 2008, 49–51, 55).[15] The petition campaign succeeded in raising the visibility of the issue among political parties in the run-up to the national elections for prime minister in January 2001. At approximately the same time, another separate health movement, this one led by fellow Rural Doctor and Sampran Forum member Amphon Jindawattana, sought to provide further momentum to the drive for universal coverage. Dr. Amphon's campaign aimed to promote a draft National Health Bill, which would serve as a legal blueprint for a broader health reform involving decentralization, expanded community participation in health care decision-making and governance, as well as universal coverage (although universal coverage was not its primary objective).[16]

Convening an Expert Panel to Apply Pressure from Above

The heightened attention to the issue of universal health care was not enough to guarantee that it would be a substantive issue in the 2001 political race. To raise the visibility of the issue further, the Rural Doctors drew on the resources of one of the parastatal organizations they controlled, the Health Systems Research Institute, to commission a high-level panel of experts in 2000 to explore technical and financial issues related to universal health care. Aside from Sanguan's participation and that of some of the other Rural Doctors, the panel included several other people who had collaborated with the Rural Doctors previously and were known to be sympathetic to the cause, including Chulalongkorn University pharmacy professor Yupadee Sirisinsuk, who also served as a leader in the civil society campaign for universal coverage. At the time, political parties had not taken up the issue of universal health care yet, and the panel was used as a "pressure point" in the run-up to the 2001 elections (Siamwalla interview 2009).

Notably absent were the usual international experts or consultants one might expect—which may have been a strategic calculation made by the Rural Doctors, since international experts might have suggested making changes to aspects of the proposal made by members of the committee (Pannarunothai interview 2009). Invited to chair the panel was Ammar Siamwalla, the president of the Thailand Development Research Institute who was also widely regarded as the country's most respected economist. Ammar recognized that the committee was being used to pressure politicians in the run-up to the election, but after some of the Rural Doctors suggested that the program was fiscally feasible, he agreed to be part of the team (Siamwalla interview 2009). New to issues related to health economics, Ammar was strongly influenced by the Rural Doctor who led the committee (Siamwalla interview 2009).

Panel deliberations were dominated by the concerns and agenda of the Rural Doctors, many of whom were pushing for a single-payer model of the type that some of them had observed in their time in graduate school in Britain (Chunharas interview 2009; Siamwalla interview 2009; Suebwonglee interview 2009; Tangcharoensathien interview 2009). In some cases, the shape that Thailand's program would take was defined by what panel experts did not want Thailand's health care system to become. Dr. Ammar said, "My first order of business [was] for god's sake [to] prevent Thailand from becoming like the United States. That's rule number one. . . . The system unerringly selects the most the most expensive technology without regard to cost-effectiveness" (Siamwalla interview 2009). But even more than foreign models, the doctors' ideas were shaped by their own unsuccessful attempts at making existing government health insurance programs universal. One retrospective account by an ILO consultant who had worked with the Rural Doctors for a decade and had a privileged "insider" status suggested:

> It is the failure of the social security scheme to make provision for dependents of contributors which, it is argued, precipitated the development of plans by the MOPH for the universal coverage scheme. Disappointment at the lack of progress towards [the social security scheme's] expressed goal left the MOPH with little option but to address the continued burden on the public sector health scheme as a matter of some urgency. The universal coverage scheme was a direct response to this. (Burns 2002, 14)

The inability of the Rural Doctors to advance the cause of Universal Coverage through existing policy avenues became frustrating enough that in 2000, some involved in the deliberations published an article in the international academic journal *Health Policy and Planning* that lambasted the government's voluntary state health insurance program for providing no meaningful path to universal coverage.[17] The final report of the commission referred to the rights in the 1997 constitution as a basis for the program.

Embedding the Policy in the Campaign Platform of an Innovative Political Party

While the expert panel helped give standing to a policy enterprise that might have otherwise been considered impossible less than a decade earlier, this "pressure from above" still did not, by itself, succeed in putting universal coverage on the agenda of any of the major political parties contending in the upcoming election. For much of the 1990s—from 1992 to 1995 and again from 1997 to 2001—the Democrat Party controlled Thailand's government. Known for taking a technocratic approach to macroeconomic management, the party had not been friendly to the doctors' entreaties on universal health care and, during the depths of the Asian financial crisis, had instead opted to expand marketing of the very program doctors in the movement had found wanting as a strategy to achieve universal coverage.[18] Sanguan began to look for other political allies, taking aim at political parties directly and bringing politicians and high-level bureaucrats out for visits to the Ayudhya Demonstration Project (Chunharas interview 2009).

The professional movement made more substantial inroads to putting universal health care on the political agenda for the 2001 election when former colleagues with whom the doctors had worked in the 1970s took up executive positions in an innovative new political party. The official in charge of writing Thai Rak Thai's health policy—Dr. Surapong Suebwonglee—was an old friend and colleague of Sanguan from their activist days in the 1970s at Ramathibodi Medical School in Bangkok.[19] Surapong had been one of the more radical medical activists who was forced to go underground in the 1970s. After returning to medical school after the amnesty, Surapong went on to have a very respectable career in medicine.[20] In 1996, an unsuccessful run for Senate with the Palang Tham Party provided him with the opportunity to get to know an executive in the party named Thaksin Shinawatra who would go on to form his own political party, Thai Rak Thai, just three years later (Suebwonglee interview 2009).

In addition to Surapong, the Rural Doctors' movement had another foothold in Thai Rak Thai through another one of its executives, Dr. Prommin Lertsuridej. Dr. Prommin had been vice president of the Rural Doctors' Society and had gone on to work with Sanguan in the Ministry of Public Health from 1990 to 1993 before leaving to work in the private sector with Thaksin Shinawatra's Shinawatra Group (Lertsuridej interview 2009). While Surapong and Prommin were not founding members of the Rural Doctors' Society or Sampran Forum members, they were close friends and had been some of the most committed activists back in the 1970s, having been driven to hide out in the forest after being branded as communists after the military coup in 1976.

Surapong called Sanguan because he knew that for Thai Rak Thai to be successful, it had to differentiate itself from the existing major political parties. Looking for the party to do something big, he asked Sanguan, as one of the government's leading health policy experts, what his top policy priorities were. With a foundation dedicated to promoting health having already been formed in 1999 (and controlled by the doctors), Sanguan had only one goal left: universal health care. Over the next few months, Surapong met with Sanguan several times until enough details had been fleshed out for a meeting with the party's leader, Thaksin Shinawatra (Suebwonglee interview 2009).

The meeting, which took place on Christmas Eve of 1999, involved two of the Rural Doctors working in the Ministry of Public Health—Sanguan and Wichai—along with Thai executives from the Thai Rak Thai inner circle, Thaksin, Pansak Vinyaratn (Thaksin's closest adviser), Prachuap Ungpakorn (a cousin of Jon Ungpakorn and a medical doctor), Somkid Jatusripitak (the party's lead economic adviser), and Surapong. While this description of the actors at the meeting accurately reflects the positions of the people involved, the meeting could alternately have been described as a meeting between Thaksin, a couple of his personal advisers, and three long-standing members of the Rural Doctors' Movement.

In a presentation lasting roughly fifteen minutes, Sanguan and Surapong pitched the idea of universal health care to Thaksin. Thaksin immediately recognized the program's potential appeal to voters.[21] However, he felt that Sanguan's working name for the program, Universal Coverage (or "universal health insurance" in Thai), was too jargonistic and did not clearly communicate the benefits of the program in a way that ordinary people would understand. Thaksin suggested a name for the program that he thought might resonate more effectively with voters: "20 baht to cure every disease," with 20 baht (50 cents) representing the co-pay required of patients seeking treatment for diseases (Suebwonglee interview 2009).

Having agreed to adopt the policy as part of Thai Rak Thai's campaign platform, Thaksin left it to his deputies to work out the details.[22] Surapong wanted to make sure that it was affordable to the ordinary Thai, but he also felt that Thaksin's original suggestion of 20 baht per visit did not go far enough in addressing the inevitable moral hazard problems that might result from care being so cheap, which might lead people to seek treatment more than was necessary. Reasoning that the general populace could afford the 30 baht toll at a major highway in Bangkok (Lertsuridej interview 2009; Suebwonglee interview 2009) and knowing that one hospital in the country had piloted a working scheme charging 40 baht per visit (Chokewiwat interview 2009), Surapong decided that 30 baht was a reasonable co-pay. Thai Rak Thai made its commitment to the policy public in March 2000 (Pitayarangsarit 2004, 58).

Scholars have noted that Thai Rak Thai was the first political party ever to bring to bear sophisticated polling and marketing techniques on political campaigns (Phongpaichit and Baker 2004). Indeed, the emphasis that Thai Rak Thai placed on health care has long been understood to have been a product of this polling. In actual fact, however, polling by Thai Rak Thai found economic problems to be the number one issue among concerned voters, the need for village loan programs to finance projects of local interest second, and social problems associated with the spread of illegal drugs third; compared to these three problems, the desire for greater health insurance coverage was actually very low on the list of voter priorities (Lertsuridej interview 2009).

The important role that the Rural Doctors' movement played in getting the new political party to champion the policy cannot be overstated. Drawing on their knowledge, networks, and privileged positions in the state, the Rural Doctors acted strategically to make universal health care a major issue in the 2001 elections, even though the party's own polls had led them to prioritize other issues. However, the 30 baht program replaced the number three campaign issue that polling had identified—resolving the drug problem[23]—and became the flagship issue on the party's campaign platform, standing alongside a debt moratorium for farmers (who comprised a large but untapped segment of the voting population) and $25,000 revolving loan funds for villages. Once it became clear that Thai Rak Thai's policy platform was generating support nationally, other leading political parties that had rebuffed Sanguan's previous attempts to get them to take up universal coverage suddenly adopted very similar programs, including the Democrats and Chart Thai, a major opposition party to the Democrats with a checkered past.

Implementation of the Policy as a "National Pilot Project"

The victory of Thai Rak Thai in the 2001 election provided the Rural Doctors with a breakthrough in terms of their agenda. The party that had done so much to give visibility to the issue won the right to head a coalition government. However, among some of the Rural Doctors, there was a feeling that, even though Thaksin had made the program the centerpiece of his campaign platform and had committed the government to implementing it, he did not generally support it (Sakunphanit interview 2009). As was the case in many countries, Thailand did not have a history of politicians following through on their campaign promises. To counter any hesitation by Thai Rak Thai, the Rural Doctors' movement organized themselves into five strategic areas to try to ensure an altogether different future for universal health care; the areas were political support and political movement, implementation, primary care, financial management, and technical support (Wibulpolprasert interview 2009). Ensuring that the policy would be implemented before politicians could go back on their word became the chief cause of one of the doctors.

In 2001, Dr. Mongkol na Songkhla served as the ministry's permanent secretary, the ministry's highest-ranking civil servant. While Mongkol was not a member of the Sampran Forum, he had been a committed medical activist dating back to his work in the country's poorest rural areas in the 1970s.[24] To Mongkol, the sooner that clear benefits could be delivered to the people, the less chance that the program would fall victim to the political process (na Songkhla interview 2009). He therefore sought to implement the program in less than a year—a timeframe that was much faster than any of his colleagues had championed (Burns interview 2009). Sensing some reluctance among Thai Rak Thai politicians toward the policy after the party came to power, Mongkol sought to move forward with implementation of the program as a national pilot project *before it was even passed into law,* motivated by the idea that people would "cry out" and pressure their MPs to embrace the program (na Songkhla interview 2009).

Another incentive may also have spurred Mongkol's insistence to implement the program quickly: In late 2001, he was scheduled to retire, and so a desire to secure his own legacy may have provided him with additional motivation (Suebwonglee interview 2009). The triumph of Dr. Mongkol's speedy vision of implementation was particularly impressive given that even the Minister of Public Health, who was herself a Thai Rak Thai executive, favored a much slower approach[25] (na Songkhla interview 2009). Dr. Surapong would himself later suggest that even though the hastiness of implementation would create its own problems, in hindsight fast implementation was likely a major reason that the program did not fall prey to the political process. In an interview, he reflected on the words of senior statesman and emeritus professor Dr. Nidhi Eawsriwong,

who wrote of the program in a Thai newspaper, "If we do not hurry [to implement it], we cannot implement anything" (Suebwonglee interview 2009).

A debate among the reformers ensued over the level and type of financing
method to use. A landmark meeting to finalize the details of the program at
Government House on March 17, 2001, gave two physician-health economists
from the movement an opportunity to hash out the financing issues in front
of the new prime minister. Over time pressure from Thai Rak Thai had grown
to keep expenses for the new program within the existing cost envelope (Burns
interview 2009), and the lower of two figures was accepted.[26] And it was decided
that the program would be implemented as a "national pilot project" by November in three phases according to Mongkol's plan (Nitayarumphong 2006, 94).
The implementation of the program before it became law provides a somewhat
remarkable illustration of unique powers that members of Thailand's professional movement were able to align toward promotion of the policy because they
were the ministry's top advisers on health care policy.

By April, just over two weeks after the landmark meeting at Government
House, the first phase of the pilot program was already being implemented. As
senators watched the program become implemented in the first six provinces,
politicians from other provinces where the program had not yet been implemented began to knock on the doors of Dr. Surapong and others in charge of
the project, seeking to have their provinces earmarked as next in line for implementation, so that they too might reap some of the political benefits of the program. The program was implemented in another fifteen provinces in June and
throughout the entire country by October. Yet, remarkable as the reform was in
its size and scope, a legislative bill for the program had not yet even been drafted
and would not be introduced into Parliament for debate until the fourth quarter
of that year (Suebwonglee interview 2009). When it was on November 21, 2001,
however, a first reading of the bill passed the House unanimously (377–0) after
just two days of debate (Susanpoolthong 2001).[27]

Drawing on Symbolic Resources from International Allies
to Resist Retrenchment Attempts

Just as Parliament was beginning to consider a bill that would give Thailand's new
"30 baht" program legal standing, a report funded by the World Bank arguing that
the program would bankrupt public hospitals and that the financing system would
dilute health care quality was circulated among officials in the Ministry of Public Health (Tangcharoensathien interview 2009; Wibulpolprasert interview 2009).
This criticism in the report was echoed by a World Bank economist who publicly
expressed concern over the unpredictability of its future costs (Chaitrong 2002).

To counter criticism of the program, the doctors drew on their relationships with individuals from other international organizations with whom they had worked on state projects to provide greater legitimacy to the reform. In mid-April 2002, the chief economic architect of the 30 baht program remarked to the media that "the World Health Organisation had thrown its full support behind the project" (*The Nation* 2002b). Even more significantly, the doctors drew on their relationships with representatives of the International Labor Organization (ILO), with whom they had relationships stretching as far back as their work on the country's social health insurance program in the early 1990s.

The vocal support of the ILO for the Universal Coverage program was somewhat counterintuitive. While the ILO had long been a proponent of social health insurance programs around the globe for decades, Thailand's Universal Coverage program was *not* a contributory social health insurance program but a tax-funded program in the mold of a British National Health Service. ILO support was therefore somewhat unorthodox and a direct result of relationships between members of the professional movement who served as leading experts in the ministry and their ILO counterparts.

ILO representatives began to press critics to give the program time to work after implementation problems were reported in the media (Assavanonda 2002d). But even more significant than these public measures of support was the ILO's technical stamp of approval on the program's budget estimates. During sensitive budgetary discussions, the gesture offered reassurance to politicians and bureaucrats that the program's figures were "scientifically sound" and helped to "immunize" the Doctors' estimates from criticism (Tangcharoensathien interview 2009).[28] With Rural Doctors in control of executive positions in the ministry with the support of friendly voices, the World Bank's criticisms became muted, and broader distribution of the World Bank's report was halted. Unlike the Rural Doctors' movement, members of the medical profession who opposed the policy did not hold positions in the state or have access to similarly formidable symbolic resources abroad.[29]

Reaction within the Ministry and the Medical Profession to Universal Coverage

The rapid action launched by the Rural Doctors' movement put Thailand's medical profession at a distinct disadvantage in organizing effective opposition to the policy. And implementation of the policy as a national pilot project before it became law left the profession with no locus around which to organize. When the bill received its second reading in Parliament in May 2002, it passed the House by another large margin—235–70—reflecting the fact that no politician wanted to be seen as voting against a reform that was already delivering benefits to the masses (*The Nation* 2002a). This second vote paved the way for consideration by the Senate Committee on Public Health and later the full Senate.

The Senate Committee on Public Health was chaired by a doctor with ties to a private hospital (Ongsomwang interview 2009). Under her leadership, the committee planned to ensure that the bill received full scrutiny, holding eight public forums in Bangkok and another twenty in the provinces (*Bangkok Post* 2002). Prior to this point, no significant protest campaign had been mobilized against the bill. Of all the "veto points" in the legislative process, this one offered vocal opposition groups their biggest chance to influence legislation. Some major sources of contention in the bill included a limited budget with a radical new financing system aimed at controlling costs and channeling funding away from urban hospitals and toward rural hospitals; new medical malpractice measures; merger of the program with existing state health insurance funds for workers in the formal sector and civil servants; and a new mechanism for complaints that would for the first time include citizen oversight alongside physicians (on these last three points, see Assavanonda 2002a, e). Doctors of all stripes were also concerned about new liability stemming from a new medical malpractice fund and the way it might alter the doctor-patient relations by giving patients a way to challenge their authority. The Medical Council and other professional organizations that stood to be affected, including the Medical Association of Thailand (a voluntary professional development organization) and the Private Hospital Association (representing the interests of private hospitals), succeeded at this stage in getting the complaint system and malpractice fund dropped from the bill (Assavanonda 2002a; Nontharit 2002).

The reform also prompted the spontaneous creation of two new professional organizations to protest the bill. The group Doctors for the Nation organized the first national meeting by dissidents to discuss the bill in July 2002 (Assavanonda 2002b)—more than eight months after the program had been implemented nationally and two months after the second reading of the bill in the House. While many doctors in public hospitals were aghast at the increased workload the reform had created, Doctors for the Nation's criticisms had a strong ideological bent. The organization's founder was an owner of a private clinic who stood to lose patients because of the reform, prompting him to call the program "public health care for socialists" (Nontharit 2002). Another larger opposition group, called Doctors for the Medical Profession (DMP), organized a protest by several hundred doctors who dressed in black and wore black armbands outside hospitals around the country. The DMP expressed concern over new sources of liability that could result from malpractice (Shevajumroen 2002b).

The Medical Council, which oversaw ethical standards related to medical practice, also took on an increasingly visible role as an opponent of the policy. The head of the Medical Council was an executive at Thailand's most famous medical school (where many of the Rural Doctors had graduated) and the owner of a private hospital. He publicly criticized the program on a variety of grounds: dilution of quality care through incentives that encouraged less diagnostic use and fewer specialist referrals; the raising of public expectations, which outstripped hospital capacity to provide service; the long-term fiscal unsustainability of the program; the undermining of people's incentives to take care of themselves given the availability of nearly free care; the growing use of generics at the expense of imported drugs; growing dissatisfaction among doctors working in the program; rising doctor workloads that might force many doctors into the private sector; and the rising number of complaints against doctors in the program (Assavananda 2001b, 2002f; *Bangkok Post* 2006, Santimataneedol 2003; Shevajumroen 2002b). Like Doctors for the Nation and Doctors for the Medical Profession, the main avenues through which these professional organizations channeled their dissent were conventional ones: the media, lobbying, and some limited but highly visible protests. But they lacked access to some of the unique resources that Rural Doctors in the state enjoyed.

Just one month later—a full year after the program had been implemented nationally—a law was passed that gave legal standing to the pilot program, which in the meantime had become a treasure to the country's rural poor. After two hours of debate, the bill passed 314–38 over bitter opposition by the medical profession, and provisions that had been cut by the Senate Committee on Public Health were restored (Nontharit 2002; Somsin 2002; Khwankhom and Noeykhiew 2002). A professor of medicine from one of the country's larger academic hospitals remarked that a reform that required "error-free treatment" on such a small budget was akin to holding a knife to doctors' throats (Khwankhom and Noeykhiew 2002).

Organized medicine, though, in the end was not the policy's only source of opposition. The reform also affected the national Ministry of Public Health in a way that caught many health officials by surprise, since it effectively redirected nearly the entire budget of the ministry to fund the new Universal Coverage program (Pitayarangsarit 2004, 109). The reform included important new health system changes and improvements. It introduced a new system of payment designed to help control costs and limit medical inflation; redirected funds away from urban hospitals and toward underfunded rural hospitals and clinics; created a new national complaint system, managed by one the Rural Doctors' partners, the Foundation for Consumers, aimed at empowering citizens by giving them more of a voice in their health care experience (Ongsomwang interview 2009).

It also led to the creation of a national health information database that would provide policymakers with evidence on which to base decisions about the health care system and closer relationships between rural health centers and community hospitals. And in an effort to create more transparency and accountability, it separated the functions of purchasing health care from the provision of it.

This last aspect of the reform separated the ministry from direct control over its own budget and made it accountable to a new organization, the National Health Security Office (NHSO), from whom it would receive funding to provide services. The first secretary-general of the NHSO—a new and suddenly enormously important organization—was none other than Dr. Sanguan.[30] While the Medical Council and private hospitals have retained a strong voice on the new program's Quality Control Board and have tried to ward off attempts to compensate patients for malpractice (Ungpakorn interview 2009), the combination of these changes and the speed with which they happened left some in the ministry "shell-shocked" (Burns interview 2009).

Conclusion

Remarking on efforts by villagers to organize for progressive reform, one of the key physician-architects behind Thailand's universal coverage reform said, "Since unorganized lay people can not strongly voice out or put pressure on the state, it is 'workable' for organised groups . . . to represent the local people" (Tangcharoensathien quoted in Bhatiasevi 2002, 41). His ideas reflect a broader approach taken by the Rural Doctors' movement, most popularly articulated by Prawase Wasi, that stresses the role of elites (and the state) in civil society mobilization (Phatharathananunth 2006, 6–7). While these sentiments are not intended to diminish the contributions that the masses can make to large-scale social reforms, they are certainly reflective of the path that universal health care reform has followed in Thailand.

This chapter has illustrated how a small movement of elite medical professionals succeeded in overcoming not only a country's own political inertia—which had dashed attempts at universal healthcare reform previously—but also opposition from the medical profession, the World Bank, and political parties, which had long been dominant. In the absence of a mass movement for healthcare reform by people in need, Thailand's Rural Doctors' movement acted strategically to institute universal healthcare policy over the broader opposition of a medical profession that stood against it. In the absence of the strategic actions of the Rural Doctors, there is little reason to believe that a number of critical things that enabled Thailand's Universal Coverage policy to come into being would ever have happened.

3

BRAZIL: AGAINST ALL ODDS

[The Unified Health System] would not exist were it not for the
***sanitaristas*. . . .**

—Wendy Hunter and Natasha Borges Sugiyama (2009)

In the absence of mass demands, the story of Thailand's Universal Coverage reform illustrates the way in which democratization empowered a professional movement of public-minded physicians working in the country's Ministry of Public Health. In a context of heightened political competition, Thailand's Rural Doctors' Movement drew on privileged positions in the state to institutionalize universal health care over opposition from the broader medical profession and conservative international organizations. In Brazil, we find a remarkably similar story: After democratic breakthrough in a context of heightened political competition, a movement of progressive medical professionals that occupied privileged positions in the state overcame remarkable odds and instituted a universal health care program. The strikingly similar pattern we find in Brazil provides further support for the theoretical claims developed using the case of Thailand.

Prior to Brazil's efforts to transform its health care system following the country's transition to democracy in 1985, meaningful health care access was largely confined to the country's more developed regions. In 1970, the country's southeast enjoyed more than three times the number of doctors per patient than those in the country's north and northeast (Anuario Estatistico 1973 in Malloy 1979, 111). Even as late as the mid-1980s, Brazil's health system was characterized by exclusion (Shankland and Cornwall 2007, 166), and the country was well on its way to earning the distinction of being the most unequal nation in the world (Victora et al. 2011, 2042). In 1987, two years after the country's first civilian president was elected in more than twenty years, immunization rates for polio and measles in northeastern states like Ceara still hovered around 25 percent, and not even a third of the state's municipalities had a doctor or nurse, much less a clinic; mayors sometimes had an ambulance and kept a small in-home dispensary of prescription medications to dole out in exchange for promises of political loyalty (Tendler 1997, 21). Health care facilities were heavily concentrated in urban middle-class neighborhoods, with often nothing at all in poor communities and rural areas (Weyland 1996, 179). In other words, health care access was stratified between the formally employed and the poor, who received little, if any, publicly provided care at all.

Where state-run programs did exist for the rural and urban poor, frequently they were vertical programs that focused on single issues such as malaria eradication and provided little in the way of curative services or engagement with the local population (Shankland and Cornwall 2007, 166). The state-run social insurance programs that provided care to workers in the formal sector did so in a manner that was geographically uneven and left the majority of the population without access to care or with minimal benefits (Malloy 1979, 138–39, 168). Where benefits were delivered, they were often given by the military as a way to coopt the labor movement and dampen the possibility of social protest (Malloy 1979).

However, not long after its transition to democracy, Brazil staked its claim as a leader in the industrializing world by providing expansive health policies to all of its citizens through two new policy commitments: first to a decentralized universal health care program known for its participatory governance mechanisms in the Unified Health System, or SUS, in 1990, and later by starting an AIDS treatment program that would be recognized as a model for the industrializing world in the years that followed. While these programs—and particularly the country's universal health care program—would take time to reach their full potential, these impressive policy achievements occurred in spite of factors that would seem to have predisposed policymakers to reduce state commitments to health care, rather than increasing them: Brazil was one of the first countries in the region to transition to democracy in the 1970s, so democracy's prospects and the emancipatory potential of policy remained uncertain, with no real guiding template to offer politicians or citizens.

Even basic "rules of the game," including a date for the first direct presidential election, were not set until 1986, one year after the country's first civilian administration was elected by an Electoral College run by elites (Keck 1992, 27). Prior to the formation of the Workers' Party (PT) in the early 1980s, the country had no mass membership party in the European social democratic tradition, which scholars usually point to as typical sources of universalistic social policy, and the much weaker Brazilian Communist Party had been outlawed since the 1940s, with its candidates frequently running on the tickets of other parties (Keck 1992, 8, 179). A powerful and entrenched private medical industry held vast influence over the workings of the health care system and preferred maintenance of the status quo (Weyland 1995), and popular movements of the lower classes were weaker historically in Brazil than in many of its neighboring countries (Mainwaring 1989, 171).

Brazil's economic situation would have seemed to make it an even more unlikely candidate for universal health care. Between 1981 and 1990, the country experienced negative economic growth at an average of –0.7 percent (Friedman and Hochstetler 2002, 28). Inflation had increased from 40 percent in 1979 to 200 percent in 1985, reaching historic levels by 1988, with average incomes declining by 10 percent between 1979 and 1984 (Fishlow 1989, 83). By 1990, Brazil had the world's largest foreign debt, at $112.5 billion (Biehl 2007, 54) and between 1980 and 1991 undertook seven structural adjustment packages (Parker 2003, 180). As if these factors weren't constraining enough, the expansion of state commitments took place even more improbably against a backdrop of massive debt and austerity measures that led per person federal spending on health to plunge from $83 in 1989 to $37 in 1993 (Biehl 2007, 59) and hyperinflation of around 2,500% (Friedman and Hochstetler 2002, 28).

The country's political culture was not friendly to universal health care either. In a political system where presidential politics dominated over the priorities of political parties and the legislature, Brazil's first two presidents were not leftists but conservatives, with José Sarney having been a former leader in the political party associated with the junta under military rule and Fernando Collor de Mello having promoted a neoliberal agenda aimed at scaling back the state. Furthermore, corruption and scandals rather than innovative policy arrangements would mark both administrations: Clientelism reached its zenith in the Sarney administration, while Collor himself would be impeached on corruption charges and removed from office.

More broadly, Brazil's commitment to universal health care was embraced at a time when 90 percent of Brazilians voted for individuals, rather than political parties espousing coherent platforms that reflect stable party membership, firm ideological commitments, and overall party discipline (Ames 2002, 42, 65, 69, 148, 160); when the country's political system provided politicians with incentives to eschew policies that would further the national interest in favor of pork-barrel politics that would deliver resources to the regions they represented and which favored personalized exchange supporting the interests of the elites; when the conservative nature of political parties was underscored by the fact that more members of Congress owed their political beginnings to the pro-military party during the period of military rule than they did with the opposition (Ames 2002, 29); and when the Health Ministry, which would play a lead role in overseeing these new policies, was itself in disarray, "rotten with patronage" (Ames 2002, 30–31).

Yet expansionary health care reform in Brazil succeeded largely due to the efforts of a professional movement known as the sanitaristas. Quite unlike the rural and urban poor whose needs they served, the sanitaristas were themselves public health professionals. As in Thailand, the movement occupied positions in the state and promoted transformative change from those positions. However, they did so in a political-economic context that might be regarded as more unfriendly to expansive reform than Thailand was. While both cases might be regarded as successes, the sanitaristas advanced transformative reform using different strategies than did the Rural Doctors in Thailand.

Instead of getting a political party to take up the policy in its campaign platform and implementing the policy before it became law as a national pilot project, the sanitaristas succeeded by putting the policy on the political agenda by embedding principles and mandates that would guide the program's implementation in the 1988 Brazilian constitution. Then, owing to rules that allowed state ministries to propose bills to Congress, the sanitaristas played key roles in crafting legislation, which was then forwarded to Parliament, and lobbied policymakers to support it. While a more far-reaching version of the legislation ran into opposition in Congress, a compromise bill nonetheless succeeded in advancing the largest transformation in the history of Brazil's health care system. And although the program has taken time to live up to its promise due to the many problems I have regaled, the implementation and accountability strategies promoted by the sanitaristas have ensured that the program has become more robust over time, providing substantive medical care to millions who did not have it before.

The character of Brazil's transition to democracy in many ways mirrored Thailand's transition. As in Thailand, the military presided over a period of economic success and exhibited less repressive tendencies than some other authoritarian governments of the era. While the regime and its paramilitary forces did perpetrate disappearances, arbitrary detention, and murders, as took place in other Latin American countries at the time (Keck 1992, 25), Brazil's junta did not bolster its rule using the kind of systematic racial segregation and oppression that South Africa's apartheid government used to control the black population.

The transition (*abertura*) from military rule in Brazil was very gradual and controlled by the military, eventually leading to elections and the development of a new constitution. Political liberalization began in the 1970s at the behest of the dictatorship according to careful plans, but once underway, the movement "acquired a logic of its own" (Codato 2006, 17). Under the system imposed by the military leaders in 1965, just two political parties competed with one another (Mainwaring 1986, 9), with elections relying on an electoral college that was "highly manipulated" (Skidmore 1989, 7, 34). The conservative National Renewal Alliance (ARENA), the official government party, was subordinate to the military, while the Brazilian Democratic Movement (MDB)—which had actually been created by the military—was the official party of the opposition (Mainwaring 1988, 96–97). And while the military regime maintained the institutions of Parliament during its rule—even though they were little more than "ornamental" vessels, with real power centralized in the executive branch, which remained under military control—the share of votes in legislative elections that went to the government steadily decreased up to the early 1980s (Codato 2006, 8, 13).

In 1976, elections between the MDB and ARENA at the municipal level led the opposition party, MDB, to take over some mayoral posts, which enabled the first members of a movement of medical professionals to obtain positions as directors of municipal health secretariats (Dowbor 2011, 10). However, this occurred at a time when most other organized civil society groups had been weakened under dictatorship (Niedzwiecki 2014, 41). "Popular" (poorer) classes were largely excluded from serving in representative institutions, and peasant movements and labor unions proved to be more visible than urban movements in their political activity, although labor unions themselves were a product of corporatist arrangements that were tightly controlled under the military, which privileged economic development and social stability over strong representation of class interests (Mainwaring 1987, 133–34, 141, 149; on corporatism, Keck 1992, 63; Weyland 1996, 55). It was only after General Ernesto Geisel initiated the liberalization process in 1974 that greater space for social movements opened up and new popular and autonomous social movements developed over the next several years (Mainwaring 1987, 134, 149). Despite this, the political activities of the state's representative institutions (as well as clientelistic relations within the state), though subordinated to the executive, continued to function (O'Donnell 1988, 289). And in this respect, the serious role that elections and political parties played in political life set Brazil apart from most of the authoritarian governments in Latin America at the time (Mainwaring 1988, 91).

Toward the end of military rule in the late 1970s, there was an upsurge in activity by popular movements, including notable strikes by the Greater São Paulo auto workers' union, as well as a growth in peasant unions, neighborhood associations, and (amid rapid economic modernization) movements that developed around concern for urban services (Mainwaring 1986, 10). However, organizational linkages among civil society organizations, including unions, were generally weak, informal, and short-lived (Keck 1992, 51). In the 1980s the number of voluntary associations in major urban areas increased substantially, challenging traditional dynamics that responded not to the needs of citizens but clientelist patterns (Avritzer 2000, 65–66). Massive demonstrations for direct presidential elections were a part of this resurgence of popular participation, with thirty thousand people taking part in an initial demonstration in Curitiba in January 1984 and over a million gathering in Rio de Janeiro and São Paulo just three months later in April, in spite of warnings from the regime (Mainwaring 1986, 15). These grassroots movements put workers' rights and participation on the political agenda as early as 1979 (Keck 1992, 66) and played at least a partial role in the military's decision to allow a civilian president to take office (Mainwaring 1987, 135). However, in the mid-1970s broader human rights demands were being articulated more vigorously (Skidmore 1989, 11). And a different kind of movement, with a character and channels of influence quite different from the existing blue-collar peasant unions and neighborhood associations, would emerge as a particular force in a democratizing Brazil.

Origins of Brazil's Professional Movement for Health Equity

Brazil's modern sanitary (or "public health") movement was comprised of public health professionals who identified with leftist ideology and emphasized the importance of making a difference in expanding access to health care, especially in rural areas (much like Thailand's Rural Doctors). The movement was born during the leftist Goulart government of the early 1960s and was mobilized more forcefully during the 1970s under the shadow of Brazil's military junta (Falleti 2010, 47). At a time when medical schools in the country were stressing the importance of public health more forcefully, self-identified members of the movement were graduating from medical school and allied professional programs and were heading into government service at the local, state, and federal levels to work on these issues.

The *sanitaristas*, as they were called, drew inspiration from Italy's 1978 *riforma sanitaria* (Brown 1984, 76–77), a transformational health care reform that sought to address the ills of a system that had historically been marked by inequalities and fragmentation; the reform was modeled on Great Britain's National Health Service, which provided everyone with the same access to care (Weyland 1995, 1710). Several of the movement's members were part of the banned Brazil's communist party (PCB), which envisioned progressive health reform as part of a broader movement toward socialism (Falleti 2010, 48; Weyland 1995, 1710). The movement had its roots in the country's universities (Escorel 1999, 18)—in particular, the FIOCRUZ National School of Public Health in Rio de Janeiro (Shankland and Cornwall 2007, 167)—but brought together doctors working in the country's Preventative Medicine Departments, union-organized physicians, doctors working in the country's medical schools, and medical students (Dowbor 2007, 4).

In the context of an undemocratic state, the movement pressed loudly for broader democratic and equity-enhancing reforms, albeit to little real effect under the military government. Pervasive clientelism led many social movements in the 1970s to rely on relationships to facilitate change at the local level, and in the broader context of military control these movements rarely pushed for broader demands that involved redistribution on a national scale (Weyland

1996, 158). Decentralization of decision-making was one of the modern sanitary movement's major aims and was articulated politically as early as the 3rd National Health Conference of 1963 (Falleti 2010, 47; Sugiyama 2007, 63, 129, 164). However, the absence of basic medical services in large parts of the country made universalizing access to health care a major priority of the movement.

The distribution of medical services in Brazil was highly skewed toward developed urban areas, particularly the south and southeast, and the government's main social insurance program outright excluded or otherwise provided minimal benefits to some 52 percent of the population (Weyland 1996, 97, 132). Although the military regime extended a thin measure of social insurance to the rural, unemployed, and self-employed through the Assistance Fund for Rural Workers (FUNRURAL) in 1971, largely to coopt rural pressures for change (Falleti 2010, 44), in practice it provided the rural poor with minimal protection, while leaving urban informal workers excluded from coverage entirely (Weyland 1996, 91–92). While the program exempted rural beneficiaries from payment for services, many saw it as a hollow and underfunded gesture, as the program's provider network was so limited (Malloy 1979, 120, 133). Still, for all its flaws, it represented "the most important redistributive change ever made in Brazilian social security" (Weyland 1996, 91–92).

The *sanitaristas* envisioned substantially improving and expanding the program to cover the entire population while extending basic prevention and primary health care programs to the poor (Arretche 2004, 167). However, proper reform would involve not only correcting the distribution of health services but also addressing the country's skewed investment in expensive (urban hospital–based and often private) curative care over preventative care. For almost two decades beginning in 1960, spending on medical assistance in the social insurance program for workers, which was mostly curative, increased by over 60 percent, while spending on prevention struggled to stay even or declined (Malloy 1979, 137). To address this at the local level, the *sanitaristas* worked to open a network of rural health outposts in areas that had neither public nor private services through a program called the Program of Internalization of Health and Sanitary Actions (PIASS) in 1976 (Falleti 2010, 50–51). They also sought to create legislation to decentralize the system and empower state and municipal health authorities (who might know the needs of the local population better), control the runaway costs of curative treatment, and curb excessive reliance on private providers and extend regulation over them. In that regard, programs such as PIASS simplified services and reduced costs while at the same time diverting resources from programs that went toward private and hospital-based care, integrating treatment and prevention, and encouraging popular participation in health care (Dowbor 2009, 5–6).

Amid a broader context of repression, the *sanitaristas* worked to find space to exchange and debate ideas that were not threatening to the regime, such as Community Health Studies Week, held annually since 1975 (Dowbor 2009, 4), and held rallies and meetings in the context of larger scientific meetings (Dowbor 2011, 10). According to *sanitarista* Gastão Wagner de Souza, the experiences of "working close to the people on the periphery, in the slums, among workers and, consequently, working in primary care" was extremely important (quoted in Fleury 1997, 135). However, in promoting ideas about how public health should work in a democratic nation, the *sanitaristas* promoted ideas on behalf of people in need in scientific and official spaces that were quite unfamiliar and inaccessible to ordinary citizens. As Judith Tendler writes, "The debates [advanced by the *sanitaristas*] had taken place far away from the civil society of the communities . . . although many of the participants in the debates had led or worked in programs in such communities in the past" (1997, 155).

In 1976, the *sanitaristas* founded the Center for Brazilian Health Studies (CEBES) as a bulwark against the military regime, whose policies were often denounced in the center's influential journal *Saude em Debate*; CEBES became "the home for an ideologically assertive group—a 'guerrilla headquarters' of sorts—that set itself up to sell ideas, raise consciousness, and use political power to achieve its goals" (Adler 1986, 691). From this base, they worked with congressmen to develop the National Health Policy Symposia, started in 1979, where they put forward reform proposals (Dowbor 2009, 4). In addition, they established annual municipal health meetings as venues for protest and encouraged the development of municipal health secretary positions, many of which would come to be occupied by *sanitaristas* (Dowbor 2011, 9).

With the landmark 1978 Alma Ata Conference on Primary Health Care and the formation of the Brazilian Post-Graduate Association for Public Health (ABRASCO) the following year, the ideas and organizational power of the movement began to consolidate itself. Producing and disseminating progressive ideas, occupying positions of power within the state, and lobbying Congress became their three-part strategy (Falleti 2010, 49). Their lobbying of the lower house of Congress in 1979 resulted in the first symposium on national health policy, during which the leading members of the public health movement presented a paper outlining its vision for a universal health care program (Falleti 2010, 49).

Policymaking in Brazil's New Republic

The *sanitaristas*' political activism on health care in 1979 coincided with broader steps toward political liberalization taken by the military regime. That same year, reform of the two-party system and restoration of a multi-party system began, in part due to the growth of the opposition party MDB, whose power the regime sought to dilute (Mainwaring 1988, 96). Direct elections for state governorships were held in 1982—the first such elections in nearly twenty years—with the opposition notching wins in most major and several minor states (Mainwaring 1986: 9, 11). After popular protests, an amendment that would have allowed direct elections for the presidency (Diretas Já) was defeated in the National Congress in 1984, owing to the lack of opposition control of the houses of parliament (Mainwaring 1986, 15). However, in a context of new political party competition and some defections from the old regime, the centrist opposition party, the Brazilian Democratic Movement Party, or PMDB (the new name for the MDB), won the presidency through a vote that took place within the country's electoral college—which itself had been established in 1982—on January 15, 1985, by a margin of 480 to 180 votes, and reestablishment of direct presidential elections soon followed (Codato 2006, 8, 14; Mainwaring 1988, 97; on the establishment of the electoral college, Mainwaring 1998, 529).

The government that won the election in 1985 was to be led by Tancredo Neves and José Sarney. Neves was a moderate who had been an important figure in the opposition to the military junta that took power in 1964 but was viewed as acceptable by the military (Mainwaring 1986, 1, 24). Neves explicitly assured the military of continued representation and access to resources in the post-military government as well as moderate policies (Hagopian 1990, 158). However, when the seventy-four-year-old Neves fell ill and died before he could assume the presidency, Sarney—the former head of the party that supported the military government—became the president (Codato 2006, 14). As a former leader of the establishment party, Sarney, along with his colleagues, had helped to put an end to the Amendment for Direct Elections; some leading commentators at the time suggested that the concessions initially made to the center-right by Neves and the marginalization of social movements and the left suggested that the Sarney administration would not take up redistribution and social justice as major concerns (Mainwaring 1986, 31; 1989, 198). Rather, representing a "triumph of traditional Brazilian ways of doing politics," exclusion of the popular sectors—and the needs of the poor—continued (Mainwaring 1989, 195).

Although the end of the dictatorship put more focus on political parties (de Souza 1989, 379)—as potential aggregators of constituent interests—military members and conservative politicians connected to the military retained significant influence in the new government (O'Donnell 1988, 287). Indeed, in the first years of democracy, more members of Congress started their political careers as members of the pro-military ARENA party than with the opposition MDB (Ames 2002, 29). The Sarney government upheld many of the priorities of the military and protected some of its positions and access to resources in the state, with the pervasive clientelism having damaging effects on state responsiveness and the authority of democratic institutions (Hagopian 1990, 157–59; O'Donnell 1988, 292). However, the constitutional convention occurred on his watch, producing a new constitution in 1988 followed by two direct presidential elections in 1989 and 1994 (Mainwaring 1998, 529). Whereas a lack of effective challenge to the African National Congress (ANC) characterized the politics of democratic transition in South Africa, between 1982 and 1990 the effective number of political parties more than doubled in both the Chamber of Deputies (the lower parliamentary chamber) and the Senate in Brazil (Mainwaring 1998, 538–39).

At the same time, legislation was passed in 1985 permitting parliamentary representatives to deviate from the line of party leaders, which led to reduced party discipline, greater incidence of party-switching and personalized appeals, and higher electoral volatility overall (Mainwaring 1998, 537–38).[1] Between 1987 and 1990 alone, some 40 percent of deputies in the lower house switched parties (Ames 2002, 148). Whereas South Africa's ANC would dominate its nearest competitor in the 1994 elections by over forty points, due in part to these dynamics capture of the electorate in Brazil was much more widely dispersed: While not winning, the left-wing Workers' Party—which sought to challenge Brazil's elitist political tradition—and the populist Democratic Labor party had showings in the 1985 election that suggested a bright political future (Mainwaring 1986, 34; on the Workers' Party, Mainwaring 1988, 99). The Workers' Party (PT), in particular, would go from winning just one mayoral election in 1982 and 1985 to taking a surprising thirty-one contests in 1988 and would come within five points (42.75% versus 37.86%) of beating conservative Fernando Collor de Mello in the runoff for the 1989 presidential election (Keck 1992, 157, 160).

While these factors by themselves did not encourage the development of programmatic campaign platforms designed to appeal to the electorate with broad-based social policies like universal health care (political parties at the time had been described as "ideologically malleable"), they did prevent any one party from dominating all the others (Mainwaring 1988, 92). However, these factors and the historical dominance of the executive left political parties to play a weak role in the representation of constituent interests and policy formulation; in this context, elections often amounted to a choice between personal leaders rather than ideas or policies (Mainwaring 1988, 93, 98). These dynamics meant that "the major political parties of the New Republic were prevented from becoming genuine transmission belts of non-elite interests as a result of the political pacts struck with traditional political elites during the regime transition" (Hagopian 1990, 159). Congress passed virtually nothing on its own initiative in major areas of social policy, and Brazilian presidents frequently worked around Congress rather than involving them by issuing thousands of emergency decrees, which took effect but required either the approval of Congress in thirty days or reissuance by the president (Ames 2002, 4–5). Just as before the transition, Brazil's political system concentrated power in the executive (de Souza 1989, 382), leaving technocrats with an unusual degree of influence on major policy decisions (Weyland 1996, ch. 7). While these circumstances did not provide popular movements with any particular advantage in the new order, they did provide leverage in policymaking for professional movements who would come to occupy strategic positions in the state in newly democratic Brazil.

Democratization and the Changing Role of Civil Society

Prior to the transition from military government, the notion of citizenship as a package of rights belonging to members of a nation had never existed in Brazil before (Mainwaring 1987, 148). Since 1985, civil society in Brazil's new democracy has used the master frame of citizenship to mobilize around political, social, and economic exclusion and to make new claims on the state; in this context, efforts by the Workers' Party and provisions in the 1988 constitution (in particular Article 29) led to the formation of local councils to involve citizens in policy formulation and implementation, alongside spectacular growth in the NGO sector (Friedman and Hochstetler 2002, 27, 29–31). This discourse married the notions of universal rights and active citizen participation and led to the formation of inclusionary new processes aimed at creating a new and very different Brazil (Shankland and Cornwall 2007, 175). The constitutional provisions provided governments at the municipal level with the economic resources and political autonomy needed to create and maintain innovative decentralized and deliberative participatory governance, which has helped to transform the processes by which budgets are made and public goods are distributed (Wampler and Avritzer 2004, 291; on participatory budgeting, Baiocchi 2005). These new processes played an important role in helping to challenge established patterns of political patronage and replace them with governance mechanisms responsive to the citizenry, although clientelism based on personal exchange has continued to remain a defining feature of Brazilian life and politics (Wampler and Avritzer 2004, 292).

In the immediate aftermath of the transition, clientelistic relationships and the influence of rent-seeking special interests actually grew more entrenched and greatly diminished state capacity (Weyland 1996). Elitism and exclusion continued to characterize the country's political life after 1985; NGOs did not succeed in developing a mass base, and close relationships between the state and some social movements presented a new spin on the old pattern of clientelistic relationships based on personal ties (Hochstetler 2000, 14). And while the country's transition was not marred by particular violence, the continued elitism and exclusion that characterized Brazilian politics, combined with the holdovers from the old regime, marked Brazil's transition as a "highly conservative" one (Keck 1992, 251). Even the opposition governors at the state level who came into office in the 1984 election and the first presidential administration in 1985 were widely thought of as disappointments by most movement leaders (Mainwaring 1987, 132).

Sanitarista Influence in the New Republic: Promoting Reforms from Inside the State

Reorienting the Health Care System

Amid the gradual opening taking place in the early 1980s and a fiscal crisis that led to a dramatic decrease in health care expenditure, efforts to address the health system's fragmentation and centralization began. A commission established in 1980 recommended a three-stage approach to addressing challenges in the health sector, which included a pilot Integrated Health Actions (AIS) program, followed by a Unified and Decentralized Health System (SUDS), with a transition to a Single Unified Health System (SUS) (Lewis and Medici 1998, 270–71). The imprint of the *sanitaristas* on these proceedings was clear from the beginning in the design of the AIS program and throughout the broader program of transformation. Based on preexisting CEBES proposals, AIS went into effect in 1984 and came out of the National Health Policy Symposia, which had been a bulwark of the *sanitaristas* (Dowbor 2009, 7). The program diverted money away from the old agency in charge of the country's social security program, the Instituto Nacional Assistência Médica Previdência Social (INAMPS)—which was known for its clientelism—and toward health care provision at the local level, going further than the earlier PIASS program in decentralizing health services (Dowbor 2009, 6). Due largely to the *sanitaristas'* control of the institutions in charge of health policy, AIS saw a rapid expansion of implementation at the municipal level and a deepening of commitment to the program's guiding mandate (Dowbor 2009, 7).

The presidential victory of José Sarney in 1985 allowed public health experts in the *sanitarista* movement to make further inroads into prominent positions at the highest levels of the federal bureaucracy. Hésio Cordeiro served as a member of the new government's Action Plan Coordination Team, charged with putting together the new government's policy program (Dowbor 2011, 12), before becoming head of the country's social security agency, INAMPS.[2] The appointment of Eleutério Neto as director of the Planning Department in the Social Security Administration marked one of the first high-level *sanitarista* appointments (Falleti 2010, 52–53). However, the capture of other important posts by *sanitaristas* soon followed, including the appointment of José Felipe to head of the medical services division of the social security agency; meanwhile, Sergio Arouca, who had also advised PAHO (and later served as representative to the WHO) became head of Ozwaldo Cruz Foundation, the country's most important research institute (Nunn 2009; Weyland 1996, 159). All in all, *sanitaristas* would come to fill many posts in the new government (Dowbor 2011, 12), and *sanitarista* leaders would run for office themselves and eventually form the Sanitarista Party or caucus in the Chamber of Deputies, where they would take control of the Chamber's health committee (Niedzwiecki 2014, 42). In the absence of mass demands for transformative change—and a political context in which fierce competition among political parties and politicians reigned but the policy-making role was ceded to the executive organs of the state—the capture of key positions in the state would allow the *sanitaristas* to be particularly influential in the early years of Brazil's new democracy. *Sanitaristas* drew on positions in the local and state levels to challenge the status quo held in place through clientelist arrangements, to provide legitimacy to their efforts, and to blunt opposition (Falleti 2010). Between the national election in 1985 and the constitution that would come into being in 1988, the *sanitaristas* held eleven different mobilizing events aimed at institutionalizing their agenda (Dowbor 2011, 11).

Hésio Cordeiro's position as head of the social security agency, in particular, facilitated opportunities for the *sanitarista* efforts to decentralize and universalize access to health care and to limit the influence of the private sector in health care. In 1987, a new and more radical SUDS program was taken up based on a proposal put forward by Cordeiro; the program led not only to greater municipalization of health services but also to a dramatic scale-up in public sector funding by INAMPS and a dramatic downturn in contracts awarded to the private sector (Dowbor 2009, 7). The program took decentralization a step further with the transfer of INAMPS facilities and staff to state health secretariats, with the goal of transferring responsibility for care to the municipal level under SUS (Lewis and Medici 1998, 271).

With a strong base in the state bureaucracy, the *sanitaristas* embarked on further efforts aimed at promoting greater equity in the system and reorienting health care away from curative service, which relied principally on expensive private hospitals, and toward publicly provided health promotion and prevention efforts. To redirect resources in a more progressive way, they tried to chip away at the privileged position of private providers in the Brazilian health care system, which operated on a fee-for-service basis[3] as contractors to the social security program for workers in the formal sector vis-à-vis INAMPS (which was now under the leadership of Hésio Cordeiro and which held 85 percent of the country's health resources) now under the leadership of Hésio Cordeiro (Weyland 1996, 161–62; on INAMPS resources at the transition, Dowbor 2011, 12). Using their new powers as leading state bureaucrats, they convened a commission in 1985 to discuss new arrangements for hospital contracting not just with the Brazilian Hospital Federation (dominated by for-profit hospitals), with which INAMPS had previously worked in the military years, but also with the Confederation of Philanthropic Hospitals, a group of nonprofit health care organizations. The movement's aim in doing so was to divide their voice and weaken their bargaining position (Weyland 1996, 161). While a new deal with the Confederation of Philanthropic Hospitals initially appeared to have achieved the goal of weakening the bargaining position of for-profit hospitals, the Hospital Federation soon flexed its muscles. Providing two-thirds of publicly funded hospital care gave them the power to resist and ultimately defeat the new institutional arrangements that the professional movement sought through their divide-and-conquer strategy (Weyland 1996, 161–62).

Despite this setback, Arouca, a communist party activist who had also been a researcher at the National School of Public Health in Rio, led a group of sanitaristas that convened the 8th National Health Conference in 1986. While previous conferences had been closed to all but "technocrats and power-brokers," in the context of the post-military new democratic space in Brazil, the 1986 conference brought together activists and professionals devoted to health in local communities from across the nation (Cornwall and Shankland 2008, 2175). The conference took place amid growing demands for public services in the new democracy and in the context of growing fears over the AIDS epidemic in Brazil. Over four thousand people, representing all walks of life related to health and health care attended the conference, including significant blocs representing the medical industry, amid a sea of one thousand delegates that was evenly split between government and civil society (Falleti 2010, 54). *Sanitaristas* had been at the center of this effort to broaden the profile of attendees at the conference as a means of encouraging wider participation from society and implicitly increasing the standing of their own agenda (Dowbor 2011, 13).

Initiated by the *sanitaristas*, these National Health Conferences brought together citizens who used health care services and representatives from civil society organizations and government together every four years to discuss and debate the problems, challenges, and needs of the health care system (Dowbor 2011, 14). In these meetings, the *sanitaristas* sought "to speak in the name of others," while also giving citizens new opportunities to add their own voices to the deliberations (Dowbor 2011, 14). However, at the 1986 conference and others subsequent to it, the strategy of the *sanitaristas* was to attend the conference in large numbers in order to overwhelm opposing voices and to provide force and momentum to the policy goals articulated by the movement (Arretche 2004, 171). Organizing prior to the conference by the *sanitaristas* helped to build alliances across local and state groups and provided the movement with a strong and credible voice. The effectiveness of their mobilization efforts enabled the *sanitaristas* to propose the establishment of a new National Sanitary Reform Commission with representation by ministries with health-related missions and stakeholders from society, with the aim of drafting health policy proposals that would be subsequently submitted to the Constitutional Assembly (Dowbor 2011, 13). Some of the most radical *sanitarista* proposals at the Health Conference aimed at upending the exclusionary status quo in the health care sector through the nationalization of private health care providers and pharmaceutical companies (Shankland and Cornwall 2007, 169). As a result, the three issues of health as a right, reform of the national health system, and health sector funding received important attention at the conference (Falleti 2010, 54–55). And largely due to the influence of the *sanitaristas*, the conference affirmed the principles of decentralization, participation, equity, and universality and declared health to be "the duty of the state and the right of the citizen" (Cornwall and Shankland 2008, 2175). These proceedings then were sent to the Constitutional Assembly in early March 1987, at a time when the Assembly's work was just beginning (Dowbor 2011, 13).

Enshrining Important New Provisions in the 1988 Constitution

The *sanitaristas* that had been so involved in the 8th National Health Conference of 1986 again articulated the movement's proposals in as well-organized a fashion as any group at the 1988 constitutional convention (Falleti 2010, 54–55). The convention was conducted in a more open and transparent manner than typical state business, which usually favored clientelistic interests (Weyland 1996, 167), and the constitution that would result from these deliberations was referred to popularly as "the Citizens' Constitution" (Cornwall, Cordeiro, and Delgado 2006, 144). However, much like the process that marked the production of Thailand's 1997 "People's Constitution," it was primarily elites who would leave a lasting impression on the proceedings. And as in Thailand, the professional nature and strategic actions of an elite movement of medical professionals would set their contributions apart from other popular grassroots movements. Operating inside and outside the state, they advised left and center-left constitutional delegates during the process, who took up positions in key committees through a process of self-selection and proposed norms in keeping with the movement's agenda (Weyland 1995, 1706–7). In addition, *sanitaristas* directly held some fifty-eight of the parliamentary positions related to health at the assembly (Niedzwiecki 2014, 36). At the top of their agenda was a strongly public universal health care reform, which they called the Unified Health System, that would integrate curative and preventive care and reduce the role of private providers from dominant players in Brazil's health care system to a provider of "last resort" (Weyland 1995, 1706–7). The success of the professional movement in organizing to embed principles that reflected their values in the constitution was ultimately reflected in the final text of the constitution: All five provisions in the constitution related to health in large part mirrored the movement's proposals (Dowbor 2011, 11). However, a conservative bloc in the Assembly managed to preserve the legitimacy of the private sector's role in health care (Melo 1993, 136).

The movement's successes galvanized private sector opposition which succeeded in watering down initial proposals, and, in particular, provisions dealing with state regulation of the private medical industry and efforts to curb expenditures on curative care, which represented a large share of the private sector's business (Weyland 1996, 168). However, the movement sought to consolidate their gains and strengthen their position in the process by introducing a "people's amendment" on health reform through the use of a petition. The *sanitaristas'* petition drive aimed to give universal health care a firm place on the political agenda by requiring that the constitutional assembly consider the measure if it obtained a sufficient number of signatures; however, the drive obtained just 54,133 signatures (Weyland 1996, 168–69). In the context of other popular amendments on public education and land reform, which had respectively garnered some one million and three million signatures, the petition campaign underscored the lack of mass demands for transformative health care reform (Gomes 2011, 194). In-fighting among the *sanitaristas* over which ministry should control INAMPS, which was in charge of administering the state's social security program for formal sector workers, and broader control of the health budget contributed to this weakening of the sanitaristas' efforts (Weyland 1995, 1707). However, as challenging as these problems were, they further underscored the elite character of the movement, whose problems were quite unlike those faced by popular grassroots movements working from below.

Even though the professional movement was not able to achieve all of its goals, its success in enshrining the principles of universalism and decentralization in the constitution put universal health care as a right of citizens on the political agenda in the years to come. Although an entrenched private sector succeeded in ensuring that it would continue to play a role in the new order, its role was to be circumscribed and made "supplementary" under the new arrangements (Weyland 1995, 1707). While these important symbolic victories at the constitutional convention were nontrivial, since the language agreed on set guidelines and mandates for the organic laws that would follow, there remained significant legal room for interpretation over the meaning of the new constitutional language, making the legislative process the next logical site of contestation (Weyland 1995, 1707). Private providers, now well acquainted with the *sanitaristas'* efforts to marginalize them at the 1986 National Health Conference and the 1988 constitutional convention, turned their focus to the legislative process.

Drafting Legislation from Inside the Health Ministry

With a mandate set for a universal health care policy by the constitution, the political battle turned to the process of creating legislation. Here, the Sarney government proved to be something of an obstacle for the realization of a universal health care law, first delaying the project of creating a bill and later providing no stable funding mechanism in the bill's early days (Gomes 2011, 219). However, despite the president's tepid response, Brazil's Health Ministry was endowed with the power to draft a bill on behalf of government for consideration in Parliament. While an alternative bill that reflected the interests of the private medical industry and politicians in the social security agency was drafted by INAMPS, it was the Health Ministry that held the power to decide which version to submit to the legislature. Keenly aware of this power, *sanitaristas* within and outside the state played a role in drafting a bill that emphasized public provision of health care and regulation of private providers (Weyland 1995, 1707). Although some compromises were made in the bill that the Health Ministry ultimately submitted to Congress in mid-1989, the *sanitaristas'* imprint on the bill was clear in that both the existing medical industry and INAMPS officials opposed it (Weyland 1995, 1708).

The private sector—and officials within the ministry overseeing the country's social health insurance program—marshaled a significant lobby to attempt to weaken the compromise legislation that went before Parliament. The *sanitaristas*, for their part, were suffering from a new strategic disadvantage, having seen most of their appointments to high-profile positions in federal government come to nothing under the conservative Collor administration in 1990. Adding to these woes, their earlier success in pushing through a decentralization agenda also effectively channeled focus away from broader national policy issues (Sugiyama 2007, 131). Exhausted from their earlier efforts and having lost many of the advantages that high-level office provided, the *sanitaristas'* efforts to counter the lobbying campaign of the medical industry came to nothing (Weyland 1995, 1708).

However, politicians from the center-left party PMDB supported the reform as they saw that it would increase the popular appeal of their party (Weyland 1996, 159, 170).

Although progressive MPs outnumbered the conservative opposition that was more likely to side with the medical industry, the law's opponents engaged in obstructionism, forcing conservative and progressive MPs to come to a compromise. This compromise granted the private sector and the ministry, which had overseen the old social health insurance program, a significant role in a new decentralized order—a far cry from the "supplementary" role that the *sanitaristas* had desired (Weyland 1995, 1708). Private providers were also guaranteed a voice on the National Health Council, ensuring that it would play a direct role in health policy-making in the future (Weyland 1996, 170). These provisions played an important role in contributing to the continued dominance of private providers in state-run health care programs: In 2008, almost twenty years after the law's passage, just 35 percent of beds were provided by public hospitals, while private contractors provided the other 65 percent (Kepp 2008, 877). The structure of the new law also at least initially left the system dependent on revenue from social security taxes—an artifact of existing clientelist arrangements and a circumstance that would leave it starved for funds during its first several years as the country navigated the economic crisis (Weyland 1995, 1708). Even the new health minister contributed to the weakening of the reform by diverting funds away to patronage activities, including new hospital construction, rather than prevention and health promotion activities and the extension of community clinics in rural areas (Weyland 1996, 172). President Collor likewise struck a blow against the law on behalf of clientelism by using his powers to veto the parts of the law that would have made federal funding transfers to states and municipalities automatic; instead, his vetoes allowed the president to retain significant discretionary control over funding transfers for a time (Weyland 1995, 1708). However, the new law was significant in granting power to municipal authorities to manage the new decentralized system, which would be financed and coordinated by the federal government (Nunn 2009, 48).[4] It replaced the existing decentralization program, SUDS, which had been piloted just three years earlier with the full-scale Unified Health System, in which decentralization was given even greater importance and the Ministry of Health had a central role (rather than the Social Security Ministry, which had overseen the exclusionary contributory system of the past) (Shankland and Cornwall 2007, 170).

In spite of the significant shortcomings of the new law, the achievements embodied in the reform were remarkable for what they represented: a shift away from an exclusionary health care system based on contributory principles to one that offered free access to health care based on a legal right (Arretche 2003, 332).

As a result, hospital use increased by an incredible 53 percent between 1987 and 1991, the year after the SUS laws were adopted (Lewis and Medici 2008, 277).[5] Yet these achievements are all the more spectacular when read against the political and economic context of the time. The realization of the right to health care in Brazil, a fledgling democracy struggling to redefine its major social institutions after decades of military rule, took place against a backdrop of massive debt, hyperinflation, austerity, corruption, and conservatism.

Owing to these facts and the Collor administration's resistance to the Unified Health System legislation, decentralization was one of the few meaningful aspects of the reform that was institutionalized in the program's early years. But even these efforts were slow in coming, as the health minister at the time, Alceni Guerra, eager to keep traditional avenues of patronage open, did not want to see his old agency, INAMPS, folded into the Health Ministry (Weyland 1996, 171; Parker 1994, 37).[6] The INAMPS infrastructure, however, was eventually turned over to the Ministry of Health in 1990 and a deadline set for its closure (in 1993) after the *sanitarista* movement and local health officials applied pressure on the Collor government (Arretche 2004, 169).

While political compromises and the country's economic situation in the early 1990s left the SUS weak and imperfect for much of its first decade, the new program was finally given stability and financial support beginning in the mid-1990s. Funding for the SUS did not improve substantially under the crisis-ridden administration of Itamar Franco (1993–1995), which had its hands full dealing with hyperinflation, but the health budget received a 30 percent increase after President Fernando Henrique Cardoso assumed office in 1995 (Font 2003, 105), and two different health ministers—Adib Jatene and José Serra—advocated for improved funding of the SUS during Cardoso's tenure (Shankland and Cornwall 2007, 172–73).

Three associated policy changes that enhanced the financial viability of the program were made during Cardoso's tenure in office. First, the Provisional Contribution on Financial Transactions (CPMF), a tax on commercial revenues, began directing significantly greater funding to the SUS in 1996, channeling some $6.7 billion dollars into the health care system in 1998 alone, and accounting for 42 percent of total health expenditure that year while growing in subsequent years (Font 2003, 105).[7] Second, implementation of the 1996 Basic Operational Norms (NOB) in 1998 provided greater incentives for the provision of public health and preventative services (Arretche 2004, 175–78). And a constitutional amendment in 2000 provided a more lasting solution to the system's persistent funding problems during the country's earlier periods of financial crisis (Font 2003, 105). However, spending on health would do little more than remain steady once Lula's Workers' Party (PT) took the reins in 2003 (Hunter 2011, 315).

Creating a Practical Strategy to Extend
Health Care to the Masses

"SUS best takes care of those who need primary health care."

—Pedro Cardoso, Professor of Public Health Management, Rio de Janeiro National
School of Public Health (Kepp 2008, 877)

While the strategic actions of the *sanitaristas* in the late 1980s were a primary
reason for the agenda-setting constitutional provisions and enabling legislation
that brought the Unified Health System into being in 1990, the practical problem of how to bring health care to the people remained a major challenge of the
1990s. The 1988 constitution increased the proportion of federal transfers to
municipalities and required that 10 percent of revenues be directed to health:
Between 1994 and 2002, owing in no small part to the new system of fiscal transfers, municipal responsibility for primary care increased dramatically, from just
22 percent to almost 100 percent, a remarkable transformation (Shankland and
Cornwall 2007, 169). However, in practice many mayors spent less than the mandated amount due to the absence of effective enforcement mechanisms, and clientelistic practices frequently continued to prevail (Tendler 1997, 21).

Unlike the Thai case, health care infrastructure was in many cases not immediately ready when Brazil's new universal health care policy was adopted. And
in the context of an increasingly decentralized health care system in which
many decisions related to the shape and organization of health care programs
were left to municipal governments, decision-making and responsibility at the
local level played an incredibly important role. So to ensure that the program
would be implemented effectively, the *sanitaristas* again played a major role.
After the impeachment of President Collor, in 1994 they created a strategy called
the Family Health Program to universalize access to health care, in addition to
new avenues for citizen participation that would provide them with an arena
to mobilize, promote accountability, and make demands (Dowbor and Houtzager 2014, 152–53). Once again, occupation of positions in the state—most
notably, the Department of Primary Care, which oversaw the Family Health
Program—proved crucial for the success of the program's rollout (Dowbor and
Houtzager 2014, 156).

Brazil's Family Health Program had its origins in an emergency employment
program developed in the northeastern state of Ceara to respond to the region's
periodic droughts in 1987 (Tendler 1997, 22). The Health Agents Program, as it
was called, was the brainchild of a *sanitarista* who was invited to implement his
vision for a rural preventative health program after a new governor took power
in 1987 (Tendler 1997, 155). The program focused on maternal and child health
(Macinko and Harris 2015) and accounted for just 3 percent of the budget of

the larger emergency employment program and was given permanent funding status in 1989 (Tendler 1997, 22). The Health Agents Program recruited and trained relatively low-skilled workers, 80 percent of whom were women (and all of whom resided in the communities in which they worked), as "health agents" using a rigorous selection process administered by the Department of Health and supervised by nurses who were hired and paid by the municipality (Tendler 1997, 22, 24). The 7,300 agents were responsible for disease prevention activities as well as basic curative services, including applying sutures, giving injections, dressing wounds, providing advice on how to treat flus and colds, and getting sick children hospital care when needed (Tendler 1997, 38, 45). The basic curative services provided by the health agents frequently led to breakthroughs in prompting more difficult behavioral changes that had consequences for health. As one agent explained, "I first earned the respect and trust of families by treating wounds or giving a shot . . . so that now families listen to me when I talk to them about breastfeeding, or better hygiene, or nutrition—things that don't show immediate results" (quoted in Tendler 1997, 39).

The division of labor between different branches of the government helped to break some of the patterns of patronage that might have been created if the program had been solely overseen and managed by the municipalities, and the merit-based recruitment process (amid a broader context of clientelism) succeeded in creating a strong commitment among health agents[8] (Tendler 1997, 27–29). In addition, the discretion and responsibility given to nurses, who played a supervisory role in the program—and the respect accorded them by members of the community—was a stark contrast from the inferior status normally accorded to nurses in urban hospital settings (Tendler 1997, 36). These dynamics helped contribute to a situation in which health workers regularly exceeded their mandates (Tendler 1997, 41).

While municipal governments had the power to choose what kind of health care program to adopt following the advent of the Unified Health System, the Family Health Program (PSF), as a federal program implemented by municipal governments, served as one important model that quickly achieved national prominence for rapidly extending basic health care services at the primary care level to Brazil's poorest rural areas (Dowbor and Houtzager 2014, 143). Initially, within the *sanitarista* movement, there were divisions on whether the program represented "poor policy for the poor" or truly quality universal primary care; however, significant debate took place within *sanitarista*-created institutions (CEBES and ABRASCO, and later the National Health Councils, to be discussed shortly), and the demonstration of the program's success over time dampened early criticisms (Sugiyama 2008, 96, 98). Building on the original template of the Health Agents Program, the Family Health Program relied upon a slightly more skilled health team that included a doctor, a nurse, a nurse's assistant, and approximately five lay health workers to serve communities of up to one thousand people each (Macinko and Harris 2015). These health teams were intended to replace clinics and hospitals as places for citizens to go for their for primary health care needs (Sugiyama 2008, 93).

To ensure that access to health care could be rolled out quickly, PSF allowed the contracting of medical staff through universities, NGOs, charities, and community organizations, which aimed to overcome some of the time-consuming and costly processes involved with hiring civil servants to staff up a new program (Dowbor and Houtzager 2014, 153, 155). This design put the *sanitaristas* into conflict with some other members of the health profession, including the health workers' unions as well as some segments of a community-level popular health movement (Dowbor and Houtzager 2014, 154). But while community groups played a role in negotiating the implementation of PSF and in holding the government accountable, the "popular health movement" for the most part did not mobilize pressure from below and instead acted more as a "bystander" than a "dissident" or "strategist" (Dowbor and Houtzager 2014, 156, 159).

Rather, several of the *sanitaristas* who were members of center and left-leaning parties, including the PSDB and PT, played a key role in the expansion of the program, once again underscoring the elite professional-led character of the policy's implementation.[9] While *sanitarista* organization proved to be somewhat uneven across the country (Shankland and Cornwall 2007, 173), they used their political ties to expand implementation of the Family Health Program at the municipal level dramatically (Dowbor and Houtzager 2014, 153). Between 1998 and 2014, the program expanded from about 2,000 Family Health Teams covering roughly 7 million people, or 4 percent of the Brazilian population, to 39,000 teams serving 120 million people, or 62 percent of the population in 2014 (Macinko and Harris 2015). Although the program provided greater financial incentives to extend access to health care in small and medium-sized cities, mayoral candidates in some of the country's urban municipalities where health care access remained tenuous, including São Paulo, saw the electoral promise that PSF represented along with the potential to extend coverage to 60 percent of the population in just four years (Dowbor and Houtzager 2014, 153–54). Yet even after the program failed to pay the political dividends to which politicians had initially staked their hopes and political priority shifted toward investment in urgent and emergency care in large cities like São Paulo, PSF continued to grow, albeit at a slower pace, aided by new demands from lower-income groups (Dowbor and Houtzager 2014, 155). Much as with Thailand's program, once the program was implemented, citizen interest in it helped to continue to sustain it.

Engaging Citizens and Ensuring Accountability through New Governance Mechanisms

Alongside universalism and decentralization, participation was another key principle that the *sanitaristas* had advocated for at the 8th National Health Conference in 1986 and subsequently worked to write into the 1988 constitution and 1990 Unified Health System organic laws (Shankland and Cornwall 2007, 167–68). To invest citizens in the new reforms, the *sanitaristas* promoted the development of health councils, which meet monthly, in the country's states and municipalities (Cornwall, Cordeiro, and Delgado 2006, 144, 146).

The first health councils that would serve as a template were developed in eastern São Paulo in 1979, where the *sanitaristas* worked together with the poor to bring visibility to the problem of quality health services (Avritzer 2009, 119, 122). A popular movement soon developed nationally in 1981 and promoted the idea of autonomous councils independent of the state that would oversee matters related to health policy; with *sanitarista* involvement, a hybrid design would emerge that involved state sponsorship and civil society participation and would be promoted at the Constituent Assembly and ultimately reflected in the 1990 Unified Health System law (Avritzer 2009, 121–25).

Complemented by a regular series of state, local, and national health conferences, these health councils aimed to provide organized civil society groups with a space to discuss the operations of the health sector with state officials and hold them accountable for how money was spent in the country's twenty-three states and five thousand municipalities (Shankland and Cornwall 2007, 166). Although participatory budgeting processes have received much greater attention in the literature, these deliberative bodies, which by 1999 included some twenty-seven thousand councils at the municipal level (of which four thousand specifically concerned health), have in fact proliferated to a much greater extent than the PT-led participatory budgeting processes (Schönleitner 2004, 1). Pioneered once again with the support of the *sanitaristas*, their wide reach into all levels of Brazilian government, involvement of hundreds of thousands of citizens, and status as institutions that had the power to make binding decisions led them to take on a great amount of political importance (Shankland and Cornwall 2007, 174).

The Basic Operational Norms (NOBs) that govern the SUS require that at least 50 percent of council representation come from actual users of the health care system (including representatives from civil society organizations) and make federal transfer of resources contingent on the existence of councils (Schönleitner 2004, 6; on civil society, see Coelho 2004, 35). Another 25 percent of council representatives are drawn from health workers and 25 percent from service providers and health managers (Victora et al. 2011, 2044). This representative schema has not meant that councils have been immune from the influence of party politics (Cornwall, Romano, and Shankland 2008, 28) or a "lingering authoritarian political culture" (see Coelho 2007, 35). At times, municipal governments have made significant decisions related to health policy without consulting the councils in spite of their role in providing oversight on health sector matters (Coelho 2004, 34–35). Likewise, technical rather than popular discourse by health professionals and bureaucrats have sometimes dominated these forums (Coelho et al. 2002), and popular participation has sometimes been uneven, with a vocal minority sometimes dominating debate (Cornwall 2008, 520; on inequalities, Dal Poz and Pinheiro 1998). In some cases, the allocation of council representation by civil society groups has reflected preexisting state–civil society relationships and have excluded popular voices (Coelho 2004, 36). In spite of all these drawbacks, by the late 1990s these forums had become important places for citizens to make new demands (Shankland and Cornwall 2007, 168). More broadly, the forums built "a bridge into the community," providing opportunities for "people to grow" and bring "'new faces, new people' to engage with the state," becoming key institutions implicated in the reproduction of rights-based ideology (Shankland and Cornwall 2007, 176–77). Above all, the citizens involved in the forums have—quite apart from the background of the *sanitaristas* who promoted the policies—come from the lower income strata in Brazil (Cornwall 2006). And part of what has taken place at these forums has involved education of the newly involved citizenry in the value and importance of preventative medicine and primary care as opposed to ambulances and acute curative services (Shankland and Cornwall 2007, 178). In this way, even a deeply participatory project like the Health Councils has involved a measure of paternalism, in spite of the *sanitaristas*' aim for the Councils to be instruments that provide societal oversight of the health sector (see Shankland and Cornwall 2007, 178).

The 2003 National Health Conference—named after communist *sanitarista* Sergio Arouca, who had been based at FIOCRUZ—nonetheless brought with it the promise of a new National Health Plan informed by the five thousand participants in the conference and the three hundred thousand people they represented—to that point one of the most diverse showings of participation in the country's many health fora (Shankland and Cornwall 2007, 183). Nearly half of the participants were women, 40 percent were black, and less than a third had university education, highlighting the degree to which participation in health sector affairs was increasingly becoming an affair that no longer involved just professionals but also ordinary citizens (Cornwall 2008, 2177).

More than ten years after the founding of the SUS, the broadening of participation in health sector governance was also signaled by raucous confrontations between different civil society groups over issues such as abortion services at the conference, which brought the feminist health movement and the Catholic Church into conflict (Shankland and Cornwall 2007, 183–84). Similar developments at other levels of the health system signaled the growing vibrancy of health councils as important fora of deliberative debate and decision-making for the formerly excluded. Some health conferences at the municipal level taking place at the same time brought health workers into communication with newly elected council members, approximately half of whom had only primary education (Cornwall 2008, 515). Although they have been largely unsuccessful and marked by a lack of consensus on their role and mandate, there have even been attempts to further broaden community participation by building local health councils at the neighborhood level[10] (Cornwall, Romano, and Shankland 2008, 27) as well as new National Health Conferences devoted to specific issues, such as indigenous health (Cornwall and Shankland 2008, 2178).

Conclusion

By many counts, the effects of the important new health rights in Brazil can be measured in several ways: citizens registered with the Family Health Program receive medicine free of charge at their local health centers (Macinko and Harris 2015). The percentage of pregnant women who received at least one antenatal consultation increased from 60 percent to 84 percent between 1990 and 1996, and the percentage of births attended by trained staff increased from 73 percent to 88 percent over the same period (WHO 2005 in Shankland and Cornwall 2007, 164). DPT3 (diphtheria, pertussis, and tetanus) immunization coverage—another simple measure of health care access—increased from 69 percent to 96 percent from 1992 to 2004 (WHO 1995, 2005, 2006 in Shankland and Cornwall 2007, 164). SUS is the largest public system for organ transplants in the world, and upwards of 80 percent of the transplants, surgeries, and other high-risk procedures took place in public hospitals and SUS affiliate hospitals as of 2003 (Font 2003, 104). The expansion of access to health care represented by the Unified Health System reform and its associated programs has led to reductions in infant mortality (Macinko et al. 2006; Aquino et al. 2009), adult mortality (Rocha and Soares 2010), and unnecessary hospital admissions (Macinko et al. 2010). The life expectancy of Brazilians increased from 67 to 72 years between 1991 and 2005; infant mortality decreased from 32 to 22 deaths per thousand infants between 1997 and 2004; and the number of health care professionals increased from 1.1 to 1.4 per thousand people between 1990 and 2005 (Ministry of Health 2006 in Falleti 2010, 59). Use by the poorest households increased by nearly 50 percent by 2007 (Shankland and Cornwall 2007, 164), and public opinion polling in some large urban areas has shown that people in the bottom two quintiles who rely most on the SUS have positive views of it (Falleti 2010, 59).

These remarkable changes, which took place at a time when the political and economic context did not favor change, help to explain why Brazil's *sanitarista* movement has been called "one of the most influential political forces to emerge from the dictatorship period" (Shankland and Cornwall 2007, 173). This chapter has illustrated the role that a movement of public health professionals who occupied positions in the state has played in putting universal health care on the political agenda in the country's 1988 constitution; drafting laws from positions in the Health Ministry; devising an implementation strategy to bring health care to the masses; and creating participatory accountability mechanisms to ensure that Brazil's universal health care policy is more than just a policy on paper but one that meets the needs of millions of citizens in practice.

4

SOUTH AFRICA: EMBRACING NATIONAL HEALTH INSURANCE— IN NAME ONLY

There was no real uncertainty about the outcome of the 1994 election.

—Hermann Giliomee, former president, South African Institute on Race Relations (1998, 131)

Before apartheid fell, access to health care in South Africa was not a right. The country's health care system was deeply segregated, and the vast majority of the country's minority-white population relied on private health insurance to gain access to quality health care through the country's network of private hospitals and clinics. The vast majority of blacks, by contrast, were left to depend on traditional medicine and a crumbling, racially segregated public health care system that provided care to people with low incomes, with admission and fees governed by an unevenly applied means test.

Perhaps even more so than in Thailand or Brazil, a constellation of factors would seem to have predisposed South Africa to make major new commitments to expand access to health care and make health care a right of all citizens at apartheid's end in 1994. A fast-growing AIDS epidemic and the abysmal legacies left by the apartheid regime marked health care as a sector in need of particular attention by the rapidly rising African National Congress (ANC). And indeed, plans laid out in the government's 1994 Reconstruction and Development Programme (RDP), which formed a cornerstone of the ANC's campaign platform for the 1994 elections, referred to the need to transform the health system inherited from the apartheid regime. But even prior to the development of the RDP, an organized professional movement of doctors and health economists had been vocal in laying the groundwork for a universal health care program that would serve the needs of all citizens. Given these factors, the unrivaled majority of the ANC, the party's close relationship to the South

African Communist Party and trade unions, and the rise of visionary leader Nelson Mandela to power, one might have expected to see a particularly aggressive effort to expand access to health care in the wake of democratic transition in post-apartheid South Africa.

Proposals for bold new single-payer health reforms included a new National Health Service in the British mold, in which universal health care was publicly financed through taxes and publicly provided by salaried doctors; care would be provided as an equal right to all without regard to income. These proposals involved either nationalizing the country's private health care providers or, less radically, allowing them to operate alongside the public health care system. Proposals for a new National Health Insurance system were also considered that would provide insurance coverage to all and for the first time promised to give the masses access to the country's elite private health care system, which for the most part had served the white population exclusively.

While the ANC-led government did build over a thousand clinics and take up two important incremental reforms promoted by an organized movement of medical professionals dedicated to expanding access to health care (making comprehensive care available to pregnant women and children under six free through the public system in 1994 and basic primary health care free for all in 1996, also through the public system), it embraced the more transformative reforms advocated by the movement in name only. It chose instead to continue to allow the majority of the population to rely on an overburdened and understaffed means-tested public health system. For over twenty years, with few exceptions, this circumstance has not changed.

The role that neoliberalism has played in explaining public policy in South Africa is of course important in understanding the ANC's direction (Bond 2000; Williams and Taylor 2000; Decoteau 2013). While the grand plans laid out by the ANC in the RDP foretold a social democratic future for South Africa, the government's adoption of the neoliberal Growth, Employment and Redistribution (GEAR) economic program in 1996 privileged the importance of maintaining stable macroeconomic conditions, stimulating economic growth, maintaining low inflation and taxes, and reducing deficits over the expansion of social policy and investments aimed at redressing and correcting the ills of apartheid.[1] Increasingly conscious of how the new South Africa would be perceived by international capital, the country's leaders sought to eliminate any suggestion of threat to the business climate, including taxes that might accompany the introduction of major new social policies. Applying this lens to the shortcomings in the ANC's policies in the health sector offers critical and important insights. However, I suggest it is incomplete.

This chapter makes an argument grounded in political incentives rather than ideology. It advances the claim that the major reason South African officials resisted

particularly striking. And while the progressive doctors who championed the cause of health equity in South Africa were, by and large, white, Indian, and Coloured (a peculiar apartheid-era racial construct), the professional movement ran up against a broader medical profession that was dominated by whites, who in the mid-1970s accounted for some 93 percent of all medical doctors in the country (van Rensburg 2004, 329). Owing to historical oppression, there were very few black African doctors. In the 1980s, the majority of the medical profession in South Africa belonged to the Medical Association of South Africa (MASA) (Neser 1989, 115). MASA had been implicated in the discriminatory practices perpetrated by the government and had not only failed to uphold professional standards but also worked regularly with the repressive apartheid state security apparatus (Moodley and Kling 2015).

While HWO, HWS, and HWA shared a broad vision for building a movement of health care workers and tried to bring nonprofessional health care workers into the fold as well (Pick et al. 2012, 403), the National Medical and Dental Association (NAMDA) was founded in 1984 as an association of doctors and dentists that aimed to address health inequities and to assist in the dismantling of apartheid (Coovadia 1999, 1505). One of the most highly visible movement organizations of the time, NAMDA was formed over concerns related to the issues faced by black doctors in the practice of medicine, racial relations within the profession, and physician involvement in the death of physician and activist Steve Biko (Monamodi 1996, 362).[3] While it was not ostensibly formed in opposition to MASA, its commitment to a free and democratic society put NAMDA into direct conflict with MASA, which purported to represent the medical profession as a whole (*Critical Health* 1983, 16). NAMDA members argued that MASA "provided a bulwark against criticism of the health inequities of this evil [apartheid] system" through the legitimacy it conferred on the state as a professional group of doctors that took no firm stance against it (Mji et al. 1989, 116).[4] However, the professional movement represented in organizations like NAMDA stood as a definite minority within the broader medical profession: as late as 1988, some twelve thousand of the country's twenty thousand medical doctors belonged to MASA, while NAMDA members were estimated to number between five hundred and fifteen hundred (Neser 1989, 115).[5]

By the late 1980s, some consolidation among professional movement organizations took place. A landmark NAMDA conference in April 1987 brought together ninety-one delegates from around the country for the first time to share experiences and a plan to advance the cause of primary health care. This event spurred the creation of the National Progressive Primary Health Care Network (NPPHCN), which would convene a second national consultation in September 1987 attended by 350 medical professionals and would later send a delegation to the United States to consult with grant-making organizations about the prospect of funding (NPPHCN 1989, 3–4).

NPPHCN was formed to advance a more equitable health experience in South Africa and advocated for a publicly provided National Health Service (like the one in Great Britain) in which all had access to health care and the community participated in it (NPPHCN undated a). Funded by the U.S.-based Kaiser Family Foundation, the organization was recognized for having laid the groundwork that made some of the post-apartheid government's work on health care possible by organizing communities, educating and training health workers, producing and circulating information about primary health care, and building an alliance of professionals with a coherent vision of how health care should be reorganized. NPPHCN's goals and strategies referenced the WHO's visionary Alma Ata conference that popularized the idea of Health for All, human rights, and more specifically, the right to health, imagining health care facilities as the "moral and political duty of government" (Jinabhal 1989, 26–27; Health Focus Memo undated).

Just as NPPHCN was drawing diverse organizations under one umbrella, the HWA and HWO were also doing their part to consolidate divisions within the professional movement. In the late 1980s, they joined together to form the South African Health Workers Congress (SAHWCO). Although composed of medical professionals, SAHWCO aimed to position itself as a member of the broader mass movements that were gaining momentum at the time: It was an affiliate of the United Democratic Front (one of the largest grassroots organizations, formed in 1983) and became a member of the broader Mass Democratic Movement[6]—two of the most important umbrella anti-apartheid organizations (HWO 1988, 2). Like many of the other professional movement organizations of its time, SAHWCO drew on Marxist ideas in taking the apartheid regime to task for its racist policies. Literature put out by SAHWCO drew linkages between the evils of apartheid and the inequalities of capitalism, which they argued had particularly deleterious consequences in the health sector. Against a backdrop of social injustice, these organizations sought to promote a rights-based approach to health, with the struggle for democracy inextricably linked to the right to health:

> we in the health sector (being aware of the devastating effects of apartheid and capitalist greed on the health of all South Africans) are attempting to research and debate the value of Constitutionalizing the right to both health and healthcare. (SAHWCO 1989b)

Hoping to inform the creation of a new constitution in South Africa, professionals in SAHWCO conducted research on constitutional rights to health and health care in forty-eight different countries (SAHWCO 1989b).

By the late 1980s, at least rhetorically, the apartheid government had incorporated many of the movement's ideas related to primary health care into the government's 1986 National Health Plan and 1989 Strategy for the Development of Public Health. The apartheid state recognized the need for a partnership between the state and the private sector to create a more substantive primary health care program that was universalistic (SAHWCO 1989a, 1–2, 8). However, such measures can also be read as part of a broader government campaign to "win hearts and minds" through socioeconomic development for the very poorest amid a broader backdrop of extreme repression (Coovadia 1999, 1507). Apart from public pronouncements, the more emancipatory and empowering aspects of primary health care that might threaten the existing order were sidelined (Friedman interview 2008). And the professional movement remained highly critical of the state's weak commitment to primary health care as well as MASA's attempts to gain credibility and legitimacy in the eyes of the international community through engagement with professional movement organizations (Health Policy Sub-Committee Minutes 1991, 5).

In 1990, NAMDA, OASSA, SAHWCO, the National Education Health and Allied Workers Union (NEHAWU), the ANC, and other professional movement organizations worked with a number of partners abroad to host the International Conference on Health in Southern Africa in Maputo (*Critical Health* 1990, 2; NAMDA 1990, 1). Over time, these interactions led organizations, like NAMDA and SAHWCO, to forge greater linkages and to develop policy together (Health Policy Sub-Committee 1991, 1).

While supportive of the ANC, as the apartheid era drew to a close the professional movement at times wavered on whether it would lead on issues related to health policy or would defer to the ANC. SAHWCO consulted with the ANC, the United Democratic Front, and the country's most important trade union association, the Congress of South African Trade Unions (COSATU) at the time of its founding to develop unified positions (SAHWCO 1990b, 1). However, in some discussions involving the state, MASA, and the professional movement organizations, the movement consulted the ANC only in passing, deferring to the ANC when needed to make negotiated agreements binding (Health Policy Sub-Committee 1991, 1, 4). This wavering, however, melted away following the calls for unity after Nelson Mandela was released from prison in 1990 (SAHWCO 1990b, 1). NAMDA, NPPHCN, OASSA, and SAHWCO developed closer connections and elaborated a joint policy program (Joint Working Group for Health Policy 1991, 1).

Two years later, in 1992, there were more mergers of professional movement organizations, including SAHWCO, NAMDA, OASSA, HWS, and the Overseas Medical Graduates' Association under the rubric of the South African Health and

Social Services Organization (SAHSSO) (Pick et al. 2012, 405). Like the organizations that preceded it, SAHSSO espoused the goals of health care as a right of the people and a duty of the state, informed by community involvement (SAHSSO undated). A joint NPPHCN/SAHSSO Policy Conference in December 1992 issued a thirteen-point call to the government, among other things, to ensure that no one is denied care on the basis of lack of ability to pay; to provide free care to children under 6, pregnant women, and the elderly with communicable diseases; and to increase financing for health care through a range of measures, including hospital fees based on ability to pay. Both NPPHCN and SAHSSO would play important roles in supporting the work of an ANC Health Desk that was established in 1992 (Health Systems Trust 1995, ch. 5), and prominent members of the movement who would go on to play important roles in the post-apartheid government's health ministry, such as Manto Msimang-Tshabalala, played important roles at the conference.

In practice, members of the different professional movement organizations often held overlapping memberships and were also members of the ANC. Noddy Jinhabhal, who for many years managed the School of Family and Public Health Medicine, and Eric Buch, who served as the General Secretary of NPPHCN and also Deputy Director-General for Health Care in Gauteng Province, for example, were both members of the ANC Health Committee and NAMDA. Manto Msimang-Tshabalala was a member of NPPHCN and would later become minister of health in the second ANC government led by Thabo Mbeki (NPPHCN 1991). Ivan Toms served as Secretary of the NPPHCN while active in the ANC and in the AIDS movement. Some members of SAHSSO also held executive positions at NPPHCN.

Putting Universal Health Care on the Agenda in the Final Years of Apartheid: The Role of Medical Professionals

As early as the mid-1980s, members of the professional movement began to advance more concrete proposals for a racially inclusive universal health care program that would address the deep health inequities that had come into being under apartheid rule. In 1985, Solomon Benatar, a physician and head of the Department of Medicine at the University of Cape Town, submitted a letter to the editor of the MASA-controlled *South African Medical Journal*, arguing for the need for a British-style National Health Service (NHS) that would rely on funding from taxes to provide care for all through a public system (Benatar 1985, 839). This was followed by no fewer than twenty-seven letters of support and opposition from members of other university faculties and other interested parties in just the next two years (Abdullah 1987, 4).[7] These calls stood on the shoulders of earlier efforts to build a tax-funded NHS to serve the health care needs of all South Africans before apartheid came into being in the 1940s (McIntyre and van den Heever 2007, 72).

Apart from equity concerns, the push for expansive health reform was spurred by other motivations, including population pressures and unrest resulting from high unemployment and recession, the high cost of care, the need for cost containment, and the recent trend toward privatization (Klopper 1986, 293, 295). At a time when contribution rates to medical schemes were rising 30 percent in a single year and there was a widespread recognition of a growing crisis within the private sector (Broomberg 1991, 1), these calls for a National Health Service emphasized better funding of a public health care system that could provide health care to everyone, while at the same time allowing the private health care system to continue to exist but to wind down over time due to "the unpredictable nature of the market . . . and left to collapse under the weight of its own limitations" (Zwarenstein 1990, 32). While Britain's program was dominated by public providers, many of the calls for a South African NHS generally aimed to sidestep conflict that would be provoked from nationalizing health care and eliminating private practice (Benatar 1985; Zwarenstein 1990). However, some of the measures proposed included radical steps, such as eliminating a tax rebate on employer contributions to employee medical schemes, which was projected to lead to a 20 percent increase in the budget for the public health system, and moving public employees, which comprised about a third of all medical scheme members at the time, into publicly provided health care arrangements (Zwarenstein 1990, 32).

Other proposals by members of the professional movement called for the adoption of a National Health Insurance (NHI) program (Broomberg 1991; de Beer and Broomberg 1990). While it is important to emphasize that the proposals at this time were made by analysts whose experience with health systems design was somewhat limited, they deepened the emerging policy conversations that were going on by tackling thorny political issues that so far had been avoided and critiquing the shortcomings of existing plans. They also found the doubling of health expenditure required to make an NHS viable unrealistic (amid other future government priorities) and instead took direct aim at "the progressive eradication of the two-tier [public and private] health care system" through the creation of a centralized mechanism of funding through the state (de Beer and Broomberg 1990, 146).

Over time, some analysts involved the debates came to favor NHI, which had been used successfully to cover everyone in Canada, over a British-style NHS

(Thomas and Gilson 2004, 281)—which, in its most extreme form, would have involved making doctors in private practice salaried employees of the state. However, the NHI proposals were radical in their own right because they explicitly recognized the role that the entrenched system of medical schemes had played in the development of South Africa's unequal system of health care services and suggested that private health insurance had an uncertain future in such a new system. As one prominent proposal at the time stated:

> This means, by definition, an end to the medical aid system as we know it. Private health insurance could only be permitted to pay for services not available within the package of care paid for by the national insurance system. The exact process by which the medical aid funds were dismantled, or incorporated into the national health insurance system, would need to be negotiated and is also beyond the scope of this paper. (de Beer and Broomberg 1990, 146)

Future proposals by the same authors took a softer view of the role that private health insurance could play in the transition toward the development of a national health insurance system. While NHI would eventually involve "public and private *provision* of health care . . . integrated within a public financing mechanism," the authors argued that in the near term, shoring up the collective purchasing power, risk-sharing capacities, negotiating ability, cross-subsidization capacity, and co-ordination functions of medical schemes were necessary first steps to the incorporation of medical schemes into a national health insurance program (Broomberg 1991, 4). This approach to universal health insurance coverage—providing coverage to everyone regardless of whether or not they had actually contributed through taxes—recognized that NHI was not something that would happen overnight but involved making private health insurance coverage mandatory among the population groups that could afford it (what is frequently called social health insurance) and gradually extending coverage to more and more citizens as new groups were made to purchase coverage, as citizens joined the formal sector and could contribute, or as poorer citizens were extended subsidized coverage.

Several of these proposals came out of the Center for the Study of Health Policy (later the Centre for Health Policy, or CHP) of the University of Witwatersrand, South Africa's most prestigious university. Very generally, CHP promoted efforts to make South Africa's health care system more unified and integrated through either an NHI or NHS model that envisioned a gradually diminishing role for private health care (van Rensburg 2004, 103). Many of the health professionals working at CHP had been active members of NAMDA, such as Cedric de Beer and Max Price (who would go on to become dean of the health sciences at the University of the Witwatersrand and later vice chancellor at the University of Cape Town). Just as CEBES had been a focal point for health activism under dictatorship in Brazil, so too had CHP explicitly worked to promote health equity and universalism in the provision of health care in South Africa. And like the *sanitarista* movement of Brazil and Thailand's Rural Doctors' movement, many in South Africa's professional movement held the private sector with suspicion, a view also held by many ANC members.

At the International Conference on Health in Southern Africa in Maputo in 1990, the ANC Chief Representative "unequivocally condemn[ed] the [apartheid] regime's programme of privatizing health services . . . aimed at limiting the options of available to a democratic, non-racial government . . . [and] starving the state sector of resources" (quoted in *Critical Health* 1990, 7). And in another early formulation of the ANC's plan for health care in a post-apartheid South Africa—sounding surprisingly similar to the some of the earlier proposals detailed here—a future South African National Health Service would tolerate a well-regulated private sector with a longer-term vision of having most health care provided through the public system (ANC 1990, 4–6).

Democratization and the Transition to a New Order

Democratization in South Africa brought with it an end to the system of racialized segregation and oppression that apartheid represented and the promise of a new and inclusive South African government committed to ending neglect of the majority that had for so long existed in the country. On February 11, 1990, nine days after the ruling National Party announced an end to the ban on the ANC, the country's charismatic leader, Nelson Mandela, was released from prison; the following year, Mandela was elected president of the ANC and engaged in talks to end the rule of minority whites (Nelson Mandela Foundation 2015). These actions represented important first steps on the road to "profound political changes" (Fourie 2006, 84).

During apartheid, members of the professional movement to expand access to health care worked as academics in universities and grassroots service providers as well as in exile far away from the levers of state power. But following elections in 1994 and the ANC's ascension to power, many of these professionals would come to occupy positions of influence of the highest order in the new government. The groundwork that they had laid in their advocacy for universal health care and the development of concrete plans—and the absorption of many of the movement's most important people into executive positions in government—would have seemed to have positioned the government to begin to address the deep inequalities wrought by the apartheid government's policies of intentional neglect of the public health care system and the needs of citizens more broadly.

However, the character of democratic transition in South Africa unfolded quite unlike that in Thailand or Brazil. Systematic racial segregation and oppression by a white minority government for over half a century, the imprisonment of the visionary Nelson Mandela for twenty-seven years, and the leading role of the ANC in the underground struggle for a new order prefigured electoral outcomes in South Africa in a way that was quite unlike patterns of political competition in Thailand or Brazil. Whereas the democratic transition was marked by fierce political competition in the other two countries, because of these dynamics in South Africa the ANC was the obvious heir apparent, and no other party seriously challenged the ANC in the country's first democratic election.

Immediately following legalization of the ANC in February 1990, polls suggested that the party could pick up more than 60 percent of seats in a national election, and these projections held under different kinds of electoral scenarios (Giliomee 1995, 92) and remained consistent over time (Giliomee 1998, 131). When elections were held in 1994, the ANC predictably dominated, capturing over 62 percent of the vote, with the second-place—and quickly fading—National Party receiving just 20.4 percent and the third-place Inkatha Freedom Party receiving just 10.5 percent of the vote. These incredible disparities would only grow wider in the two subsequent national elections in 1999 and 2004 (Alvarez-Rivera 2014).

However, the taken-for-granted nature of the party's ascendant status was reflected not only in the views of ordinary voting citizens but also in the outgoing National Party government's stance toward the ANC. It was the ANC with whom the National Party carried out secret bilateral negotiations on security issues in the three years after the party was legalized (Giliomee 1995, 96–97). While the negotiated 1993 interim constitution assured the National Party of holding cabinet seats and one of the two deputy president positions, more general sentiment at the time suggested that a close contest—which would have suggested election-fixing by the National Party—would not have been accepted (Giliomee 1998, 131). This is not to say that a new government's post-election posture was completely free from risks amid a fragile new political order, but it does point to the relative certainty that key actors—in particular, voters and the outgoing authoritarian regime—felt about the likelihood of the ANC's ascendancy in the early 1990s when preparations for democratization were being made.

Actual election results in 1994 not only conformed to these expectations but also found that voting ran almost entirely along racial lines, with the ANC winning 90 percent of the vote among the three-quarters of the electorate that were African (Giliomee 1995, 103). This left six opposition parties to split the 36 percent of the vote not won by the ANC—a number that would later grow to eleven splitting an even smaller percentage of the vote (33.15%) in 1999 (Southall 2001, 2). Among black Africans, only a small Zulu professional class and rural Zulu-speakers did not line up with the ANC (Giliomee 1998, 131). In fact, so complete was the ANC's domination at the polls that two years after the first elections one survey would suggest that nearly half of black voters would "support and stand by my political party and its leaders even if I disagree" (Johnson 1997, 9, quoted in Giliomee, Myburgh, and Schlemmer 2001, 163). This "certainty of majority" of the ANC ensured that even shifting coalitions built around interests would be muted, and political opposition would remain on the periphery (Giliomee, Myburgh, and Schlemmer 2001, 163). By 1999, even the small group of Zulu opposition, which had gathered under the banner of the Inkatha Freedom Party, won just over 10 percent of the vote in the 1994 elections, and fiercely criticized the ANC, would become "just another component of the ANC's broad church" (Schrire 2001, 142).

The domination of the ANC at the polls was, however, not just a product of inspiration provided by Nelson Mandela's visionary leadership, or its alliance with the trade unions (Giliomee 1998, 131), but was also a product of widespread intimidation that made campaigning by rival parties in townships all but impossible (Giliomee 1995, 103). While its massive mandate—and the legacy of struggle that it had overcome—provided the ANC with a degree of moral authority, elements of the party used this authority to clamp down on dissent and narrow debate by labeling critics of its policies racist (Giliomee, Myburgh, and Schlemmer 2001, 169). In this context, even prominent members of the ANC, such as physician activist and former University of Cape Town vice chancellor Mamphela Ramphele, have pointed to a growing fear among the country's intellectual elite about criticizing the abuses and mistakes of the ANC for fear of being cast "anti-liberation" (Southall 2001, 18).

This censorship extended not only to critics outside the party but also to those who resisted adopting the line held by top brass within the party. The government's commitment to the neoliberal Growth, Employment, and Redistribution program (GEAR) in 1997 marked one of the first tests not only of disagreement between the ANC and its partners in the South African Communist Party and the country's largest trade union, COSATU (McKinley 2001, 191), but also within the ANC itself. Debate over GEAR was kept out of public view, with concerted efforts made by the leadership to crack down on dissent vis-à-vis threats of economic and political marginalization (McKinley 2001, 190–91). Such internally directed intimidation sparked some frustrated and alienated parliamentarians to talk publicly about a "climate of fear" where "internal democracy [within the party] gets crushed" (Davis quoted in McKinley 2001, 191).

Party loyalty has at times been used to quash effective oversight of the executive branch in parliamentary committees; in one instance, a popular ANC MP, Bantu Holomisa, was actually expelled from the party—and thereby ejected from Parliament—after accusing a cabinet member of past corruption in the apartheid era (Mattes 2002, 25, 27). And a 2001 ANC National Executive discussion actually took "enemies within" the movement as its focus (*Mail and Guardian* 2002 in Lodge 2004, 200). Over time, these efforts to centralize power have directed their attention downwards toward the provincial and local levels through national party structures, which now nominate candidates for provincial and local executive positions rather than branches of the party at those levels (Mattes 2002, 25).

While one writer has suggested that the ANC's "crushing victory" in the 1994 national elections "provided powerful incentives for the organization to free itself from the formal and informal commitments to govern in a spirit of national unity" (Giliomee 1995, 104), the benefit of hindsight suggests that the ANC has avoided taking the same kind of steps as Robert Mugabe in Zimbabwe. The National Party did depart from the Government of National Unity in 1996, some three years before the end of its term, and receded into the background of parliamentary politics (Giliomee 1998, 128). While such departures have not freed the party from a commitment to unity, the ANC's dominance has paradoxically freed it from following through on some of the more difficult mandates that professional movements had succeeded in embedding in ANC policy statements—universal health care chief among them.

Movement Transition and Efforts to Institutionalize Policy in the New South Africa

After the transition to democracy, in spite of the deep neglect of people's health care needs by the apartheid regime, the most vocal voices for reform did not come from the masses. Even before apartheid fell, the largest and most representative grassroots social movement organization, the United Democratic Front, which claimed to represent over two million—mostly poor—people was dissolved in 1991 and incorporated into the ANC (Ellis 2015, 210; Robins and Colvin 2015, 259). Once the ANC formally came to power, an early survey of the issues that led people to protest found that health care rated fourth out of five public goods (after housing, education, and public safety); by 1999, it rated dead last, falling behind public services (Klandermans 2015, 247). However, the lack of organized mass demands for health care should not be read as a lack of need. The sorry state of health care infrastructure left by the apartheid regime, the steady migration of white medical expertise out of the country, and the growing AIDS epidemic meant that the need for effective health care was particularly dire. In the absence of mass movements that would give voice to people's health care needs amid a host of other pressing concerns, movements of well-organized professionals, knowledgeable about the health care system, advocated for transformative reform.

After the 1994 elections, some members of the professional movement were absorbed into the new government.[8] At the same time, members based in universities gained influence based on their pre-1994 activism and commitment to improved health equity (Thomas and Gilson 2004, 283). The campaign promises that had been made in the ANC's Reconstruction and Development Plan (RDP) and supported by movement organizations like those already mentioned became official policy (Bond 2004, 89). And a new technocratic organization, the Health Systems Trust, which was formed in 1992, established a working relationship with government to assist in addressing the problems in the country's fragmented health care system by developing a new uniform and standard system based on districts (HPCU 1995, 1–2). While the professional movement organizations that had for so long championed universal health care did not immediately die out after the ANC came to power, they did have to renegotiate their relationship with government and other social institutions. In this context, the delicate relationship between MASA and NAMDA was something that had to be renegotiated entirely. Meanwhile, organizations such as NPPHCN continued to contribute to the building of new and better health legislation over the next few years, as former executives of NPPHCN now in government drew on the expertise that those in the movement who remained outside of government could provide. And increasingly, new international voices that had for the most part stood outside national policy conversations during apartheid now began to join the longstanding advocacy efforts of the country's professional movement.

In 1994, UNICEF and World Health Organization officials were flown in to support efforts by the ANC to draft a National Health Plan for South Africa. The plan, which was intended to guide future policy development, drew on some of the longstanding ideas promoted by the movement, among them free health care for pregnant women and children under six and the development of a national health insurance program. The plan suggested that principles such as equity, universalism, and the right to health be enshrined in a National Health System that would unify the fragmented system of health care that had been created under apartheid (ANC 1994). Soon after the transition, a number of other important policy decrees were made and commissions formed that suggested that the government was not only taking up the ideas of the professional movement but doing so in a swift and serious way.

On May 24, 1994, less than a month after the national elections, the new government announced that it would begin offering free health care for children under six and pregnant women. The adoption and quick implementation of this important incremental reform by the ANC—which had been advanced by NPPHCN and SAHSSO before but had not been expressed as important priorities by citizens in national surveys—provided powerful evidence of the early influence of the professional movement on policy. The free health care policy resulted in a predictable rise in attendance in public hospitals but was not accompanied by any budget increase, which led to further strain on the already overburdened public health care system (McCoy and Khosa 1996, 157–59, 161). At approximately the same time, the ANC embarked on a major new clinic-building program that resulted in the creation of five hundred new clinics that collectively delivered health care access to five million people by 1998 (Mandela 1998).[9] More broadly, amid tight budget constraints, efforts were being made to equalize spending and the distribution of resources among the nine provinces that were being fashioned out of the old apartheid administration—staggering changes, given that approximately 70 percent of the country's specialists worked in just two provinces at the time (van den Heever interview 2008).

But even while the ANC made efforts to introduce these sweeping changes, serious questions over how to transform the crumbling and underfunded public health care apparatus into a system that could deliver the kind of comprehensive care envisioned by the professional movement increasingly fell into the domain of the more technocratic wing of the movement, housed at the country's universities. Coloring all of these discussions was a concern over what to do with a bloated private health care system that soaked up so much of the country's financial resources but served so few. In addition, the dramatic change represented by the ANC had prompted many of those white doctors who could obtain visas to practice abroad to leave the country. Recognizing the many difficulties that would need to be overcome, the new health minister, Nkosazana Dlamini-Zuma, and her director-general, Olive Shisana—who was instrumental in founding the School of Public Health at the University of the Western Cape—made attempts to jump-start discussions on more transformative efforts to address the inequities in the health care system. Over the next several years, deliberations on National Health Insurance would animate much of the work of the ministry under their leadership.

Deepening Discussions on National Health Insurance

Even before the Government of National Unity was elected in 1994, the ANC Health Desk invited John Deeble, architect of the 1975 Australian Medicare reform, to South Africa to discuss national health insurance options with the ANC in 1992 and to inject further ideas into the policy conversations that were already occurring in the country (Sidley 1994). Once in power in 1994, the health minister convened a Health Care Finance Committee to explore different options related to implementing some kind of compulsory insurance, including social health insurance for workers in the formal sector and national health insurance for everyone (Department of Health 2011a, 13). The most sweeping idea—a form of national health insurance—which had been championed by Deeble and offered the greatest redistributive potential, appealed greatly to the minister but had been rejected by the other committee members over concerns related to its viability (Thomas and Gilson 2004, 283). Yet, for affordability reasons, Deeble's plan—which involved the contracting of both public and private providers—promised to provide everyone with access to basic primary care and only the most essential medicine, foregoing comprehensive coverage of the kind of complex services usually provided at hospitals (McIntyre and van den Heever 2007, 78).

The committee, which lacked left-leaning trade union representation (but did include a representative from the medical schemes), recommended the more conservative option of introducing a social health insurance program that would require workers in the formal sector and their dependents to obtain health insurance with the objective of gradually expanding coverage to other groups over time (Department of Health 2011a, 13; on the trade unions, Thomas and Gilson 2004, 283). While the committee's preferred option did not promise to provide coverage to everyone—as NHI theoretically did—casting shadows over the discussion was the relatively small tax base represented by workers in the formal sector, which would presumably be drawn on to fund the program. In many other (but not all) countries, the path to NHI had involved the gradual extension of compulsory insurance coverage to more and more sectors of the population over time, usually with subsidized coverage provided to those who could not afford to make contributions to fund it. Eventually, the different funds into which people contributed were merged into a more efficient single fund administered by the government.

However, the demographics in South Africa differed dramatically from industrialized countries like Canada, where most of the country's adult citizens worked in the formal sector. Not only was the percentage of people who worked for tax-paying businesses in South Africa small, but an extraordinarily high percentage of people were unemployed. This is not to say that social health insurance would have had no value in addressing *some* of the underlying problems of inequity: Compulsory social health insurance would enable some formal sector workers without coverage to become covered by requiring them to purchase insurance, and some of the money from that purchase could be directed to support efforts to improve health care for the poor through the public health care system (McIntyre, Doherty, and Gilson 2003, 51). But this gave rise to sober commentary about the prospects of national health insurance by people involved in discussions at the time, "as universal insurance coverage [in South Africa] is improbable given high unemployment rates, NHI would probably have to begin with people in formal employment and their families, with the state continuing to provide services directly to the rest of the population" (Bachmann 1994, 27).

Upset by the lack of support for his plan, Deeble went around the committee and convinced the minister of the program's viability, and the committee was urged to alter its findings, which it refused to do; when his plan was leaked to the press (possibly to stop it from moving forward), a furor ensued over the plan's details (Thomas and Gilson 2004, 283). Some of the flashpoints in the proposal included the size of the tax increase that was required, the plan's cap of three primary doctor visits a year, and its proposal to force general practitioners in private practice to participate in a program with caps on payment (Sidley 1994).

Despite the furor, having developed some conviction in the Deeble plan, the health minister pressed onwards and convened a second commission, the Committee of Inquiry on National Health Insurance, in 1995 to cost out the program and create a detailed plan for implementation of NHI or a publicly provided alternative (Thomas and Gilson 2004, 283–84). On its face, the prospects for advancing NHI looked brighter initially when the co-chairs that were selected for the committee were Jonathan Broomberg, a South African academic who had advanced some earlier proposals for NHI while at CHP, and Olive Shisana, the minister's director-general and a staunch advocate of NHI. However, some of the assumptions that underpinned the Deeble proposal were thought to be unrealistic, in particular the impact of the program on primary care physicians' salaries in the private sector, which might lead doctors to leave the country in droves (van den Heever interview 2008). More generally, the enormous and very rapid changes represented by the plan, coupled with questions about how the proposal's details would work and the ministry's uncertain administrative capacity, gave ample cause for a wide range of stakeholders to worry.

Broomberg's threatened resignation over concerns with the Deeble proposal led the terms of reference for the committee to be changed, directing it instead to focus on developing a universal primary health care policy and considering different insurance options as a secondary concern (Thomas and Gilson 2004, 285). The committee's findings ultimately echoed those of the earlier Health Care Finance Committee, proposing a more limited social health insurance program for workers in the formal sector (Department of Health 2011a, 13). However, with primary care services to be provided through the public health care system, this committee's plan differed slightly from the 1994 version in that compulsory insurance coverage for formal sector workers only needed to cover hospital services, theoretically bringing down the cost of the newly mandated insurance coverage (McIntyre and van den Heever 2007, 78).

Parliamentarians in the National Assembly Portfolio Committee on Health praised many of the report's recommendations but also expressed concerns about health being treated as a commodity under a national health insurance system that utilized both public and private providers (Committee Submission on the Report of Inquiry into a NHS System 1995). More generally, the recommendations were applauded for their efforts to address the problem of health inequity, although Treasury expressed concern over the program's tax implications (Thomas and Gilson 2004, 285), in the context of a predicted 3.4 billion rand (US$934 million) shortfall over the next five years (*Weekly Mail and Guardian* 1995, 4). One important stakeholder that did endorse the proposal, however, was the Representative Association for Medical Schemes (RAMS), which supported the idea of compulsory health insurance for workers—since it would mean more business for the industry—but which also expressed serious reservations over a proposal to remove the tax subsidy to medical schemes, the savings from which would be redirected to finance primary health care efforts (van der Linde 1995, 722–23).[10]

With the deliberations of the committees in mind (and the actions of the professional movement before them), the ANC decided to sidestep the bigger and more complicated decisions related to health insurance and how best to incorporate private providers into the state's strategy for ensuring access to quality health care. Instead, the government opted for a quick win by announcing a policy of free primary health care for everyone in the country's public clinics. Until that point, a means-tested fee structure had governed admission to the country's public hospitals and clinics (Castro-Leal 1996, 25). The country's highest income earners (and those with medical schemes) were not deemed eligible to use state facilities but were allowed to use them for a fee upon request (Health Systems Trust 1995, ch. 14). While the means test was often not applied by clinic and hospital administrators when needy patients showed up at medical facilities, blacks' use of public hospitals and clinics fell well below international standards (Schneider and Gilson 1999, 95). The policy represented an attempt to live up to some of the provisions in the country's new 1996 constitution, which stated that everyone should "have access to health care services" (Government of the Republic of South Africa 1996). However, by 2008, the poorest South Africans continued to face problems accessing public hospitals at the provincial, central, and regional levels relative to wealthy South Africans (Ataguba and McIntyre 2013: 40–41), and by 2016, some 5.5 million people who do not have medical scheme coverage still fell outside the means test (van den Heever 2016, 3).

The decree nevertheless amounted to another important policy commitment that built on the ANC's earlier 1994 policy of free comprehensive health care for children under six and pregnant women. However, like the 1994 policy before it, the 1996 policy seemed to involve few budget considerations; the announcement during the parliamentary budget speech took many by surprise, as the financial impacts of the preceding 1994 policy had not yet been carefully analyzed (McCoy and Khosa 1996, 162–63). The policy's adoption again gave fresh evidence of the influence of the professional movement, with NPPHCN and others having advocated free primary health care in the years before the fall of apartheid. But in opting for the easier policy and stopping short of any broader transformative change, the ANC-led government's decision also illustrated the luxury that a forty-point win over the party's nearest challenger provided: The party could essentially afford to stall major decisions with sticky political implications until later.

Two years, 1997 and 1998, came and went with three developments related to efforts to transform the health care system. In 1997 the Health Ministry published the "White Paper for the Transformation of the Health System," which aimed to provide further support and guidance to the ANC's efforts to promote health equity and unify the disparate health systems inherited from the apartheid government. At the same time, the ministry also established a small Social Health Insurance Working Group, whose work was largely internal to the Ministry of Health. The Working Group was tasked with designing a compulsory social health insurance program for workers in the formal sector that could be used with public hospitals, but—at the urging of the minister—again reconsidered some of the issues related to NHI. However, interest in a broader social security program that would include health coverage, discussed at the national conference of the ANC and supported by COSATU, temporarily redirected the ministry's efforts (Thomas and Gilson 2004, 285–86). Passed in 1998, the Medical Schemes Act provided overarching regulation of the medical schemes industry, which had operated in an unregulated environment. It was not until two years later that the Taylor Commission was formed; it would take up the issue of National Health Insurance in the context of a more broad-reaching social security program.

The Dilemma of Expanding Coverage but also Entrenching Private Health Insurance

The Taylor Commission dealt with a wide range of issues, most notably exploring options for a comprehensive social security program with a health component. Related to health system reform, the commission recommended establishment of a social health insurance program for formal sector workers (just as the 1994 and 1995 committees had recommended) in addition to two new programs: a state-sponsored medical scheme dedicated to serving the low-income market *and* compulsory coverage of civil servants (Report of the Committee of Inquiry into a Comprehensive System of Social Security for South Africa 2002).[11] While COSATU had initially supported development of a comprehensive social security policy that would include a health component (Thomas and Gilson 2004, 286), it began to see compulsory health insurance as a counterproductive policy that threatened to entrench the private system of medical schemes that had been responsible for inequitable development in the first place (Bisseker 2001, 36). In addition, COSATU objected to SHI over the potentially high contributions workers—particularly low-income workers—would be forced to make (Makgetla interview 2008).

While the proposals for expanding insurance coverage through an SHI program for workers in the formal sector again went nowhere, the proposals of the Taylor Commission did lead to two important developments that expanded the population's access to health care. Prior to the introduction of the Government Employee Medical Scheme (GEMS) in 2005, many civil servants could not afford medical scheme coverage; GEMS addressed this gap by providing subsidized insurance coverage to the nation's nearly two million civil servants (GEMS 2015). The program led to a predictable rise in the number of medical scheme beneficiaries; by 2007, a full 25 percent of medical scheme beneficiaries were government officials, with only a few using their new health insurance coverage to access care at the nation's network of overburdened public hospitals (Hassim, Heywood, and Berger 2007, 169, 190).

That same year, Johnny Broomberg—now an executive at Discovery Health, one of the country's largest medical schemes—was appointed to lead a process to explore development of a Low Income Medical Scheme (LIMS) program, which aimed to make private health insurance available to around 2.5 million low-income people in the formal sector (Broomberg interview 2008). Interestingly, the LIMS program—which would have represented a substantial expansion in the number of people using medical schemes—had the support of government to move forward. However, a change in the government midway through the process—and resumption of the old NHI discussions—led the window of opportunity that had opened for LIMS to close (Broomberg interview 2008).

In many ways, GEMS and LIMS represented the partial but ultimately unsatisfying realization of the dreams of government officials who had been involved in the NHI discussions that had gone on for more than a decade. By extending access to the country's well-regarded private medical facilities through these medical schemes, more than four million of the country's citizens stood to benefit. These policies collectively promised to take the country several steps closer toward insurance-based universal coverage. However, they also stood to further institutionalize inequity. With official unemployment rates hovering around 25 percent (the unofficial rates were much higher),[12] the provision of insurance coverage to 4 million when approximately 40 million lacked it threatened to further entrench inequity and the very private institutions that had been responsible for the bifurcation of health care in South Africa in the first place.

Toward National Health Insurance?

The 2007 National Conference of the ANC at Polokwane proved to be significant in the story of health care expansion in South Africa for many reasons. First and foremost, in a significant defeat to incumbent President Thabo Mbeki, his deputy Jacob Zuma was elected president of the party. The victory marked a shift to the left within the party and foreshadowed Mbeki's eventual resignation in 2008 to make way for Zuma as the head of the new government. Amid the changing political winds, the South African Communist Party (SACP) and COSATU emerged with a stronger voice (Johnson 2009), and a policy resolution was passed at the conference that reaffirmed "implementation of the National Health Insurance System by further strengthening the public health care system and ensuring adequate provision of funding" (ANC 2007).

The Polokwane resolution signaled a redoubling of efforts around NHI by the ANC and would lead to even more concrete commitments in the run-up to the 2009 national election. However, it also marked continued muddiness within the party over just what kind of reform the government was going to pursue. NHI systems typically involved public financing of private health care when administered through a single centralized state fund or, prior to the merger of funds into a single fund, the financing of private health care through multiple private nonprofit funds. And yet the ANC's Polokwane resolution suggested that it aimed to address not the public financing of private health care but the strengthening of the means-tested public health care system.

Following the resolution, in an odd echo of the past, the ANC convened a task team to consider implementation of NHI, much as had been done thirteen years earlier in 1995 to discuss implementation of the Deeble plan. However, unlike the earlier government committees, this task team was convened by the ANC rather than the government. Amid the new political environment, the SACP and its trade union allies in COSATU dominated the committee (Johnson 2009). Discussions centered on finding ways to harness the surplus in the private health care market so that it might be used to benefit the whole of society (Hassim interview 2008). More specifically, the task team focused on finding ways to redirect the tens of billions of rand per year that 8 million South Africans spent on medical schemes to help provide better quality health care to the 41 million people who did not have them (Johnson 2009). In other words, while the ANC resolution at Polokwane had focused almost exclusively on strengthening the public system, the major focus of the task team's work centered on ways to open the private system to use by the masses, using the money that was currently being spent by corporations and individuals to do that. The committee ultimately recommended that citizens should have the right to use public or private facilities as they wish in a scheme that drew on an additional R100 billion, financed largely by the rich (Johnson 2009).

A lawyer who was involved in an NHI task team that was set up reportedly resigned after raising concerns about the constitutionality of NHI, prompting members of the task team to question her status as an ANC member (Paton 2009). A prominent health economist involved in the proceedings remarked, "The proposals that were discussed were ludicrous. There were so many things that were technically wrong that it was difficult to know whether to walk away or try to engage them" (van den Heever quoted in Paton 2009). Yet at the same time that some team members involved in the process were giving voice to the impractical nature of the proposals, voices leading the committee were denouncing critics and raising expectations of the public related to the immediacy of the program's implementation.

Blade Nzimande, the general secretary of the SACP, for example, said in speeches to groups of unemployed citizens that poor South Africans would soon be able to use private hospitals and suggested that the party would "wage war" on NHI opponents (quoted in Johnson 2009). At the same time, in what had become indicative of the party's approach to debate, internal criticism of the technical aspects of the task team's proposals was earning critics the labels of being "imperialist" and "anti-transformation" (Paton 2009). And yet, as opposition MP Mike Waters wrote, "Often the only concrete information coming out of the process is from people such as health economist Alex van den Heever, who have removed themselves from the process because of their concerns about it" (quoted in Politics Web 2009).

The ANC's 2009 National Elections Manifesto would do little to clarify the ANC's seemingly schizophrenic position and at the same time made even more concrete the tight timeline for the program's implementation. The manifesto stated that the ANC would

> introduce the National Health Insurance System (NHI) system, which will be phased in over the next five years. NHI will be publicly funded and publicly administered and will provide the right of all to access quality health care, which will be free at the point of service. People will have a choice of which service provider to use within a district. In the implementation of the NHI there will be an engagement with the private sector in general, including private doctors working in group practices and hospitals, to encourage them to participate in the NHI system. (ANC 2009)

While the language used in the manifesto and other statements at the time conveyed that the implementation of NHI was imminent, precisely how the government would coax private providers to participate in a scheme that would likely pay them little relative to what they were making or what role medical schemes would play in the new program was left largely unaddressed. However, in suggesting that NHI would be publicly funded and administered, the implication was that medical schemes would be abolished and that the remaining private providers would agree to what the government would pay them.

Such profound and immediate changes, however, carried immense risks. First and foremost, they amounted to the destruction of the country's established private health insurance industry and set both private providers and insurers on edge. Like them or not, the medical schemes had demonstrated a capacity for managing risk and financing health care in a competitive environment—a capacity the government had not yet developed and would be difficult to develop quickly. Second, by the mid-2000s, an increasingly powerful black middle class was relying on medical schemes to access the private health care system. While just 8 percent of blacks were using medical schemes, up from less than 4 percent in 1986, by 2010 the total number of blacks using medical schemes eclipsed the number of whites who did so (Innovative Medicines South Africa 2011, 2–3; *Mail and Guardian* 2010a; Price 1989, 126). While the percentage of whites with medical schemes still dwarfs the percentage of blacks with medical schemes, the racial dimensions of medical scheme participation were changing in ways that no longer made insurance coverage an issue that benefited whites only—and made medical schemes increasingly difficult to abolish. Third, the question of what would happen to the private clinics and hospitals in South Africa if medical schemes were abolished loomed over everything. A massive outflow of the country's most advanced medical expertise—even if it benefited only a small but growing proportion of the population—threatened to set the country back in terms of its base of human resources and capacity in the medical field, rather than help it move forward.

Reaction to the New Momentum for an Old Project

In a surprising early showing of support for the ANC's efforts, the South African Medical Association (SAMA)[13] affirmed its endorsement of an NHI model that included a role for both public and private sectors (Mustago 2008, 32) and increased funding for the public sector (Gantsho 2008, 27). However, many private providers and medical schemes considered the reform to be radical and fundamentally against their own interest, so SAMA's show of support led to divisions within its membership. Fracture within the profession developed between general practitioners, who served as providers of basic primary care, and specialists, who dealt with more complicated and expensive care and were more highly compensated for their work. Once again, at the center of these divisions were the medical schemes themselves, which had come to pay general practitioners an increasingly small share of total medical payments over the previous decade—a situation that had led primary care physicians to see alternatives, such as NHI, in a more positive light than in years past[14] (Thulare interview 2008).

Rather than agree to contracted rates of remuneration, specialists, by contrast, wanted to maintain the generous "fee-for-service" system they currently used in which they billed private health insurance for services, so they set up a new association to protect their interests. The South African Private Practitioners Forum (SAPPF) effectively replaced the Specialist Private Practitioner Committee within SAMA, which had stopped functioning in November 2008 due to the exodus of specialists from SAMA (SAPPF 2010). While specialists comprised only about 4,000 of SAMA's membership of over 17,000 (mostly private) doctors, the vast majority (an estimated 3,500 or so) were interested in maintaining the traditional relationship between specialists and medical schemes (Thulare interview 2008). As had been the case since the inception of modern medical practice in South Africa, racial dynamics continued to underlay the dynamics of the profession, albeit in new ways: While black nurses and some GPs led efforts to provide care at the primary level in largely black rural areas, mostly white specialists continued to provide services in urban areas. Reflecting these dynamics, the founding executive committee of the SAPPF was all white (SAPPF 2011).[15] While these racial dynamics were important, the fracture that occurred within the medical profession over NHI might be even more precisely characterized as a situation of mistrust and suspicion between private doctors and the department of health under the leadership of the ANC. The department of health was fundamentally concerned that the private sector—in particular, specialists—were unnecessarily driving up costs, and conversely, the private doctors held deep worries about the state's ability to manage and administer financing for health services effectively and to its satisfaction under an NHI (Thulare interview 2008).

While divisions between specialists and general practitioners were primarily responsible for the disintegration of SAMA as an inclusive association representing the interests of the medical profession as a whole, tensions in that mission and SAMA's role as a labor union affiliated with COSATU, which had had a strong hand in the push for NHI, were also to blame. COSATU had attempted to manage differences that might arise between the official positions it adopted and those of its affiliates by allowing union affiliates some freedom to stake out different positions. So while COSATU favored a publicly funded and administered NHI with both public and private providers, SAMA favored a kind of social health insurance, or modified NHI approach, in which two to three medical schemes played a role administering the program (Thulare interview 2008). These different preferences—which centrally bore on physician autonomy and pay—threatened to unravel the unified medical profession and COSATU's influence as a powerful political broker in discussions. Aquina Thulare, the secretary-general of SAMA at the time of the push for NHI at Polokwane in 2007, was also a member of the South African Communist Party, and although she had stated that she was "acting on behalf of COSATU," her support for NHI created tensions within SAMA and ultimately led to her contract not to be renewed by the SAMA Board in 2009 (Paton 2009; also Bateman 2009). Kgosi Letlape, chairman of SAMA and South Africa's first black ophthalmologist, likewise regularly espoused views that led to tensions with SAMA membership, where there was a general perception that he was "anti-private practice." These tensions eventually contributed to his departure as well (Bateman 2009).

Just as tensions surfaced within the medical profession in this debate, the medical schemes association, formerly RAMS and now known as the Board of Healthcare Funders (BHF), likewise showed some fracture and political realignment toward the policy as well. Importantly, Discovery Health made the decision in late 2008 to withdraw its membership from the BHF, reportedly because of the BHF's stand against NHI. Johnny Broomberg, who had played such an important role in the 1995 Committee of Inquiry, was an executive at Discovery, one of the market leaders in private health insurance in South Africa. Its withdrawal may be alternately read as a signal that it sees the move toward NHI as imminent, necessary, or ultimately beneficial to its interests or, more cynically, that it sees little to be gained in fighting a program that will never be implemented. In a further display of realignment toward the policy, at least some in the health insurance industry suggested some willingness to give up the R10 billion subsidy given to the industry through tax subsidies, if medical schemes were still allowed to play a role in it. Further reflecting the uncertain political environment and industry's desire to demonstrate to ANC officials their willingness to participate, a BHF representative stated, "We think we will be able to play a very meaningful role" in NHI (Clarence Mini quoted in Gentle 2009).

While the equivocation and immediacy inherent in new NHI discussions played an equal role in the creation of an uncertainty that caused major stakeholders to take new positions, the most immediate effect of the ANC's extended vacillation on whether or not to move forward on the most radical options on the table was the somewhat unstable reproduction of the status quo—a private health care system that, while increasingly serving the black population, served an exclusive minority and an overwhelmed means-tested public system that served the majority. In that context, incremental reforms that served to stabilize the private health insurance industry and increase the number of beneficiaries using medical schemes, such as the 1998 Medical Schemes Act and the 2005 GEMS program, further entrenched medical schemes and cemented the public-private divide,[16] while policies for free health care in the public sector (without additional budgets or staffing) only served to overwhelm further the public system.

In 2009, new health minister Dr. Aaron Motsoaledi appointed a twenty-five-person commission to advise him on the development of NHI (Malan 2011). The strongly progressive bent of the committee was perhaps nowhere more evident than in its inclusion of Dr. Aquina Thulare—the communist former head of SAMA who had been dismissed by the SAMA Board over her advocacy for NHI—as a special adviser to the minister of health (*Financial Mail* 2009). And on August 12, 2011, the ANC-led South African government took its most concrete step yet to move forward with NHI by issuing a Green Paper on National Health Insurance, which called for implementation in three phases over fourteen years.[17] Under the proposal, health care services would be purchased from public and private providers and would include nearly six hundred contracted private general practitioners in eleven pilot districts beginning in early 2013 and the rollout of a centralized state fund by 2014/15 (Matsoso 2013). Medical schemes would be allowed to continue under the new program. However, tax breaks for members of medical schemes would be eliminated, and people who purchased medical scheme coverage would be required to pay a new tax contribution to the NHI fund (BBC 2011; Childs 2011; *Mail and Guardian* 2011b).

The publication of the Green Paper led to more than one hundred submissions to the minister of health and a conference that explored international experiences with universal coverage (Matsoso 2013). In addition, the new momentum around NHI led to new government financial commitments designed to support rollout of NHI, including R1 billion ($123 million) to initiate the NHI pilot projects in ten different districts around the country; R2.7 billion ($333 million) to upgrade public health care infrastructure; R1.4 billion ($172 million) to improve child and maternal health care services; and R117 million ($14 million) to set up a new Office of Health Care Standards and Compliance that would play a role in overseeing the program (AllAfrica.com 2012a, c; BuaNews 2012; Khumalo 2012; *Mail and Guardian* 2011a; Malan 2011).

While these developments provided some basis for thinking that the government might have finally embraced transformative health care reform, they had to be set against the otherwise sobering fiscal picture. In April 2009 provincial health departments were some R7.5 billion ($800 million) in arrears (Parker 2010). Projected estimates suggested that the health care budget would have to more than double to R255 billion ($36 billion) by 2025 to support national health insurance (*Mail and Guardian* 2011b), while at the same time more than tripling its output of doctors and finding some way to keep them in the public sector (AllAfrica. com 2012b; Malan 2011). The hospital workers' union even suggested that the new system would have to feature a role for foreign doctors, given the staff shortages in the public sector and the eighty thousand new positions national health insurance would require (*Mail and Guardian* 2010b).

Amid the incongruence represented by intense rhetoric and these broader realities—and despite the fact that official government timelines suggested that a White Paper produced by the ministry and Parliament that would give national health insurance legal standing should have been produced by 2011 (Department of Health 2011a, 47)—perhaps somewhat tellingly, by September 2015 still no White Paper had been produced. In the interim, some suggested that even the health minister at the center of recent NHI efforts knew that a full-blown national health insurance system is unrealistic (Malan 2011). More broadly, economists involved in the discussions have estimated that the achievement of national health insurance in South Africa could take as long as thirty years (van den Heever interview 2008), while estimates in some of the government's own policy documents have suggested much longer time frames.[18]

Yet, politicians at the highest levels continued to talk regularly about National Health Insurance—and sometimes a National Health Service—in confusing ways, as if the plan was clear and implementation imminent. As President Jacob Zuma said in 2014, "We are currently working hard to bring into operation the National Health Service (NHS) . . . that will ensure that quality health care is available to all regardless of economic or financial means" (quoted in *Mail and Guardian* 2014). The incongruity led one serious observer to comment, "I think that there's a commitment to NHI, but very few people really know what they mean by that. So it's seen as a kind of panacea by people who . . . seek a quick fix" (Heywood interview 2008). If history is any guide, this continued double-speak suggests that embrace of the major policy initiative championed by the professional movement more than twenty years ago will continue to take place in name only.

Conclusion

More than in Brazil or Thailand, the substantial legacies of neglect left by the apartheid regime meant that the ANC started from a much weaker position when it came to power as leader of the Government of National Unity in 1994. At the same time, the ambitious goals it set for itself were in many ways more substantial than the types of transformative health care reforms pursued in Thailand or Brazil, where tax-funded reforms sought to extend access to health care to the disenfranchised primarily through the public system. In Brazil, the Unified Health System reform created a British-style National Health Service, offering equal access to health care for all. In Thailand, transformative reform created the Universal Coverage program, which provided access to health care for any citizens not already covered by the state's health care programs for workers in the formal sector and civil servants and their families. While private providers were granted the opportunity to serve as contractors to the new programs, in neither case did reforms attempt to restrain private practice or to do away with private medical insurance. By contrast, in South Africa, in at least one version of the reform proposals that have been articulated, the ANC explicitly took aim at eliminating the role of an established private health insurance industry that served a sizable portion of the population and replacing it with a public financing mechanism.

In spite of the party's failure to implement national health insurance, it is worth noting that some of the ANC's policy accomplishments have been substantial and reflective of a party aspiring to institute radical redistribution along the lines of a Scandinavian welfare state: By 2009, some 27 percent of the population received welfare grants, financed by the 11 percent of the population with incomes sufficient to pay income tax (Johnson 2009). However, in the area of health reform, I have shown that the ANC embraced only incremental reforms: Access to comprehensive care was made free for pregnant women and children under six in 1994 and access to primary health care was made free for all citizens in 1996. The adoption of these policies illustrated the influence of a movement of well-organized medical professionals. However, as technically uncomplicated reforms that were undertaken without a great deal of planning, they left aside some of the more contentious issues involved in embracing some of the radical ideas for more transformative health care reform espoused by the movement.

In the context of unrivaled electoral success, I have argued that the ANC could afford to ignore more radical and transformative health care policies that involved greater uncertainty and "bigger lifts" politically. Caught between an ideological desire to address health inequity immediately and the reality of what immediate implementation would mean, the luxury of a loyal constituency meant that the ANC could afford to convene commission after commission for two decades and embrace technically more challenging proposals for a National Health Insurance system in name only, without having to embrace the risks that would come with implementing them suddenly. This policy of talking about National Health Insurance reform endlessly but in practice doing very little has created a large amount of uncertainty within the health care industry and even led to divisions within the medical profession. It has also meant that some of the ideological concerns that have animated recent debates—including, most centrally, worries over further exclusion from coverage that have come with the privatization of health care coverage—have not been fully confronted. Amid this policy of non-confrontation and avoidance, ironically, health care in South Africa has become more reliant on the private sector with the introduction of the GEMS program in 2005. At the same time, even more recent changes not discussed here have made it easier for low-income populations to purchase medical schemes, further encouraging the citizenry's reliance on private services.[19]

While a National Health Insurance system has been talked about endlessly and is now even being piloted, the content of South Africa's pilot NHI program departs from typical understandings of NHI and has at least so far avoided the hard choices—and major risks—involved in making the resources of the private sector available to the public. In the process, the ANC's stewardship of South Africa's public health care system has in many ways taken steps backwards, with the nurse-to-population ratio actually *declining* substantially during the ANC's reign and little evidence of concrete efforts to address the human resources crisis (Coovadia et al. 2009, 830). In the words of some prominent analysts, "There has been a notable lack of progress in implementing the core health policies developed by the ANC, and some disastrous policy choices" (Coovadia et al. 2009, 832). In the interim, public inquiries have found "massive corruption" in provincial health departments (Schulz-Herzenberg 2007, 60). And much like the United States, in the absence of grand strategy, expanded coverage of the population by insurance has inched forward with the help of small, incremental government policies, like the GEMS program—all largely in spite of the government's broader proclamations about NHI. In other words, the "American health care nightmare" that some members of the professional movement expressed concern about more than twenty years ago (Broomberg 1991, 4), which combines high and rising costs with incomplete population coverage, has come to pass.

Greater political competition in South Africa may eventually lead to changes in the way the ANC approaches transformative reform in health care and other areas. While new parties—most notably, Congress of the People in 2009 and the Economic Freedom Fighters (EFF) in 2014—have mounted small challenges to the ANC, the party's forty-point win in the 2014 elections suggests that it still maintains the same sort of electoral dominance that it did twenty years ago. The greatest opportunities for change to the status quo may come from fractures within the party's own ruling alliance and growing unhappiness in the wider populace over the ANC's failures in the delivery of basic services. In 2014, the National Union of Metalworkers of South Africa (NUMSA), COSATU's largest union affiliate, publicly announced that it would not back the ANC in the 2014 elections and called for COSATU to leave the governing alliance with the ANC and SACP (Marrian 2014). COSATU responded by expelling NUMSA, leading seven other unions to boycott COSATU executive committee meetings in response (Duncan 2014). While these stunning developments obviously did not affect the ultimate outcome of the 2014 election, they do suggest growing discontent with the ANC. Some have even suggested NUMSA's moves to create its own labor party with a more seasoned leadership than EFF may spell more serious challenges for the ANC in the future (Campbell 2014). More broadly, growing numbers of citizens have taken to the street to protest disruptions in basic delivery of services, like electricity, a phenomenon that has caught the attention of the ANC's leadership as it weighs its prospects in future elections (Hunter 2015).

For its part, the ANC has admitted such failures as well as the need to address corruption within the party—the latter of which government officials have at times proven to be overly sensitive in addressing (Hunter 2015), as with other criticisms directed toward the party so many times before. ANC General Secretary Gwede Mantashe has stated publicly, "Except for the impact made by social grants, we are making little progress. . . . This is serious as the patience of our people is running thin, particularly in the face of agitation for discontent" (Mantashe quoted in Hunter 2015). However, if past election results and the policy history of the health sector are any guide, then small incremental reforms rather than riskier and more uncertain transformative reform will likely continue to be the ruling party's approach.

Part II
ACCESS TO AIDS MEDICINE

5

THAILAND: FROM VILLAGE SAFETY TO UNIVERSAL ACCESS

How did a small and submissive developing country in the global community become the "Talk of the Globe" as Jack the Giant Killer?

—Thai AIDS Activist (quoted in Kijtiwatchakul 2007, 5)

Thailand succeeded in gaining control of an AIDS epidemic through an HIV pre-vention campaign, in which both state and civil society organizations played an important role. While the epidemic peaked in the early 1990s with over 140,000 new infections in a single year, HIV prevalence today stands around one percent (Loos 2015, 217). Some estimates suggested that Thailand's epidemic could have been fourteen times worse in the absence of the country's prevention efforts (Brown and Peerapatanapokin 2004). AIDS, however, still left an indelible mark on the country's landscape. As of 2005, over a million adults in Thailand had been found to be HIV-positive, and over half a million had died (Limpananont 2005, 3).

Thailand's commitment to scale up access to life-saving combination antiretrovi-ral therapy in 2001 came at a time when debate over the right of countries to produce generic versions of trademark medication still raged at the international level—and more than two years before the South African government would make similar com-mitments. And while the Global Fund to Fight AIDS, Tuberculosis, and Malaria would provide a small amount of support in the early years of Thailand's program to provide access to antiretroviral drugs, it would not be long before the country would assume financial responsibility for the program in its entirety. Even more importantly, the country's decision to invoke compulsory licenses—which entitled the government to create generic formulations of patented medications for a small royalty fee under legal provisions in the WTO's Agreement on Trade-Related Aspects of Intellectual Property Rights (TRIPS)—on the first-line AIDS drug, efavirenz, and the second-line AIDS drug, lopinavir/ritonavir, was a ground-breaking moment for an industrializing country. Thailand's declarations in 2006 and 2007 subsequently inspired other countries that already were known for progressive essential medicine policies, such as Brazil, to take even further steps to guarantee their citizens' access to pharmaceuticals.

As was the case in the health care domain, the expansion of access to treatment for AIDS in Thailand had its roots in the efforts of a longstanding movement of medical professionals. But whereas the professional movement that aimed to expand access to health care was composed of progressive doctors, the professional movement that aimed to expand access to life-saving pharmaceuticals was composed mainly of pharmacists who developed expertise in the law (the Drug Study Group) and medical professionals in the state (Rural Doctors in the Ministry of Public Health and executives in the Government Pharmaceutical Office).

In the 1970s and 1980s, when the country was governed by the military and the health care system was still being developed, many of the movements' efforts were trained at the community level. However, when the military government finally relinquished control over the "rules of the game" with the advent of democracy in the early 1990s, Thailand's movement of legally engaged medical professionals was suddenly empowered to pursue major social changes through avenues that had previously been closed to them. Working with technically savvy international partners, the advocates improved their knowledge of intellectual property law, which set them apart from ordinary citizens and led them increasingly to become a resource to which the broader AIDS movement turned. In this changing context, the professional movement gradually turned their attention toward matters of state pharmaceutical policy and began to have an impact on the national stage.

This chapter highlights the critical role played by a movement of legally minded medical professionals in expanding access to treatment for AIDS in Thailand. At a time when democratic deepening led mass citizens' movements to become more active, complicated matters of pharmaceutical policy remained still largely the exclusive domain of experts. Although activists in Thailand's AIDS movement initially opted to forego campaigns for ARV access due to the high cost of medication, the life-and-death stakes of pharmaceutical policy would gradually lead them to undergo a process of "expertification" and to develop competency in matters related to patent law.

Working with partners abroad, the Drug Study Group and activist medical professionals in the Ministry of Public Health, steeped in knowledge related to legal barriers to pharmaceutical access, played a central role in that educational process. In a political context that increasingly placed importance on citizens' rights, the knowledge promulgated by this professional movement would empower AIDS organizations to use the courts to challenge pharmaceutical companies' rights to *drug patents, to promote the use and production of generics by the state, to address concerns related to the cost of AIDS medication that would initially prove to be a stumbling block for the drugs' inclusion in the government's universal health care program, and to resist pressure from hegemonic powers like the United States. This professional movement would build state (and civil society) capacity and promote greater awareness of Thailand's right to declare compulsory licensing of AIDS medication within government agencies, providing the legal justifications for the country's landmark decisions in 2006 and 2007. While most were not in need of these life-saving medicines themselves, Thailand's professional movement of legally trained pharmacists and doctors would play a key role both in providing the broader AIDS movement with greater knowledge related to patent law and in the institution of landmark policies in Thailand.*

While the Rural Doctors' movement took aim at expanding access to health care beginning in the 1970s, a sister organization of the Rural Doctors' Society—the Drug Study Group—was taking up the problems of drug safety and accessibility at approximately the same time. During Thailand's brief window of democracy in the 1970s, at a time when student movements were burgeoning and universities were sites of radicalism, the Drug Study Group (DSG) was organized by a group of faculty and students of the pharmacy department at Thailand's most prestigious university, Chulalongkorn University. Founded in 1975, the DSG was composed of academics working on issues related to drug use and access and consumer protection (Wibulpolprasert et al. 2011). But whereas the Rural Doctors' Society moved its operations into the countryside when medical students graduated and took positions as directors of hospitals in rural areas, the DSG continued to use the Chulalongkorn University Faculty of Pharmacy as its main base for the next twenty-five years.[1]

Recognizing the lack of medicines in the rural countryside and the frequent misuse of those medicines that did exist, starting in 1976 the DSG committed itself to "research into and the promotion of safety in medicinal use" (Ondam 2004, 280). In April and May of that year, the DSG initiated a survey and found that over 77 percent of drugs obtained from drugstores and village shops came in the form of a small drug kit called *yaa chud*, which contained antibiotics, steroids, and tranquilizers; the kit was typically used for all kinds of pain without reference to specific diseases or toxicity (Drug Study Group 1984, 8). Concerned over the misuse of dangerous medications and aware of the fact that 80 percent of Thais used drugstores as their first line of medical care (rather than seeing a doctor), the DSG set out to ban the sale of *yaa chud* and other dangerous drugs. The DSG also made recommendations to the government on the country's National Drug Policy and attempted to promote further development of production capacities of basic pharmaceuticals in Thailand to reduce dependence on transnational pharmaceutical companies and to develop guidelines for appropriate technology transfer in the area of pharmaceutical production (Drug Study Group 1984, 8–10, 15).

During the 1980s, the efforts of the DSG gradually became more and more entwined with the work of the Rural Doctors' Society to expand access to health care. Sumlee Jaidee and Chanpen Wiwat, professors from the Chulalongkorn Faculty of Pharmacy, were involved in the Primary Health Care Coordinating Network, and Chanpen Wiwat served as chair of the Thai Development Support Committee for a time, which had been a collaborative endeavor with the Rural Doctors' Society (*Thai Development Newsletter* 1986a, 2). At the same time, other Chulalongkorn Faculty of Pharmacy professors, such as Niyada Kiatyingungsulee, served as respected advisers to the Thai Development Support Committee and lent credibility and legitimacy to their efforts. Rural Doctors involved in the movement to improve access to health care in the countryside were also engaging with the concerns of the DSG and experimenting with innovative ways of pooling resources from groups of hospitals within regions to purchase pharmaceuticals from drug companies in larger batches at lower costs (Kijtiwatchakul and Daechutragun 2007, 163). One of those Rural Doctors who would go on to play an important role in Thailand's antiretroviral access story was Dr. Mongkol na Songkhla, who had also been responsible for implementing Thailand's Universal Coverage so quickly. His early efforts at drug pooling had the effect of lowering drug prices by as much as 30 percent, making medicines more accessible for those who needed them in the countryside (Kijtiwatchakul 2007, 43).

New Dynamics in the Transition to Democracy

With Thailand's transition to civilian rule in the early 1990s, new voices gradually began to enter the political sphere. Although the share of GDP deriving from agriculture had declined to nearly single digits, agriculture still employed 60 percent of the country's workforce; however, the construction of large-scale dams had led to extensive destruction of the country's farmlands, fisheries, and forests (Missingham 2003, 17, 19–20). In the country's northeast, where the Rural Doctors' Society and Drug Study Group had spent so much time working in the 1970s, grassroots networks of farmers, concerned about the commercialization of agriculture, deforestation, and environmental degradation, began to meet and set up small-scale farmers' organizations (Phatharathananunth 2006, 69–73; also Missingham 2003, 36–38). While the concerns of farmers were varied and multisectoral, agricultural issues dominated their agenda; a new organization to represent the country's poor—the Assembly of the Poor (AOP)—was founded in 1995 with the goal of representing the poor very broadly, although the majority of its work focused on the problems of the country's rural northeast (Phatharathananunth 2006, 143). Land and forest conflicts formed important parts of the AOP's agenda; health issues typically related to industrial hazards and occupation-related diseases (Phatharathananunth 2006, 144). Forests and land issues dominated the kinds of grievances brought forward by members (91 grievances), followed by dam-related issues (15 grievances), while members filed only one grievance related to work-related and environmental illnesses (Missingham 2003, 45–46).

Large-scale demonstrations by AOP in Bangkok in late 1996 and 1997 brought the government into dialogue with the movement, but despite winning several unprecedented agreements from government, few resolutions actually materialized, and many were actually reversed when the conservative Democrat Party came to power in 1997 (Phatharathananunth 2006, 159–62). These dynamics illustrate the general issue focus of the increasingly organized but often ineffectual rural poor. Needs related to health care and medicine, including treatment for infectious disease, were not a major concern of growing rural movements. Rather, they were articulated by progressive medical professionals concerned about the rural poor.

As the era of early AIDS treatment was just beginning, the purpose and aims of the DSG took a marked turn away from drug safety and toward expanding access to essential medicines. The 1980s saw the United States put increasing pressure on developing countries to increase protection of intellectual property as part of multilateral trade negotiations (Wibulpolprasert et al. 2011). As part of this campaign, the U.S. government in 1985 came to Thailand to enter into trade negotiations, offering Thailand tax concessions in exchange for better protection of U.S. patents (Limpananont interview 2009). The head of the U.S. House of Representatives Subcommittee on Commerce distributed a white paper that urged the Thai government to protect the patents of American pharmaceutical companies and to protect the Thai people from potentially dangerous generics by passing new patent laws and enforcing old ones (*Thai Development Newsletter* 1986b, 23). At the time, the DSG did not know much about patent law or why the U.S. government wanted the Thai government to change the nation's patent law, which had been in effect since 1979, so researchers like DSG co-founder Jiraporn Limpananont began to study the issue intensively (Limpananont interview 2009). They conducted a research project, which found that amending the patent law would lead to a 72 percent increase in the price of imported drugs to

Thailand while hindering development of a domestic pharmaceutical industry (Wibulpolprasert et al. 2011).

Once the ramifications of patent law changes became clear, the pharmacists in the DSG knew that in order to move government policy, they would need allies in the NGO world to protest the policy, and they also knew that in order to make NGOs credible actors on the issues, they would have to "make NGOs stronger and make them aware of the information but it's quite technical, quite complicated. When we talked about the patent law, everyone just said the same thing. . . . [they] did not get it" (Limpananont interview 2009). To address these challenges, members from the DSG held a seminar in 1987—not coincidentally, the same year that AZT (zidovudine) would be approved to treat AIDS in the United States. The seminar called attention to the effects of pharmaceutical patents on Thai people, and the DSG subsequently published a story in the Thai Development Support Committee's *Thai Development Newsletter*, pointing to the growing efforts by the U.S. Pharmaceutical Products Association to get developing countries to protect drug patents (*Thai Development Newsletter* 1987, 36). However, the pressure by big pharma—including claims by the pharmaceutical industry about the severity of losses in Thailand due to weak intellectual property protections—eventually led Thailand in 1992 to amend its Patent Act, which had previously only protected process (rather than product) patents[2]; the resulting Act would commit Thailand to protection of product patents a full thirteen years before the WTO TRIPS accord would require it do so (Chan 2015, 83), and it would extend the life of patents in Thailand from fifteen to twenty years (Limpananont 2009, 140). As Drug Study Group pharmacist Jiraporn Limpananont recounted, "Thus, Thailand lost a total of 13 years in which it could have significantly developed its domestic drug industry, producing new generics . . . and expanding their market to the ASEAN countries" (quoted in Chan 2015, 83).

As early as 1993, the Drug Study Group, along with the Rural Doctors' Society and the fifteen other member organizations of the Primary Health Care Coordinating Network, published a letter in the country's leading English newspaper, the *Bangkok Post*, strongly condemning the pressure placed on the Thai government by the U.S. Trade Representative. This pressure was aimed at getting the Thai government to do more to protect the patents of U.S. pharmaceuticals (particularly those related to HIV/AIDS) and to prevent the country from invoking compulsory licensing on AIDS-related medication (*Thai Development Newsletter* 1993, 69). These early advocacy efforts amounted to one of the earliest stands by a professional movement or NGO in the developing world on the issue of patent protection, coming even before the multilateral agreement that established the World Trade Organization was signed in 1994.

Growth of the AIDS Movement and the Limited Possibilities for Treatment

This transition into work on HIV/AIDS by the Drug Study Group in the early 1990s—when the epidemic was at its peak in Thailand—coincided with the transition of another important professor-cum-activist with whom the DSG and the Rural Doctors' Society had worked in the 1970s and 1980s into work on HIV/ AIDS. Jon Ungpakorn had founded a national network for sharing experiences and technical skills on matters related to HIV/AIDS—the Thai NGO Coalition on AIDS (TNCA) in 1989.[3] Echoing the efforts of others around the world, the early efforts of AIDS NGOs in Thailand centered on combating stigma and discrimination and building solidarities nationally among local support groups (Suwanphatthana et al. 2008, 22, 28–31). TNCA sought to increase the political visibility of the problem of HIV/AIDS by organizing public demonstrations; by lobbying government on AIDS related policy; by developing a subcommittee designed to coordinate the coalition's work with political parties and committees in Parliament; by establishing a Human Rights Centre on AIDS, which investigated cases of discrimination and promoted an awareness of the rights of people affected by HIV/AIDS; and by serving as a participant in the country's National AIDS Prevention and Control Committee. In one particularly vivid example of the way in which TNCA seized on HIV/AIDS as a human rights issue, the organization sent letters to the House Committee on Human Rights in the Parliament calling for investigations of human rights violations (*Thai Development Newsletter* 1995, 67; 1996, 50–51).

A passionate advocate for social causes, Jon Ungpakorn's work on HIV/AIDS deepened further in 1991 when he founded the AIDS Access Foundation with volunteers from the Thai Volunteer Service to help fill gaps in the Thai governmental response to the epidemic through the promotion of counseling, education, and testing. During this time, his relationship and work with the Drug Study Group would expand substantially over issues related to drug access (Ungpakorn interview 2009). As a result of these and other efforts, by 1992 the government position on the rights of infected people stood in alignment with those of NGOs, manifested in the basic principles laid out in the 1992–1996 National AIDS Plan and the 1995–1996 National AIDS Action Plan (Ungpakorn 1994, 65).

However, while the government's position on the rights of HIV/AIDS patients was taking a progressive turn in the early 1990s, its commitment to treating patients with the one drug available at the time that could slow the progression of the disease—AZT—remained far from universal. The government initiated a small pilot program beginning in 1992 that provided AZT free of charge to three thousand low-income patients at a cost of $20 million over four years. When a 1996 report by a team of researchers in the Ministry of Public Health exploring the use of antiretroviral medication in Thailand found that treatment by one or two drugs, such as AZT or ddI,[4] increased life expectancy by just six months, the ministry began to reconsider its support for the program (*Bangkok Post* 1995; Sakboon 1999, 13). Ultimately, the ministry terminated the program and redirected patients to clinical research programs while exploring more cost-effective policies, such as using AZT to prevent mother-to-child transmission (Thanprasertsuk et al. 2004 on Tantivess and Walt 2008, 328–29). For its part, the World Bank encouraged the country to devote its resources to prevention rather than treatment. At a seminal conference on HIV/AIDS in Asia and the Pacific in 1995, senior World Bank economist Nicholas Prescott remarked, "The ministry has to reconsider the cost-benefit of this programme" (quoted in *Bangkok Post* 1995). By 1999, at a time when pharmaceutical prices remained cost-prohibitive, just 5 to 10 percent of infected patients had access to the two main AIDS drugs available in Thailand—ddI and AZT (Sakboon 1999, 13).

Following the groundswell of social movement activity that paved the way for the restoration of democracy in 1992, the AIDS movement began to occupy a more prominent place on the national stage. In 1995, the 3rd International Conference on AIDS in Asia and the Pacific in Chiang Mai served as a focal point bringing together the country's fifty-two PLWHA groups for the first time to share their experiences and form the basis for a larger national network. As these formerly local support groups of people living with HIV and AIDS (PLWHA) began to consolidate into larger regional groups, the broader movement gave voice to more forceful ideas grounded in the language of human rights. At the meeting, for the first time representatives from the fifty-two PLWHA groups articulated their aspirations and demands in the form of a "yellow paper" delivered to government; while this historic "yellow paper" included ideas, such as the right of the infected to receive health care without consideration of the cost-effectiveness and the right to treatment of opportunistic infections such as TB, the AIDS movement was conscious of the high cost of antiretroviral treatment and *did not* demand universal access to AZT (Suwanphatthana et al. 2008, 22, 28–31), which cost 287 baht per pill in Thailand at the time (Loos 2009, xx).

Although the life-saving benefits of combination antiretroviral therapy were made known at the International AIDS Conference in 1996, the primary focus of activists living with HIV/AIDS in Thailand before 1997 was "on earning a living and on self-care, and as a result, many patients died sooner than they should have" (Wisartsakul 2004, 25). AIDS NGOs lacked expertise in patent law, and the AIDS movement emphasized treatment of opportunistic infections, largely because nearly all antiretroviral medications in Thailand were patented, leaving treatment unaffordable (Wisartsakul 2004, 26, 29). Médecins Sans Frontières (MSF) and the AIDS Access Foundation, for example, developed a project that aimed to treat 100 percent of the pneumocystis pneumonia infections, an opportunistic infection that was the leading cause of death in AIDS patients in Thailand (Suwanphattana et al. 2008, 40–45).

Professional Movement Efforts within the State and the Growing Role of Legal Expertise

Beginning in 1996, the Ministry of Public Health's Office of Healthcare Reform, led by the Rural Doctor Sanguan Nitayarumphong, started a three-year project that aimed to enhance health equity and community involvement in health care. Access to medicine for HIV/AIDS, including treatment for opportunistic infections and AIDS itself, was identified as a major issue by the initiative, and beginning in 1997, the Office—under Sanguan—began to work with MSF, which was involved with the provision of technical support, treatment advocacy, and projects related to the establishment of district-level care standards (Ford et al. 2009, 259). However, these efforts by medical professionals within the state to link up with organizations that could help build their expertise on the issues and develop greater linkages with the broader AIDS movement were not limited to the Office of Healthcare Reform.

The Thai Government Pharmaceutical Office (GPO), which produced generic medication for the country's public hospitals, was itself also led by activists from the professional movement. After receiving her doctorate in pharmaceutical chemistry, Dr. Krisana Kraisintu had served as director of the Institute of Research and Development at the GPO since 1987. Between 1992 and 2002, Krisana's work had been focused on developing generic formulations of medications that could prolong the life of victims of HIV/AIDS, and in the 2000s her personal commitments to expanding access to medicine would lead her to work on projects that aimed to improve local production capacity in the nations that were hardest-hit by HIV in Africa (Ubon Ratchathani University 2015; also Loos 2015). Krisana's longtime deputy, Achara Eksaengsri, had been a member of a group called the Rural Pharmacists' Society that shared similar concerns as the DSG and would sometimes join Drug Study Group meetings (Eksaengsri interview 2009).

Sharing many of the concerns of members of Thailand's Drug Study Group, Krisana was contemptuous of "multinational drug companies for facilitating the dependency of weaker states and populations upon stronger ones for essential medicines and dire public health assistance" (Loos 2015, 215). Under Krisana's leadership, in 1995 the GPO produced a generic version of AZT that made life-prolonging (but not life-saving) single-therapy treatment for AIDS affordable at just eight baht per pill, this at a time when the U.S. version was five times as costly (Loos 2009, xx). The drug represented the first generic ARV in the developing world and would come to be widely used in Thai hospitals by 1999 (Loos 2015, 219). Building on this success, the GPO in 1998 launched a project to produce a generic of the Bristol Meyers Squibb (BMS) antiretroviral drug didanosine (ddI), which was stopped by threat of legal action from BMS that sought to uphold the company's patent on the drug (Ford et al. 2004, 561).

These developments led the Thai NGO Coalition on AIDS, chaired by Jon Ungpakorn's AIDS Access Foundation, to begin focusing on the issue of access to antiretroviral drugs more strongly (Kijtiwatchakul 2007, 13; Suwanphattana et al. 2008, 40–45; Wisartsakul 2004, 29). With the international support and contacts of MSF (Ungpakorn interview 2009), concerned medical professionals within the Ministry of Health, GPO, and the country's Food and Drug Administration began to work with NGOs in the AIDS movement to explore the role that patent law might play in making these costs manageable (Wisartsakul 2004, 5). The major outcome of these efforts was a decision to press the government to declare compulsory licensing on ddI, which would allow the GPO to produce the drug locally in tablet form in exchange for a very modest royalty (Wisartsakul 2004, 5).

Pharmacists from Chulalongkorn University that had been involved in these issues for years with the Drug Study Group played important roles in promoting greater knowledge on issues related to access to medicine (Suwanpatthana et al. 2008, 45–49). Initially, however, AIDS NGOs were at a disadvantage due to their lack of specialized knowledge. As the manager of AIDS Access, Nimit Tien-udom, recounted, "We need to catch up on legal details. We must know what the academics mean" (quoted in Wisartsakul 2004, 46). As AIDS Access Co-Coordinator Sangsiri Treemanka added, "Before this time, NGOs were only involved with campaigning and training, but with this issue, I had to familiarize myself with ARV medicines, patents, TRIPS and WTO" (quoted in Wisartsakul 2004, 46). In this, the Drug Study Group and their collaborators at the GPO were a particular resource.

Dr. Achara Eksaengsri of the GPO was asked to serve as a witness on the issue of patent protection in two court cases that were filed (Eksaengsri interview 2009). And DSG founder and pharmacist Dr. Jiraporn Limpananont helped train people and build capacity related to patent law. Reflecting on her role, she said, "When we gave them the knowledge, they got it so fast. They tried to understand with patent law. . . . It was very interesting when we worked with the patient group. . . . Now we can ask the infected network what is CL [and] they know what is patent law. How it started. How it changed. Why they had to edit [the 1992 Patent Law]. They all knew" (Limpananont interview 2009).

One of the AIDS NGOs' first acts in the campaign for affordable access to ddI, in November 1999, was to request legal assistance from the Lawyers' Society of Thailand (Wisartsakul 2004, 111). However, this was supplemented by traditional social movement activism and the setting up of a "ddI camp" outside of the Ministry of Public Health, staffed by one hundred members from the Thai Network of People Living with HIV/AIDS (TNP+) that called for compulsory licensing of ddI (Chan 2015, 3). GPO staff, in turn, lent moral support and joined the action (Ungpakhorn in Wisartsakul 2004, 5). And in interesting echoes of the Rural Doctors' Ayudhya Project, the Thai Treatment Action Group and AIDS Access Foundation (with funding and support from MSF) worked to develop a demonstration project at a district hospital to show how ARV provision in one community might operate successfully at the national level (Kaplan and Suwannawong interview 2009)

While control of the GPO by activist professionals would prove extremely useful for advancing the agenda of expanding access to medicines, the GPO did not hold the formal standing of being a government department that could declare compulsory licensing itself. However, it did have the power to put in a request with the Department of Intellectual Property in the Ministry of Commerce to do so, which it did in November 1999 (Ford et al. 2004, 560). The GPO's request was occasioned by the first-ever HIV+ demonstrations (the aforementioned ddI camp), who provided grassroots support to the professional movement operating in the state and who were joined in solidarity by activists in the United States who demonstrated against Bristol Meyers Squibb and the U.S. government's efforts to pressure countries which, like Thailand and South Africa, were exploring compulsory licensing policies (Ford et al. 2004, 560). As a consequence of the developments taking place in Thailand, the United States ratcheted up pressure, dispatching the U.S. Ambassador to Thailand to threaten a trade war if compulsory licensing was invoked (Glaser and Murphy 2010, 227), a prospect that scared some government officials (Limpananont interview 2009).

When the campaign to get Thailand's Ministry of Commerce (in which the Department of Intellectual Property was housed) to declare compulsory licensing was unsuccessful, the movement redirected its focus to another less conservative ministry that also had the power to declare compulsory licensing and might be more likely to act on behalf of citizens' health needs, the Ministry of Public Health (Suwanphattana et al. 2008, 45–49). In conjunction with demonstrations that had place on the ministry's campus, pharmacists from Chulalongkorn University, lawyers from Thailand's Law Society, and scientists from the GPO held informational lectures aimed at disseminating information about compulsory licensing (Cawthorne interview 2009). Meanwhile, the professional movement–controlled GPO, which was supported by MSF, AIDS Access Foundation, TNP+, and several other NGOS in the broader AIDS movement, submitted a request to the Minister of Public Health to issue a compulsory license, which also denied it due to the substantial pressure (Ford et al. 2009, 262).

Activists and public health professionals then collectively tried to provide political cover for the ministry by sending a petition letter to President Bill Clinton on January 18, 2000, asking the U.S. government not to pursue a lawsuit in the WTO against Thailand if it declared compulsory licensing on ddI; the request was supported by the Washington, D.C.–based Consumer Project on Technology, a legal aid organization founded by lawyer James Love (Ford et al. 2004, 561). Nine days later—and just one month after the WTO protests in Seattle—the U.S. Trade Representative wrote a letter stating that it would not retaliate against Thailand and affirming that the country was well within its rights to issue a compulsory license under the TRIPS accord (Ford et al. 2004, 561). A senior official in the Ministry of Commerce remarked, "Thailand has committed to the international community not to use poverty and sickness as an excuse in international trade . . . if a compulsory license were to be issued, just one million people will benefit, while the rest of the country's 61 million people will have to pay the price if the U.S. retaliates" (quoted in Ford et al. 2004, 561).

While the broader Ministry of Public Health, like the Ministry of Commerce, took no action on the issue, the movement found a department within the Ministry of Public Health that proved somewhat more willing to do something on the issue. The Ministry's Department of Disease Control—which had overseen the ministry's AIDS efforts—stopped short of issuing a compulsory license but ordered the GPO to produce it in powdered form (Kijtiwatchakul 2007, 15). While a powdered form of ddI added an important medicine to the country's arsenal of medications to fight AIDS (albeit one with more side effects), a core group of pharmacy faculty pressed on, preparing court documents for cases challenging BMs' patent of ddI, in partnership with the Foundation for Consumers and AIDS Access, with technical assistance provided by MSF-Belgium and a team of pro bono lawyers provided by the Law Society of Thailand (Wisartsakul 2004, 6–7, 44). In court proceedings related to ddI, reliance on and consultations with lawyers from the Law Society of Thailand was a regular occurrence (Limpananont interview 2009; on Law Society, Ungpakorn in Wisartsakul 2004, 7).

Building on the movement's growing confidence in legal matters related to HIV/AIDS, the AIDS Access Foundation filed a lawsuit on behalf of two HIV+ patients against BMS and Thailand's Department of Intellectual Property over BMS's claim to patent of ddI. Progressive activists in the GPO with a long history of working for the public interest testified in the case (Loos 2015, 223). The judge's October 2002 ruling stated that "lack of access to medicines due to high price prejudices the human rights of patients to proper medical treatment," setting a major precedent that drew on the 2001 Doha Declaration that affirmed WTO member states' rights to circumvent patents for public health needs (quoted in Ford et al. 2004, 560). The case was the first in which Thai patients were allowed to sue as plaintiffs, and this right was later extended beyond patients to consumers more broadly (Limpananont et al. 2009, 143). Approximately one year later—highlighting the degree to which fears over trade retaliation still held sway within the Ministry of Commerce—Thailand's own Department of Intellectual Property filed an appeal of the decision, followed by another by BMS one week later (Wisartsakul 2004, 60).

In early 2004, after more than three years of legal battles (and tellingly, before a precedent could be set in court), BMS agreed to let go of its patent on ddI in Thailand in an agreement with TNP+, AIDS Access Foundation, and the Foundation for Consumers (the main plaintiff in the case and the organization to which the Drug Study Group had given birth so many years earlier) in Thailand's Central Intellectual Property and International Trade Court (Cameron 2005, 178; Tantivess and Walt 2008, 332; Wisartsakul 2004, 48). Although the professional movement would have preferred for the case to go forward to establish a legal precedent in court, the willingness of the company to relinquish its patent at a time when AIDS patients in need of medication were already dying led the movement to accept the company's offer (Limpananont interview 2009). While NGOs would serve as plaintiffs in the case, again it was members of the DSG who provided the expertise that enabled the cases to go forward, serving as "the core group working on preparing documents for the court cases" (Ungphakorn in Wisartsakul 2004, 6).

In a second instance in which patients' groups were able "to use the [patent] law for the movement" (Limpananont interview 2009), another Thai NGO, the Health and Development Foundation, which was run by academics and lecturers with pharmaceutical knowledge, brought forward objections to the patent applications made by GlaxoSmithKline over its claim of patent of Combid, a combined version of the two antiretroviral drugs lamivudine and zidovudine (on the Health and Development Foundation, Wisartsakul 2004, 49). The objection ultimately resulted in the company's abandonment of its patent applications not only in Thailand but also in India (Limpananont et al. 2009, 144–45).

Opening Tensions between Universal Coverage and Access to Antiretroviral Drugs

While legal expertise and the courts would become increasingly central to the professional movement's project of enabling the state to expand access to HIV/AIDS medicine through the production of cheap generics, the universal health care program was the vehicle through which pharmacists in the movement envisioned that access to these life-saving new technologies would flow. In recounting the DSG's role, DSG founder Jiraporn Limpananont reflected, "We talked with infected people and said, 'We have the Health Security system [also known as the Universal Coverage program]. We should push this into the Health Security system, [which] means UC has to be responsible for ARV drugs as well'" (Limpananont interview 2009).

The country's Universal Coverage program, adopted in 2001 and enshrined in law in 2002, offered patients the promise of being able to forego jury-rigged arrangements, such as buyers' clubs to get their AIDS medication (like those featured in the film *Dallas Buyers Club*), which had also began to crop up in Thailand (Tantivess and Walt 2008, 333–34). However, the incorporation of AIDS drugs into the universal health care program presented its own new challenges.

Before rollout of the Universal Coverage program, the government had just one pilot ARV program known as ATC1, which was very small and served just 3,500 patients out of the estimated 70,000 in need. The generally low level of government commitment to the program in part reflected the high cost of ARVs (Kuanpoth et al. 2005, 167; Tantivess and Walt 2008, 336). The incorporation of high-priced AIDS medication into the UC program, however, amounted to a highly sensitive political issue. While inclusion of the drugs in the benefit package of the program might earn Thai Rak Thai some new supporters within the AIDS community, the high cost of the medication also had the potential to seriously undermine the political feasibility of the program. As Senator Jon Ungpakorn would relate, "A lot of the supporters of the universal health service/insurance bill were afraid it would collapse under the weight of having the most expensive types of treatment" (Ungpakorn interview 2009). These dynamics opened some very real tensions between members of the Rural Doctors movement who had championed universal health care and members of the AIDS movement who needed medicine.[5]

Although the AIDS movement had campaigned for Universal Coverage on behalf of the Rural Doctors, after Thai Rak Thai gained power and seemed intent on moving forward, members of the Rural Doctors' movement that had been involved in mobilizing civil society support for the UC program were now circling the wagons, suggesting that high-cost medications such as AIDS drugs should not be included. Calling attention to the sustainability problems posed by AIDS medication and other high-cost treatments, the Rural Doctor (and health economist) responsible for developing the budget for the program remarked, "How much more money would be required if the government was to pay for antiretroviral drugs for people with HIV/AIDS, chemotherapy for final-stage cancer patients and for brain surgery for accident patients who most likely will not recover?" (quoted in Bhatiasevi 2001b). The cost of expensive second-line drugs that could not be produced by the government for patients who developed drug resistance was another concern (Assavanonda 2001c).

The initial budget estimates for the UC program that won Thaksin's approval (prepared by a Rural Doctor vested in the program's success) did *not* include high-cost treatments such as antiretroviral therapy and kidney dialysis; after the March 2001 final staging meeting at Government House, the prime minister announced that the 30-baht program would not include these therapies but would cover treatment for opportunistic infections (*Bangkok Post* 2001; Bhatiasevi 2001a). Yet even after this announcement, as the UC program was being rolled out as a pilot project, the contentious battles over whether or not AIDS drugs should be included continued. So concerned with defending and protecting the viability of the fledgling new program (which did not yet enjoy legal standing) were core members of the Rural Doctors' movement that they even began to move outside of cost concerns and attempted to fashion public reasons why AIDS drugs should not be included in the program.

In some cases, these rationales had to do with the readiness of the health system and the knowledge of physicians within it ("the health care system [is] still not ready for effective treatment of HIV/AIDS, particularly if it was included in the 30-baht scheme. . . . At the moment, there are only a small number of physicians who have enough knowledge about HIV and antiretroviral drugs, their side-effects and proper dose, which is very important for HIV treatment," (Tangcharoensathien quoted in Assavanonda 2001c). In other cases, they had more to do with patient safety ("So far there has been no scientific proof that those drugs are good and safe. On the contrary, they are expensive and even cause side-effects") (Wibulpolprasert quoted in Assavanonda 2001c).[6]

Owing to their control of top positions within the ministry and the role they played in overseeing the program, the concerns of the Rural Doctors' movement held sway, and the inclusion of AIDS drugs in the benefit package was initially resisted. This, however, did not deter the AIDS movement from continuing to use rights-based approaches to put pressure on politicians to include AIDS medication in the benefit package in new ways. The AIDS movement drew on provisions of the constitution that prohibited discrimination on account of specific diseases to bolster their case for inclusion of treatments, such as ARVs and renal dialysis, which had initially been excluded from the benefit package (Ford et al. 2009, 260). And Jon Ungpakorn, the director of AIDS Access Foundation, issued a challenge to the Rural Doctor who had been responsible for coming up with the 30-baht program's budget estimates, asking him to begin work on a study to figure out the cost of including AIDS medication when the decision to exclude them was initially made (Tangcharoensathien interview 2009). Following the decision, DSG adviser and Faculty of Pharmacy chairperson Vithaya Kulsomboon—Thailand's only pharmaceutical economist—would also go on to play an important role in costing the drugs as a precursor to determining the possibility of their inclusion in the benefit package.

AIDS activists also sought to allay some of the worries of the Rural Doctors by presenting them with evidence of the effectiveness of combination therapy, in particular the substantial money that Brazil and other Western countries had saved in hospitalization costs through treatment, while at the same time pointing to the availability of cheap generic combination therapies that could be purchased from India (Tantivess and Walt 2008, 332). Practically, however, it was again the work of professional movement activists in the GPO that contributed to the expansion of access to medicine when they succeeded in developing a generic combination antiretroviral therapy dubbed GPO-vir in October 2001. This new formulation meant that the price of first-line combination therapy, which could stop AIDS in its tracks, fell from 400,000 baht (approximately $9,000) to just 14,400 baht per year (just over $320), or 1200 baht per month (just over $25); the new price was well below the level the government said would be required for the drugs to be included in the benefit package (Kijtiwatchakul 2007, 18–19; Tantivess and Walt 2008, 332).

With news of the GPO's achievement, the AIDS movement began to apply much more visible public pressure on government to include antiretrovirals in the benefit package. On November 5, 2001—just as the UC program had achieved national rollout as a pilot project—the AIDS movement sent a letter to the prime minister, the health minister, and the media proposing that the government establish a joint government-NGO commission to establish a means for integrating AIDS medication into the universal coverage program (Tantivess and Walt 2008, 332). The letter also notified the government of the movement's intentions to assemble one thousand people on the ministry campuses to commemorate World AIDS Day (December 1). The Health Ministry responded by agreeing to meet with the AIDS movement on November 28 to discuss the developments (Tantivess and Walt 2008, 332).

The pressure applied by the movement in the events leading up to World AIDS Day forced the minister of public health to agree publicly to commit to scaling up treatment for HIV/AIDS over five years (*The Nation* 2001; Assavanonda 2001a). The announcement also led to the formation of a government-civil society committee to explore the cost of including ARVs in the benefit package, a body to be chaired by Sanguan Nitayarumphong that also included the head of TNP+ and Jon Ungpakorn as committee members (Suwanphattana et al. 2008, 61). This policy reversal quickly led AIDS activists to change course and begin defending the program, which had come under heavy criticism for its many implementation problems. Nimit Thien-udom, the director of the AIDS Access Foundation, stated that "the Bt30 scheme deserved to be supported and its flaws should not be used to derail the effort to develop universal health-care coverage" (Sakboon 2002).

AIDS activists were included on four technical bodies created in 2002 designed to inform the development of the national rollout of ARV provision (Tantivess and Walt 2008, 333). They were also elected to serve on the two main boards of the National Health Security Office (overseeing governance and quality control) along with representatives from some of the eleven networks that had originally orchestrated the petition campaign for the Universal Coverage. Despite initial tensions related to financial sustainability, the strong collaboration with AIDS activists was more practically an outcome of the longstanding relationships among members of the Rural Doctors movement and the Drug Study Group and leaders of the AIDS movement, in particular Jon Ungpakorn. Collaboration accelerated when Thailand was awarded funding from the Global Fund to Fight AIDS, Tuberculosis, and Malaria to scale up its antiretroviral program in 2002,[7] with MSF and AIDS Access Foundation to play lead roles in the development of a strategy for involvement of people living with HIV and AIDS in the program (Ford et al. 2009, 261; Tantivess and Walt 2008). By 2003, 73 percent of AIDS patients on treatment in Thailand were receiving services through the Universal Coverage program, which provided all care for the cost of 30 baht per visit, once the patient paid for the initial CD4 count diagnostic test (Supakankunti, Phetnoi, and Tsunekaw 2004, 31).

Government–civil society efforts to expand access to antiretroviral medications then received a surprising boost of support from the World Bank in 2003. The World Bank had not only criticized Thailand's UC program but had also been a staunch advocate of prevention rather than treatment in Thailand, Brazil, and other developing countries for some time.[8] But a 2003 joint World Bank–Ministry of Public Health study marked a dramatic shift in policy by the World Bank. The report not only suggested that public financing of first-line combination ARV treatment was cost-effective but that provision of second-line treatment was affordable (Suwanpatthana et al. 2008, 63–65). It also argued that compulsory licensing would reduce the cost of second-line treatment by 90 percent, saving the government $3.2 billion through 2025 (Kijtiwatchakul 2007, 23). At a time when compulsory licensing remained a hugely sensitive political issue, the findings by the World Bank—which had a reputation being conservative and was frequently aligned with U.S. policy—amounted to a somewhat remarkable show of support for Thailand's efforts to make access to AIDS medication a reality.

A related study by a local research team provided further credence to the minis-try's efforts (Supakankunti, Phetnoi, and Tsunekaw 2004, 9–10).

Building State Capacity and Confidence in the Face of International Pressure

The achievement of an agreement to scale up access to AIDS drugs was a huge win for Thai citizens in need of life-saving medication. However, even as the cli-mate around access to medicine seemed to be changing in positive ways, threats to government commitments to AIDS treatment still loomed large. In particular, the effect of a potential free-trade agreement with the United States on ARV access was a major concern of the pharmacists at Chulalongkorn University. To monitor developments related to trade law that might have an impact on access to medicine, the Drug Study Group, the Foundation for Consumers, and other relevant partners formed the FTA Watch in October 2003. As part of that effort, specialists on pharmaceutical patents, like Dr. Jiraporn Limpananont, would teach introductory classes on intellectual property rights (Kijtiwatchakul inter-view 2009). In addition to publishing numerous articles and holding press con-ferences, the professional movement published two books in Thai on the issue in 2004 and drew attention to the ways in which a TRIPS-Plus agreement that went beyond the basic stipulations of the WTO TRIPS accord would further limit access to medicines and restrict the ability of the government to issue compul-sory licenses (Kuanpoth et al. 2005, 5, 32–41).

With support from a growing number of international organizations, includ-ing UNDP, UNAIDS, and the WHO, pharmacists from Chulalongkorn Univer-sity, in partnership with the Ministry of Public Health, convened a conference on the subject of "Free Trade Agreements and Intellectual Property Rights: Implications for Access to Medicine" in December 2005. The conference brought together knowledgeable lawyers, activists, and government officials from around the world (including from the ministries of health of Malaysia and India) to discuss the issue and highlighted the way in which Brazil's experience producing generic ARVs and threats to use compulsory licensing had driven down costs substantially between 1996 and 2003. The conference affirmed that entering into a TRIPS-plus agreement would irreparably harm Thailand's ability to provide access to essential medicines and recommended that Thailand consider issuing compulsory licenses for second-line ARV drugs (UNDP et al. 2006, 5–6, 21).

Pharmacists from the Drug Study Group highlighted the degree to which pharmaceutical patents in Thailand were overwhelmingly held by foreigners and disseminated knowledge related to the domestic and international laws that bore on pharmaceutical access (Limpananont 2005, 8, 15–16). At the meeting, the secretary-general of the Food and Drug Administration of Thailand affirmed that Thailand would avail itself of compulsory licensing to protect the public health and pointed to lack of knowledge and confidence on the issues as reasons that such policies had not been used in the past (UNDP et al. 2006, 17). The head of one of Thailand's largest AIDS organizations (TNP+), which was increasingly engaging with issues related to intellectual property law, added further pressure by sending a letter to the Ministry of Public Health asking for a compulsory license on efavirenz, which would save the government more than a trillion baht ($25 billion) (Chan 2015, 84).

So energizing was the conference that representatives of UNDP, UNAIDS, and the WHO collaborated in writing an op-ed that called on Thailand to ensure that health was not on the negotiating table in trade talks with the United States, which were to take place immediately after the conference. In the end, only WHO representative William Aldis came forward in signing his name to the op-ed. And it ran on the day before Thailand's free trade negotiations began in early January 2006, urging Thailand not to enter the agreement; in apparent response to U.S. anger over Aldis's use of his position as a WHO representative to speak out against U.S. trade policy, he was removed from his position one week later and transferred to another country (Kiatyingungsulee interview 2009; Kijtiwatchakul 2007, 20).

While Aldis's courageous act proved detrimental to his own career in the short term,[9] it inspired activists at the grassroots level who had participated in the conference's proceedings. Mirroring the tactics used by the movement to push for the adoption of the Universal Coverage policy in 2000, the movement sought to collect fifty thousand signatures in protest of the FTA (Wisartsakul 2004, 10). This time, many of the same NGO networks that had campaigned for the Universal Coverage program led a protest demonstration of ten thousand people against the FTA negotiations with the United States; the political salience that the issue had taken on caused Dr. Sanguan, who was now chairman of the board of the National Health Security Office, and Minister of Public Health Phinij Jarusombat to establish a subcommittee to do research in preparation of a resolution to compulsory license efavirenz, a first-line ARV, on January 12, 2006 (Kijtiwatchakul 2007, 20, 24).

The Deepening of Progressive Pharmaceutical Commitments despite Democratic Disruption

By 2006, Thailand's National Access Program for People Living with HIV/AIDS had been integrated into Thailand's UC program, and the vast majority of citizens in need of antiretroviral medication had received them. However, as of mid-2006, no decision had yet been made to invoke compulsory licensing on first- or second-line AIDS medication, which would ensure the sustainability of Thailand's ARV program. The prospects of such a decision at least immediately appeared even more uncertain following a brief military coup in late 2006. The military coup came amid widening social conflict over the excesses of the Thaksin administration, following efforts by Thaksin to avoid payment of taxes related to the sale of one of his businesses and his efforts to consolidate power over some of the country's leading media outlets. The coup led to immediate suspension of the 1997 "People's Constitution" and eventually to weakening of political parties in Thailand.

However, the greater legal knowledge that had been forged by the professional movement during Thailand's period of democracy up to 2006 translated into greater state capacity and confidence after the fact. The surprise appointment of Dr. Mongkol na Songkhla gave reason for both the Rural Doctors' movement and the professional movement dedicated to expanding access to pharmaceuticals, led by the DSG and executives in the GPO, to rejoice. As permanent secretary, Mongkol had been responsible for implementing Thailand's UC program as a national pilot project in just six months. But as a Rural Doctor in Korat province in the 1970s, Mongkol had led efforts to lower pharmaceutical costs through group purchasing. In other words, he was a patron of both causes. When Sanguan learned that it was Dr. Mongkol who had been appointed to become the new minister, he expressed his happiness over the appointment (Kijtiwatchakul 2007, 34).

And so in November 2006—after the ministers of commerce and public health previously had declined the opportunity to do so—Thailand's new minister of public health took the radical step of declaring compulsory licensing on efavirenz, which allowed Thailand to produce the drug itself and to import generic versions of the drug from India, where it was not patented (Steinbrook 2007, 544). Two additional compulsory licenses were subsequently issued on January 24 and 25, 2007, for a second-line ARV called lopinavir/ritonavir, and a heart medication called clopidogrel—under Article 31 of the TRIPS Agreement, which allowed countries to waive patent rights in cases of national emergency (Kijtiwatchakul 2007, 8, 25, 69).

The impact of compulsory licensing on the price of efavirenz in Thailand was immediate: Thailand could now import the drug as a generic from India for 650 baht—less than half of what it had cost previously; this led the pharmaceutical manufacturer, Merck, Sharp, and Dohme, to cut the prices of its trademark brand to 700 baht per person per month to compete with generic suppliers (Kijtiwatchakul 2007, 42). The move also led Abbott Laboratories to offer to reduce the price of Kaletra (the trade name of liponavir/ritonavir) if the movement would agree to lobby the Ministry of Public Health to cancel its compulsory license (Kijtiwatchakul 2007, 28). After enduring global shame for its attempts to prevent

its own compulsory license on efavirenz on May 4, 2007 (Kijtiwatchakul 2007, 39, 42). While Thailand was not the first country to invoke a compulsory license on AIDS medication—Zimbabwe, Malaysia, Zambia, and Malaysia had invoked CL on several different AIDS medications, most of them first-line drugs, in 2003 and 2004[11]—Thailand's was the first to invoke it on efavirenz, clopidogrel, and the second-line drug, lopinavir/ritonavir (WHO 2008, 38).

Under Mongkol's leadership, Thailand sought to improve the climate of access to pharmaceuticals for other developing countries. He went to Geneva to seek support from the WHO's representative body of member states, the World Health Assembly (WHA), succeeding in getting the WHA to adopt a resolution that urged the director-general to provide technical assistance and policy support to countries on issues related to TRIPS flexibilities (Wibulpolprasert et al. 2011). Thailand then became the first country to request that a WHO mission come to Thailand under World Health Assembly Resolution 60.30 of May 2007 (Wibulpolprasert et al. 2011). While the Rural Doctors who now controlled the ministry hoped for the mission to provide the country with something like a "seal of approval" for its decision to invoke a compulsory license (much as the ILO had bestowed on its budget numbers for the UC program), the WHO stopped short of doing so and instead took care only to interpret the relevant laws, due to the political sensitivity surrounding the issues (on the scope of WHO involvement, Brenny interview 2009).

The language voiced in the WHO Mission Report itself was emblematic of the WHO's growing confidence and ability to stake out a position on the issues, but it was also tempered by a sustained concern that some of its most vocal member countries (such as the United States) would find the WHO's work harmful to their own interests. The report pointed out how pharmaceutical production by the Indonesian government provided stability after private manufacturers halted production following the Asian financial crisis. It highlighted the fact that Brazil's success in fighting AIDS had been a result of its crucial reliance on local production capacity, discussed how this had improved its negotiating power for other drugs, and pointed to the experiences of Zimbabwe, Malaysia, Zambia, Indonesia, Brazil, and Thailand with compulsory licensing (WHO 2008, 38–42). The report drew attention to the fact that the WHO "advocates to Member States the importance of the TRIPS flexibilities to protect public health and promote access to essential medicines" (WHO 2008, 6). At the same time, the report was also carefully decorated with caveats, such as the following: "The report of this mission is not intended to make any evaluation or assessment of the use of TRIPS flexibilities in Thailand" (WHO 2008, 2). Attempting to sound as neutral and value-free as possible while wading into an obviously politicized subject, the report noted that the mission came at the request of the minister of public health and sought only to provide "technical information and policy option[s]," in accordance with its "terms of reference" (WHO 2008, 2, 6). However, the quiet and somewhat remarkable inclusion of William Aldis on the WHO Mission Team offered perhaps a more pointed view of where the WHO's heart was on the matter. The mission report was "widely interpreted to confirm the validity of government use licenses and their compliance with the TRIPS Agreement" (Wibulpolprasert et al. 2011).

Meanwhile, the professional movement of pharmacists continued to play a leading role in state capacity-building activities while these developments were occurring. In November 2007, the Faculty of Pharmacy and its partners in the AIDS movement organized the "International Conference on Compulsory Licensing: Innovation and Access for All" (EATG 2008). As was the case with the landmark conference before it in 2005, the conference brought together esteemed lawyers from around the world who had done pioneering work on CL, such as James Love and Brook Baker, as well as members of the AIDS movement and policymakers to discuss the issues.

Following a return to democracy in 2008, a new minister of public health, Chaiya Sasomsub, was appointed. The new minister caught the attention of the AIDS community when he suggested that the compulsory licensing declaration "might have been a politically correct decision but not legally correct" (quoted in Glaser and Murphy 2010, 229). The pronouncement led the Rural Doctors' Society to snap into action and Jon Ungpakorn of the AIDS Access Foundation to remark, "Our present health minister has no regard for public health issues. He is behaving like the commerce minister" (quoted in Glaser and Murphy 2010, 229).

The transfer of the head of Thailand's Food and Drug Administration, an outspoken Rural Doctor who had been a close aide to Dr. Mongkol and had chaired a panel related to drug price negotiations with pharmaceutical companies, prompted further concerns among members of the Rural Doctors' movement and the allies with whom it had worked closely for decades (the Foundation for Consumers and the AIDS Access Foundation) that the new government intended to weaken the country's commitment to the country's compulsory licensing policy (Treerutkuarkul 2008c). The head of the Rural Doctors' Society at the time publicly criticized the move, stating, "Dr. Siriwat's move clearly shows that the health minister doesn't want to continue the CL policy, or stand for the people as he has claimed" (quoted in Treerutkuarkul 2008c). Saree Ongsomwang, a former nurse who was also head of the Foundation for Consumers, warned that the episode bore the marks of an unfair abuse of power by the minister and urged that the case be reviewed to Administrative Court; she also suggested that Wichai Chokewiwat, a senior statesman in the Rural Doctors' movement and chairman of the Board of the Government Pharmaceutical Office and Compulsory Licensing Committee, might be next (Treerutkuarkul 2008c).

After the minister took the more substantive action of threatening to withdraw support for measures that made obtaining generic cancer drugs easier, the Rural Doctors' Society began publicly calling for his resignation (National News Bureau of Thailand 2008; Ruangdit and Treerutkuerkul 2008), while the Foundation for Consumers—inspired by some of the provisions in the 1997 constitution to increase citizen participation in politics—began a petition campaign to pressure him to step down from office (Ruangdit and Treerutkuerkul 2008), and his resignation soon followed. The turn of events was particularly sweet for the AIDS movement, which had supported the Rural Doctors' Movement's campaign for universal health care so strongly and then seen antiretroviral drugs excluded from the program's benefit package before finally being included later. Eight years after it had gathered the majority of signatures in the petition campaign to force parliament to consider universal health care, an important favor had been returned to them.

Conclusion

Thailand's transition to democracy in the 1990s occurred in parallel with the rise of an AIDS movement that sought to protect and support the rights of people living with HIV and AIDS. At a time when pharmaceutical costs remained high and the organization and capacity of the broader AIDS movement remained low, the state's commitment to treatment for AIDS remained weak, providing treatment only for opportunistic infections, such as tuberculosis, when patients' immune systems were compromised. The advent of life-saving technologies (combination antiretroviral therapy) in 1996 that could stop the progression of HIV/AIDS in its tracks added a new sense of urgency in a country that had already lost half a million lives to HIV/AIDS. However, cost pressures and a desire to maintain close trade relationships with the United States meant that embrace of those technologies was by no means a given.

This chapter highlights the indelible role played by a movement of medical professionals with knowledge of the law in helping to expand access to life-saving antiretroviral medication in Thailand. The professional movement was led by pharmacists in the Drug Study Group—in partnership with Rural Doctors working in the Ministry of Public Health and executives in the Government Pharmaceutical Office, supported by international partners such as Médecins Sans Frontières. Many of the professionals involved—pharmacists, doctors, lawyers, and economists among them—had longstanding ties dating back to the 1970s when the country had been under military rule. Working to improve medicine safety and access to drugs in the countryside, members of this movement took up positions in the country's most prestigious university and key positions in the state's health ministry. When democratization led an authoritarian government to relinquish control over the "rules of the game," the intellectual property knowledge of a professional movement would increasingly become an important resource for both the state and the broader AIDS movement.

In a competitive political environment that did not afford political parties the luxury of indulging in charlatan AIDS policy (as would happen in South Africa), these medical professionals used their knowledge of the law to train and empower the broader AIDS movement, which engaged in legal contests with pharmaceutical companies; to build state capacity and confidence related to the government's right to use compulsory licensing; and to help combat pressures that threatened to erode the government's commitment to universal access to antiretroviral drugs. At the heart of all of their contributions has been legal expertise, in particular knowledge of Thailand's patent law and the country's rights related to the production of generics under the WTO's TRIPS provisions. At a time when legal interpretations related to countries' rights remained a subject of debate, the professional movement not only helped the AIDS movement and the state gain greater confidence in this area, it also helped the country set bold new precedents related to compulsory licensing in the face of resistance that would be emulated by countries and organizations around the world. Thailand's professional movement contributed to the expansion of access to AIDS medicine by using its specialized knowledge, largely without any benefit to the people in the movement.

6

BRAZIL: CONSTITUTING RIGHTS, SETTING PRECEDENTS, CHALLENGING NORMS

> **Civil society groups used the judiciary not to ask for some sort of benefit from the state, but to force the state to comply with its legal obligations. You fortify people living with AIDS *not* by saying, "You're a victim." There are no victims, there are only citizens seeking their rights and therefore the state must recognize them!**
>
> —ABIA Attorney Miriam Ventura (quoted in Nunn 2009, 52).

In 1991—in the midst of economic crisis and just one year removed from passage of its landmark health care reform—Brazil's health minister made waves by announcing that his country would provide patients dying of AIDS with a miracle medication called AZT that could extend their lives. Brazil's commitment to provide its citizens with access to life-saving medicine set itself apart from other countries in the developing world—and many in the industrialized world. These commitments built on strong HIV prevention policies that the government had put in place earlier. And while the country's first treatment program would be a symbolic gesture more than anything—with rollout stalled by economic crisis—five years later the government would make much more meaningful commitments to provide those in need with access to state-of-the-art combination antiretroviral therapy that had the power to turn a fatal disease into a chronic illness. For its achievements, the country would go on to win international recognition as a model for the industrializing world from UNAIDS in 2000 and a Gates Award for Global Health in 2003 (Biehl 2007, 1088). But apart from awards for its domestic programs, Brazil would play an important leadership role in expanding access to HIV/AIDS medicine at the international level in staffing executive positions in the World Health Organization's AIDS program, in helping to codify and popularize a new language of human rights in treaties and conventions related to access to medicines, and in confronting governments, pharmaceutical companies, and international organizations that sought to prevent access to more affordable generic drugs.

Leading scholars have suggested that Brazil's leadership in the area of HIV/AIDS treatment has depended on "state-based activists" (Flynn 2013, 9; also Rich 2013). According to these accounts, Brazil's professional movement of sanitaristas, having occupied high positions in the federal bureaucracy, succeeded in using these positions to motivate the government to take a stronger stance on HIV/AIDS (Flynn 2013, 2015). These accounts offer critical insights by pointing to the importance of the state in providing treatment advocates with important powers. However, I suggest that the critical role that legal knowledge and expertise have played in Brazil's remarkable treatment access story has often been overlooked. As others have suggested, we must account for the role of "highly skilled activists" in these stories (Massard da Fonseca 2015, 79).

In a domain dominated by the strategic deployment of human rights discourse in legal instruments and battles over patent law, I suggest that a focus on these issues is central to understanding the roots of Brazil's success as well as the ongoing challenges the country faces. Amid competitive political dynamics that did not provide Brazilian policymakers with the luxury of entertaining dissident science (or obstructing the rollout of medication to those who needed it, as happened in South Africa), this chapter highlights the critical role that newly empowered professionals with knowledge and expertise in the law played in advancing access to AIDS treatment. In Brazil, these professionals with training in the law—sometimes lawyers, sometimes medical professionals who gained expertise through their professional work—played critical roles in leading efforts to expand access to medicine in Brazil in the wake of democratization. As in Thailand, they accomplished this by operating both from positions in the state and civil society.

From the early days, AIDS organizations in Brazil have relied on legal professionals to address workplace discrimination and later to hold the state accountable for new health rights embedded in the 1988 constitution by the movement of medical professionals known as the sanitaristas. However, until more recently, AIDS organizations frequently deferred to a movement of medical professionals (the sanitaristas) on complex issues related to intellectual property rights and patent law. These dynamics gradually began to change, however, with the recognition of the importance of patent law and the upskilling of AIDS activists who sought out legal training and engaged in processes of "expertification from below," which led to the formation of new organizations like the Working Group on Intellectual Property of the Brazilian Network for the Integration of Peoples (GTPI/REBRIP).

Amid a series of political administrations that did not question the basic science behind HIV/AIDS and a political context that increasingly emphasized individual rights, the movement of professionals with training in the law took advantage of opportunities to work inside the state and to lobby and partner with it, aligning significant legal knowledge and expertise toward the promotion of more progressive policies supportive of AIDS treatment. I argue that this interaction between the dynamics resulting from Brazil's democratization process and the deployment of legal knowledge and resources by the country's professional movement help to explain more fully the country's remarkable success in expanding access to treatment for AIDS domestically and abroad.

This account therefore underscores the influential role played by a legally proficient movement of medical professionals who embedded new health rights in the constitution that would ultimately give rise to challenges in the nation's courts; who used positions in a friendly state to draw on ties with civil society groups and international organizations to increase funding for treatment and to hold the state accountable for providing it; who provided assistance to government that would prove crucial in redefining the state's relationship with pharmaceutical companies; and who worked with the state to embed important new norms related to access to essential medicine in international legal conventions, displacing dominant legal interpretations that had privileged the interests of foreign governments and corporations. In the process, these advocates—most of whom did not need medication themselves or, as professionals, had the means to afford it—frequently drew on professional knowledge and expertise that set them apart from ordinary citizens.

Six years after Brazil's transition from democracy in 1991, with almost twenty thousand people infected with AIDS, Brazil had the highest burden of AIDS in Latin America and one of the highest burdens of AIDS in the world (Parker 1994, 28). When a visiting official from the World Health Organization stated that if nothing more were done to stop the epidemic, Brazil would have an epidemic on par with Africa, the country's president, Fernando Collor de Mello, was shaken into making the country's first national television address on AIDS (Nunn 2009, 59).

The country's first AIDS program had been formed almost a decade before in São Paulo in 1983, where AIDS had been reported within the gay community; the program grew out of an existing state program and was first organized by public health professionals, led by *sanitarista* Paulo Teixeira (Parker 2003, 147; Teixeira 2003, 184–86). Important AIDS NGOs, such as the Group to Support AIDS Prevention (GAPA),[1] the Brazilian Interdisciplinary AIDS Association (ABIA),[2] and the Group for the Valorization, Integration, and Dignity of the AIDS Patient (Grupo Pela VIDDA),[3] grew up around these efforts, with over fifty AIDS NGOs coming into being between 1985 and 1989, and a National AIDS Program (NAP) in 1985 (Parker 1994, 33, 40–41). Amid this growth, the influence of the professional movement of physicians working to improve public health, the *sanitaristas*, was unmistakable: Sanitary movement leaders such as Paulo Teixeira, Sergio Arouca, and Genia Kelson were involved in the HIV/AIDS movement, some sitting on the boards of the most influential organizations, like Grupo Pela VIDDA and ABIA, playing important roles in guiding their work (Nunn 2009, 51; Parker and Terto 2001, 22–23). *Sanitaristas* such as Hésio Cordeiro, who became the head of INAMPS, directed funding to found and support the work of organizations like ABIA and played leadership roles in the organization, connecting people to their work and directly assisting them; *sanitaristas* frequently held memberships in multiple organizations (Nunn 2009; Parker and Terto 2001, 17–18, 21–22, 29).

Setting Precedents for Expanded State Obligations

The state made some commitments to alleviate the suffering of HIV/AIDS patients through the provision of medicines to treat opportunistic infections that arose due to the compromised immune systems of AIDS patients as early as 1988 (Galvão 2002, 1862)—an extremely progressive commitment at the time for an industrializing country—although in practice these medicines were available only on a limited basis (Biehl 2007, 66). Leaders from the professional movement, like Teixeira, joined forces with prominent AIDS activists, such as sociologist Herbert de Souza (known popularly as Betinho), in calling for public provision of AZT in 1989 and 1990 after principles of universalism had been codified in the 1988 constitution but before the 1990 Unified Health System law had been passed. ABIA leaders, working in collaboration with the *sanitaristas*, castigated the conservative Collor administration and Health Minister Alceni Guerra for not providing treatment (Nunn 2009, 56).

Even more important than this public pressure and criticism, however, were the actual precedents set by the *sanitaristas* in providing access to AZT through state institutions at different levels of government. Some of the most prominent efforts were led by *sanitarista* Paulo Teixeira, whose state agency in São Paulo purchased a limited amount of AZT (enough to treat just 7 percent of the population in need in the state) in 1989 "as part of a strategy to create need, to generate demands and to spark involvement by society on the issue of antiretroviral treatment in Brazil" (quoted in Safreed-Harmon 2008, 3). These calls for treatment were soon echoed by several other notable Brazilian epidemiologists, all of which put further pressure on the federal government; INAMPS director Hésio Cordeiro (also a *sanitarista*) became a further source of pressure when he announced that he would provide treatment through INAMPS, although—amid economic crisis—these commitments never materialized (Nunn 2009, 53, 56).

As health minister in the fiscally conservative Collor administration in 1990, Alceni Guerra, a medical doctor and conservative clientelist politician who had served at INAMPS under the military government, had resisted the sanitary movement's agenda to fold his old agency into the Health Ministry and slowed down the *sanitaristas*' push for decentralization (Parker 1994, 37; Weyland 1996, 171). Yet in spite of Guerra being out of step with the *sanitaristas* on health care reform, the intense public scrutiny that had been generated around HIV/AIDS policy led Guerra to be somewhat more open to activists' demands related to AIDS treatment (Nunn 2009, 54, 57). When Guerra learned that the ministry had no AIDS drugs and that the cost of provision ($132 million) was less than the cost of hospitalization, he spontaneously announced at a media session that the government would provide the medication, justifying the decision in cost-benefit terms (Nunn 2009, 57–58). A commitment was formally signed into law in early 1991 (Biehl 2007, 66), but it was not until April that the first shipments of AZT went out to seven state governments (Nunn 2009, 58–59). *Sanitaristas* focused attention on the implementation problem, with Paulo Teixeira lamenting that just 2 percent of São Paulo's AIDS population would be able to receive medication with the supplies coming from the government (Nunn 2009, 59). These pressures and increasingly negative international attention contributed to an eye-popping expansion of the financial commitment to AIDS by the government, going from just over $640,000 in 1990 to $37 million two years later (Nunn 2009, 59–60).

Even though *sanitaristas* had reclaimed the highest ranks in the Health Ministry during the Franco government and AIDS funding by the government had increased substantially, a lack of ministerial and legislative appropriation—coupled with poor health infrastructure—between 1993 and 1995 led to a situation in which just 16 percent of patients were receiving ARVs in 1994, in spite of the government's stated treatment policy (Nunn 2009, 65; Nunn, da Fonseca, and Gruskin 2009). The government's inability to make good on its policy of providing universal access to AZT gave rise to new mobilizations that took place in the courtroom; these served to legitimize the claims made both by the AIDS movement and the professional movement (Nunn 2009, 52).

Constituting New Rights, Promoting Legal Strategies

The pioneering new rights that the *sanitaristas* had embedded in the 1988 constitution to guide implementation of the Unified Health System law would prove to be even more pivotal to the strategy and advocacy work of the *sanitaristas* and the AIDS movement in expanding access to antiretroviral medication. While the provision of legal assistance to those facing discrimination due to their HIV/ AIDS status was a prominent feature of the work of some of the earliest and most important organizations like GAPA–São Paulo and Grupo Pela VIDDA (Ventura 2003, 242; Parker 1994, 41), the AIDS movement did not actively participate in the pre-constitutional processes that led to the formation of the 1988 constitution (Ventura 2003, 244). Yet it was the legal aid programs of Pela VIDDA-Rio and GAPA–São Paulo, in particular, that played important roles in taking on strategically chosen lawsuits that aimed to protect the civil rights of people living with HIV/AIDS (Parker 2003, 160). These programs were emulated successfully in other Brazilian states (Ventura 2003, 245) and led influential lawyers, such as Nilo Batista of the National Lawyers Association, to be increasingly drawn into the work of ABIA (Parker and Terto 2001, 14–15). Attorneys played a key role in this work, representing clients in the justice system. As Miriam Ventura, director of Grupo Pela VIDDA's legal assistance program, stated, "The strategy [of] our legal department had two major fronts: First, to file lawsuits against the government, and second, to reinforce the claims with the Constitution that had been approved in 1988. This ideology and strategy was promoted by the sanitarista movement" (quoted in Nunn 2009, 51).

The first lawsuits related to HIV/AIDS aimed at pressuring government to adopt a policy of universal access to AIDS medicine began in 1990 (Ventura 2003, 244). Organizations like GAPA–São Paulo brought cases to court demanding medication on behalf of ordinary people, like schoolteacher Nair Soares Brito (Flynn 2014, 87). According to Grupo Pela VIDDA attorney Miriam Ventura, "These decisions helped to establish a broad policy of universal access to medication, which began in 1991 with the distribution of AZT in the public health network and was expanded as of 1995 with the supply of different medications that make up the so-called cocktail" (quoted in Ventura 2003, 244–45). While the effects of these early lawsuits were not immediate, the use of litigation proved to be a central pillar of the strategy of AIDS treatment activists in civil society pressuring the state to provide medicine (Flynn 2013, 8). Ventura notes that these legal mobilizations "utilized the language of human rights and the strategic application of national laws ... [and] succeeded in placing on the political agenda questions that affect the life of people living with HIV/AIDS, and in so doing altered public and state policies regarding health care" (quoted in Galvão 2002, 3). This approach drew not only on constitutional provisions that established "the right to health" but also on provisions that provided free judicial assistance to citizens who lacked resources (Biehl 2013, 423).

After researchers presented the efficacy of combination ARV therapy at the International AIDS Conference in Vancouver in 1996, Brazilian AIDS activists

(Nunn 2009, 96–97, 107). The new minister, José Serra, was an economist who brought into the ministry other economists and did much to support efforts to advance access to treatment, drawing on the vitality of the movement to insulate himself and further their agenda (Nunn 2009, 107, 140).

Prior to the 1990s, Brazil had not granted patents on pharmaceuticals (Shadlen 2009, 41). The country had, however, been a strong proponent of the formation of the WTO and had signed on to the WTO's Agreement on Trade-Related Aspects of Intellectual Property (TRIPS) agreement as the Franco government's adminis-tration came to an end in December 1994 (Biehl 2008, 3). Brazil's embrace of the agreement led to new national legislation in 1996 that would enable it to comply with TRIPS by protecting patents in all technological domains in Brazil, including pharmaceuticals. However, the legislation threatened to affect access to medicine in Brazil by going beyond TRIPS and recognizing patents that had been filed and obtained in other countries, effectively making it much easier for pharmaceuti-cal companies to maintain monopolies on brand-name drugs and, in the process, make them unaffordable to people who needed them (Chaves et al. 2008, 172).

Much like Thailand, Brazil's adoption of the 1996 Intellectual Property Law to comply with TRIPS came a full nine years before developing countries were required to pass legislation guaranteeing minimum standards of intellectual property protection (Reis et al. 2009, 21).[4] Brazil's commitment to free trade and the new intellectual property regime proved to be a predictable boon to the pharmaceutical industry. Between 1995 and 1997, the country's trade deficit in pharmaceuticals ballooned from $410 million to $1.3 billion, underscoring all the new drugs that had come to market through imports (Biehl 2008, 3). These dynamics predictably made knowledge of patent law critical for ensuring the country's ability to maintain access to affordable medicine.

The Health Ministry under Serra sought to balance the country's desire for free trade with its need to ensure access to cheap medications by using the country's relationships with international organizations that had been less friendly to AIDS treatment to the country's advantage. First, it deepened Bra-zil's partnership with the World Bank—which had promoted prevention over treatment—through a second AIDS loan in 1998 of $165 million, while at the same time concretely deepening Brazil's commitment to universal access to AIDS treatment by announcing that the country would begin to produce generic ARVs to keep costs down (Biehl 2007, 76, 216). Activists empowered by the National AIDS Program forced the government to draft legal articles that would allow for the compulsory licensing of drugs in the case of public health emergency, as allowed under the WTO's TRIPS provisions (Biehl 2007, 57), giving the coun-try the ability to import or produce cheap generic versions of trademarked medications in exchange for a small royalty fee. Using that leverage, the government actively entered into negotiations with domestic and pharmaceutical companies to reduce prices for AIDS medication. These negotiations took a more serious form in 2000 when Brazil threatened to issue licenses for generic production if drug companies didn't reduce prices. This sparked a trade dispute with the United States in 2000 and a broader global dialogue about AIDS drug pricing.

These moves came at a time when the World Health Organization and progressive international NGOs, such as the Consumer Project on Technology, Health Action International, and Médecins Sans Frontières (MSF), were playing important roles in helping developing countries to understand their rights related to compulsory licensing under WTO trade law (Chorev 2012b; Flynn 2013, 13). However, in the early 2000s, threats of U.S. pressure prevented many countries from exercising their rights under trade laws to invoke compulsory licenses and produce medicine locally or import generic medication, in spite of being well within their rights to do so. Moreover, to that point even those in the broader AIDS movement who needed medication to survive had not been fully aware of the implications of the trade laws on access to medicines. The challenge of understanding a complex body of knowledge like trade law frequently stymied activists, who were more comfortable with demonstrations and more traditional forms of social movement tactics. Mario Scheffer, a coordinator from Grupo Pela VIDDA-São Paulo, said "Negotiations and treatments have always been a very complex topic and not always very transparent for civil society. Within the priorities of the movement, it was not preferred or prioritized due to the technical level required, difficulty in acquiring information, and also lack of interest" (quoted in Flynn 2013, 12).

Longtime *sanitaristas* who had been working on these issues since the early 1990s and had developed considerable expertise in the law, such as Eloan Pinheiro and Jorge Bermudez, however, stepped in and connected AIDS activists who had been more directly involved with client work and protests with the organizational resources of the National AIDS Program and other state agencies (Flynn 2013, 12). After a twenty-year career working for transnational pharmaceutical companies, Pinheiro went to work for the government's pharmaceutical manufacturer, Farmanguinhos, in the late 1980s, eventually becoming its director in 1994 (Flynn 2014, 95–96). Pinheiro had been the head of the country's chemical workers' union in the 1970s, had played a role in the creation of the Workers' Party in 1979, and was so deeply committed to the cause of expanding access to medicine that she approved the sale of medicine to AIDS activists in 2001 for transport into South Africa in defiance of transnational pharmaceutical companies who sought to maintain their monopoly (Flynn 2014, 95).

To committed *sanitaristas* with expertise in the law, like Pinheiro, the subordination of public rights guaranteed by Brazil's constitution to patents, which protected the property of private companies, was exploitative and perverse; she felt that access to medicines was a human right, and she used her expertise to improve state capacity and leverage the law to advance those ideals (Flynn 2014, 95–97). On the country's backwards patent legislation, which did more to protect the interests of pharmaceutical companies than patients, Pinheiro said, it "was simply 'wrong'"; as head of Farmanguinhos, Pinheiro therefore set out to ensure that the country had the ability to produce generic formulations of needed anti-retroviral medications herself through processes of reverse engineering (quoted in Biehl 2004, 115). Such expertise and ability would prove critical in helping the country to resist foreign attempts to undermine the government's policy authority and in forging new international norms vis-à-vis a series of international treaties and conventions. These efforts to protect the country's access to medicine in Farmanguinhos were supplemented by the Cardoso administration's decision to give the Ministry of Health's Health Surveillance Agency the power to review and influence the patent process, starting in 1999 (Shadlen 2009, 46).[5]

In a move designed to put pressure on Brazil and rein in potential use of flexibilities provided under its own law and TRIPS, the U.S. Trade Representative began discussions with Brazil in the month before the 2000 International AIDS Conference in Durban, South Africa (Flynn 2013, 12). One month later, *sanitarista* Paulo Teixeira took an opportunity to criticize the United States for applying pressure to Brazil for producing drugs locally at the International AIDS Conference (Nunn, da Fonseca, and Gruskin 2009). At the same time, Brazilian officials at the conference presented data showing that the country had saved nearly $680 million in deferred hospital admissions between 1997 and 2000 due to the country's AIDS treatment program, fueling international interest in the "Brazilian model" (Flynn 2013, 12). Soon after that, the United States registered the dispute formally at the WTO in 2001 (Nunn, da Fonseca, and Gruskin 2009) and requested the creation of a WTO dispute settlement body (Flynn 2013, 12). Serra then personally charged Brazil's diplomat to the WTO to "find some way that no one can ever file another trade dispute against Brazil, or against any other developing country related to essential medicines" (Viana quoted in Nunn, da Fonseca, and Gruskin 2009).

Treatment advocates in the broader movement until that time had not been fully aware of the implications of trade laws on access to medicines; as one activist noted, "We were somewhat aware of patent laws when they were passed in 1996. But we really began to see the impact when the U.S. set up the panel at the WTO" (quoted in Flynn 2013, 12). In 2001, amid recognition of the emerging importance of intellectual property to the issue of access to medicine, some Brazilian civil society organizations, supported by international NGOs (OXFAM and Médecins Sans Frontières), sought to become more informed on legal issues related to intellectual property and join the increasingly formidable ranks of legal expertise operating in the higher reaches of the Brazilian state.

Together, they formed the Working Group on Intellectual Property of the Brazilian Network for the Integration of Peoples (GTPI/REBRIP) (Chaves et al. 2008, 175). The umbrella organization included AIDS NGOs as well as social movements, other NGOs, trade unions, and some professional associations (Reis et al. 2009, 30). And while the organization's focus went well beyond issues related to access to medicine and included concern for "economic, social, cultural, ethical and environmentally sustainable development," the appointment (and subsequent reappointment) of the legally savvy AIDS advocacy watchdog ABIA as GTPI/REBRIP's coordinator gives evidence of the growing importance of the law to AIDS activism in the area of health and beyond in Brazil (Chaves et al. 2008, 175–76).

GTPI/REBRIP sought to identify approaches to broadening pharmaceutical access, promoting cooperation in the Global South, impacting public opinion related to IP issues, and monitoring international fora where these issues are discussed (Chaves et al. 2008, 176), including the Intergovernmental Working Group on Public Health, Innovation, and Intellectual Property at the WHO (Reis et al. 2009, 33). The group's opposition to patents was informed by experiences with India's activist Lawyers Collective (Chan 2015, 124), and one of ABIA's first actions as head of the Working Group involved hiring two attorneys whose major area of expertise had been intellectual property rights in order to help build the case for compulsory licensing (Parker 2007, 23). This new coalition would come to play an important role on the country's subsequent clashes over intellectual property issues in 2001 and beyond. And it would play an important role in helping the Brazilian government to redesign its regulatory rules related to pharmaceutical policy (Massard da Fonseca 2015, 78–79).

While disagreement reigned among ministries within Brazil in 2001 over what position to take on intellectual property issues given the U.S. pressures, the Brazilian Health Ministry, led by Serra with Paulo Teixeira as director of the National AIDS Program, took up the high cost of AIDS drugs, such as nelfinavir and efavirenz, at international forums, including the UN Commission on Human Rights, the World Health Organization, and the UN General Assembly, working with supportive international NGOs and governments to win resolutions in support of their position (Flynn 2013, 13–14). At the same time, the Serra- and Teixeira-led government efforts involved reaching out to domestic NGOs to ensure that they would have strong support during the deliberations of the WTO Dispute Settlement Panel and price negotiations, as well as international NGOs, such as James Love's CPTech, MSF, Oxfam, and ACT-UP (Flynn 2013, 13). These efforts led to agreements for price reductions on some antiretroviral drugs with Merck and Roche Laboratories in 2001, including a 65 percent price reduction on indinavir, a 59 percent reduction on efavirenz, and a 40 percent price cut on nelfinavir (Vitória 2003, 249). The coalition-building effort by the Ministry of Health was then turned into a major public relations campaign directed against the United States, which included advertisements in U.S. newspapers like the *New York Times,* and turned the panel into a "public relations disaster for the United States," which ultimately caused the United States to withdraw the panel during the UNGASS proceedings in June, under the pretense that Brazil had not actually invoked a compulsory license (quoted in Flynn 2013, 15).

As another part of its strategy, the government—influenced by the contingent of *sanitaristas* playing a leadership role in the Health Ministry—sponsored a resolution in the UN Council on Human Rights that passed by a 52–0 vote over the vocal protests of the United States; the resolution, which amounted to "the first international human rights resolution to explicitly address the right to access to medicines" (Nunn, da Fonseca, and Gruskin 2009), built on earlier proposals the country had advanced at the International AIDS Conference in 1998 that suggested universal access to AIDS drugs should be a human right (Wetzler 2007, 1). This was subsequently followed by a "Declaration of Commitment on HIV/ AIDS" at the UN General Assembly Special Session on HIV/AIDS in June 2001, which likewise reiterated the fundamental human right of access to medicine (Flynn 2013, 14). Serra himself then went to the World Health Assembly to try to get a similar resolution passed, which would also include an international pricing database to encourage greater transparency in pharmaceutical pricing with the aim of eliminating or at least reducing the dramatic disparities in pricing around the world (Nunn, da Fonseca, and Gruskin 2009). The country's influence in the WHO would be further strengthened when Paulo Teixeira was invited by the new WHO director to formulate HIV/AIDS policy at the WHO based on Brazil's experience in 2003 (Cohen and Lybecker 2005, 225).[6] Even more substantively, the government's AIDS team played a lead role in crafting the developing country position that would affirm countries' right to produce or import generics during public health emergencies in the Doha Declaration on the TRIPS Agreement and Public Health (Nunn, da Fonseca, and Gruskin 2009). Brazil's efforts would play a key role in changing norms at the WTO at the end of 2001 when the organization affirmed that the WTO would not stand as an obstacle to national responses to HIV/AIDS (Galvão 2005, 1111).

These developments would have ramifications on the sensitive negotiations taking place domestically between pharmaceutical manufacturers and the Brazilian government, putting substantial pressure on pharmaceutical companies to reduce prices. While Merck had initially threated to sue the government over a violation of its patent on efavirenz, it eventually would agree to a price cut of nearly 60 percent, worth $39 million (Flynn 2013, 14). Negotiations with Roche would also lead to a 40 percent cut in the cost of nelfinavir, with health officials maintaining close communications with private industry in Brazil in case a compulsory license was issued (Flynn 2013, 14–15). However, some negotiated agreements, such as the one reached with Abbott over Kaletra in 2005, lowered the cost of drugs but would also have negative consequences impacting broader abilities of the state to expand access to the drug by restricting the ability of the country to invoke compulsory licenses on the drug, limiting technology transfer and investment in local production related to it, and fixing the price for six years; this decision would lead GTPI to file a lawsuit against the government, demanding that it issue a compulsory license that would decrease the price further (Chaves et al. 2008, 178). The government did go so far as to put in place preliminary agreements with Indian pharmaceutical companies to help provide for two medications that consumed 60 percent of the country's AIDS treatment budget and to arrange international support from the WHO (Biehl 2007, 1106).

In May 2005, following intense lobbying of the government to declare a compulsory license, an AIDS movement now more informed on issues related to intellectual property would make its voice heard: First, representatives from civil society who had gained greater knowledge of the law applied pressure to the government through seats on the National Health Council, which served as an influential adviser to the Minister of Health (Eimer and Lütz 2010, 144). Second, GTPI/REBRIP issued a statement on licensing AIDS drugs that was supported by 138 different organizations (Parker 2007, 23). While movement activists would unsuccessfully use both protests and lawsuits to try to push the government to issue a compulsory license on Kaletra (lopinavir/ritonavir) in 2005 (Flynn 2013, 19), the government did lay the groundwork for subsequent use of compulsory licensing by announcing that the drug was "in the public interest" and demanding that the company lower its price, which ultimately led to a lower negotiated price (Chaves et al. 2008, 171). The result of this failure to push the state to do more, however, would lead the intellectual property–focused GTPI to work with MSF to do a study assessing the capacity of local pharmaceutical companies to produce first- and second-line antiretroviral drugs, findings that would subsequently be corroborated by the Clinton Foundation and UNDP; at the same time it took actions aimed at questioning the patents of lopinavir/ritonavir and tenofavir with Brazil's patent office and ensuring that the country's congress would receive information on the impact of intellectual property–related legislation on access (Chaves et al. 2008, 178–80). GTPI/REBRIP's civil public action, demanding that the government issue a compulsory license on lopinavir/ritonavir, was the first such action in Brazil and reflected the movement's growing prowess on legal matters; while a preliminary ruling was unsuccessful, a further judgment is still pending (Reis et al. 2009, 35).

The threat of compulsory licensing that would hang over negotiations again and again would prove vital to Brazil's successful strategy of ensuring the cheap provision of medication through negotiations until 2007. The National AIDS Program director at the time, Mariângela Batista Galvão Simão, a *sanitarista*, noted that a compulsory license is "possible and . . . legal" (quoted in Okie 2006). While some have characterized these threats as "rebellious acts" by the government (Olsen and Sinha 2013, 335), these actions took place amid the government's broader compliance with TRIPS and recognition of patent rights filed in other countries that went beyond TRIPS in restricting countries' policy autonomy. The whole situation highlights the complex relationship of the state with the broader international trade regime.

The head of Brazil's negotiating team over the price of efavirenz with the pharmaceutical company Merck was none other than the country's health minister, a *sanitarista* named José Gomes Temporão (Parker 2007, 22) who had previously worked at the Oswaldo Cruz Institute and played an active role in advocacy for the SUS in the 1980s.[7] In April 2007, just as it had done with Kaletra two years earlier, the government declared access to efavirenz in the public interest (Chaves et al. 2008, 171). However, on May 7, 2007, President Lula broke from Brazil's past pattern of negotiations in making threats that it would introduce compulsory licensing and instead declared that Brazil would invoke a compulsory license on efavirenz, a drug used by some seventy-five thousand Brazilians (Biehl 2008, 5), foregoing Merck's offer of a 30 percent price reduction (Parker 2007, 23) and forcing Merck Sharp Dohme (MSD) into a $40 million loss; to legitimate the action, Brazil's declaration explicitly drew on treaties in which the right to health had been a major part—the International Declaration of Human Rights; the Convention on Economic, Social and Cultural Rights; the country's constitution; and of course the Doha Declaration (Flynn 2013, 18). The announcement was made live on television and included speeches first by the HIV+ civil society representative of the AIDS movement on the National Health Council, followed by Health Minister José Gomez Temporão, a *sanitarista*, followed by President Lula himself, the order seemingly orchestrated to impress upon viewers the role that ordinary citizens affected by AIDS had played in the decision (Parker 2007, 23). However, the country's ultimate decision to embrace compulsory licensing after threatening to do so many times before came only after Thailand's declaration of compulsory licensing on that drug in 2006 and the second-line antiretroviral lopinavir/ritonavir and the heart medication clopidogrel in January 2007 (Kijti-watchakul 2007, 25). In a letter to Thailand's Minister of Public Health, Brazil's health minister declared that "Thailand's CL is a great inspiration to Brazil" (Kijti-watchakul 2007, 42), underscoring both the changing international environment that Brazil's movement of legally minded medical professionals had played a part in creating and the role that similar movements of medical professionals with legal training were playing in helping to cement these changes internationally.

The country's use of compulsory licensing in 2007 accorded it membership in a relatively small club of just fifteen developing countries that had previously done so (Flynn 2013, 4). With the license, the cost of efavirenz dropped by two-thirds, and the cost savings to Brazil were estimated at $104 million between 2007 and 2011 (Flynn 2013, 18). While the government faced an inevitable public relations campaign from the pharmaceutical industry condemning its actions, domestic activists from NGOs like ABIA worked to combat concerns spread by the pharmaceutical industry that compulsory licensing was illegal, would lead to lower quality generics, and would threaten supply (Flynn 2013, 19). Later that same year, building on the movement's burgeoning confidence in intellectual property issues, the ABIA-led GTPI would use its growing legal standing and expertise to petition Brazil's attorney general disputing the constitutionality of laws that provided for patent protection of pharmaceuticals and other products patented overseas, including some that had been in the public domain (Chaves et al. 2008, 172, 181). And in a democratic environment no longer dominated by the military, it would use its growing legal clout to file briefs and participate in public hearings in the country's congress on bills bearing on access to medicine (Reis et al. 2009, 37–38).

Conclusion

Immediately following passage of Brazil's universal access to antiretroviral law, some 55,600 people were receiving ARVs (Biehl 2007, 69). Ten years later, that number would increase to 190,000 (Reis et al. 2009, 16). Hospitalization rates for AIDS fell by 80 percent, and overall mortality rates from AIDS fell by half during the first ten years of the country's treatment program (Olsen and Sinha 2013, 335). Brazil's progressive treatment programs would be recognized by UNAIDS and the Gates Foundation, and the country would play a leading role in helping to create a more favorable environment for access to medicine internationally, even offering technical assistance to countries in Africa to fight HIV/AIDS (Cassier and Correa 2007).

The movement of professionals with knowledge of the law played a key role in the expansion of Brazil's AIDS treatment policies. In the wake of democratic transition at a time when rule by the country's military was no longer supreme, elites with a foothold in the state and competency in the law stood particularly empowered to make major contributions to efforts to expand access to life-saving pharmaceuticals in Brazil. Drawing on these privileged positions and legal training that set them apart from the masses, Brazil's *sanitarista* movement embedded new rights in the constitution and played leadership roles on the boards of new AIDS organizations. They encouraged AIDS activists to draw on these new rights and to hold the state accountable for them through court-based legal mobilizations, even though they did not need the medication themselves. Operating from privileged positions in the state, *sanitaristas* set important precedents by directly providing access to antiretroviral therapy in an effort to press the national government to make access universal. And they used state offices to mobilize and direct international organization and civil society support to address problems in the rollout of antiretroviral medication programs. Finally, they drew on their legal expertise to help the government successfully resist pressure by foreign governments and pharmaceutical companies to protect patents and restrict access to needed medication while at the same time fashioning new conventions at the international level that made the international climate related to pharmaceutical access much friendlier to Brazil and other nations in the developing world.

In the process, AIDS organizations staffed primarily by people living with HIV and AIDS, which had for a long time deferred to medical professionals with knowledge of patent laws, gradually began to recognize the importance of the law and increasingly sought to become more conversant in intellectual property law. For some HIV+ activists, this meant participating in a bottom-up process of education and "expertification" in legal matters. However, some leading AIDS organizations, like ABIA, had for a long time relied on lawyers in legal advocacy work and simply redirected their focus to intellectual property rights and added legal staff in that area. This chapter's focus on the AIDS movement's growing reliance on lawyers and focus on the law is in no way intended to diminish the historic role that it has played in more traditional social movement activities in Brazil. However, it does highlight the importance of legally trained professionals working together to advance access to life-saving medicine. Like those legally minded *sanitaristas* in the state, lawyers in Brazil's AIDS movement frequently advocated for these changes using legal means and resources that set them apart from ordinary citizens.

7

SOUTH AFRICA: CONTESTING THE LUXURY OF AIDS DISSIDENCE

The [AIDS Law Project] and its allies in the Treatment Action Campaign and elsewhere led a legal march that vanquished many foes. They vindicated the power of popular activism in asserting constitutional rights.

—Constitutional Court Judge and AIDS Law Project Founder, Edwin Cameron (quoted in Moyle 2015, viii)

TAC has brought life to the law and the Constitution . . . TAC's use of the law has brought real improvements in people's quality of life.

—Adila Hassim, Head of Litigation and Legal Services, AIDS Law Project (quoted in Treatment Action Campaign 2010, 29)

South Africa currently has the largest AIDS treatment program in the world, with approximately half of the nation's seven million HIV+ people on life-saving combination antiretroviral therapy (Nordling 2016). This might seem to give cause to celebrate South Africa as a case of success in terms of AIDS treatment. While the AIDS epidemic's explosion in South Africa is a product of apartheid-era neglect of the problem, the properties of the disease itself, and a range of other important factors,[1] the ANC's handling of the epidemic after apartheid nevertheless contributed significantly to the spread of the disease. Under the Mandela regime, initial promise quickly turned to despair as prevention efforts faltered. Then, under Thabo Mbeki, the government would suggest that HIV does not cause AIDS, imply that ARVs are dangerous, and emphasize the use of garlic, olive oil, and beetroot for the treatment of AIDS rather than proven antiretroviral therapy.

In this context, the virus took off: In 1993, just one year before the fall of apartheid, the country's HIV prevalence rate was 2 percent; however, by one estimate, a decade later—the same year that the government finally committed to rolling out antiretroviral therapy—the HIV prevalence rate was among the highest in the world, at almost 18 percent (UNAIDS 2015). More than a thousand people were dying of AIDS in South Africa each day (Fourie 2006, 1), and the country held the ignominious distinction of having the largest infected population in the world. Worse still, an influential study by researchers at Harvard University found that if South Africa had implemented an ARV treatment program sooner that included prophylaxis for

there was a moment of flux in which any number of different political and eco-nomic futures was possible (Bond 2000, 15). The apartheid government began to put a "higher premium on human rights," and a consensus on the rights of HIV-positive workers consequently developed (Fourie 2006, 85). In 1992, the government's growing willingness to take part in important dialogues with important actors that had previously been shut out of discussions on neglected health issues was made visible at a joint ANC-government conference that sought to develop a framework for responding to the HIV/AIDS epidemic. Under the apartheid government, the number of AIDS cases in the country to that point had largely gone unrecognized, and the conference succeeded in creating the National AIDS Committee of South Africa (NACOSA), which aimed to coordi-nate the state and NGO response to the epidemic (Sember 2008, 62). NACOSA represented an important step in the country's fight against HIV/AIDS in that it marked a clear collaboration between government and civil society on AIDS, in particular on the National AIDS Plan that it would produce in 1994 (Pelser, Ngwena, and Summerton 2004, 311).

However, somewhat strikingly, medical professionals—rather than people afflicted with HIV/AIDS—were the driving forces behind the plan. Peter Busse, who would found the National Association of People with AIDS (NAPWA) in 1994 and was one of the only HIV-positive people on hand during the NACOSA meetings, recounts, "There were about 50 to 60 people there. Everyone was going around the room saying who they were and what they were doing. I suddenly realized that in this entire grouping of people that were writing the National AIDS Plan there wasn't one person who was HIV-positive" (quoted in Moyle 2015, 30). While the plan that came out of the conference was forward-thinking in many respects, its lack of attention to how the plan would be funded was one of its more unfortunate consequences (Sember 2008, 62). At the same time, as a growing number of important court cases around this time would affirm, the instruments of law—which had previously been used by the apartheid state to promote stigmatization and criminalization of victims of HIV—were increas-ingly being used to protect the rights of AIDS victims (Fourie 2006, 93).

Just as universities had been a home for professional movement activism in the health care domain, activism within the legal profession also found a home in South Africa's universities. In particular, the University of Witwatersrand proved to be an important site for legal activism. Whereas the Centre for Health Policy had provided a home for professional movement activists concerned with trans-formational health care reform, the university's Centre for Applied Legal Stud-ies (CALS) provided a space for human rights lawyers to practice their trade against a broader backdrop of repressive state control. One such lawyer working on human rights issues at CALS was Edwin Cameron, for whom the great need for greater rights protections for those living with HIV/AIDS had been brought home through the deportation of HIV-positive mineworkers (Cameron 2005, 52). As a gay white lawyer who had attended Oxford, Cameron bore little resemblance to the great mass of South Africans affected by HIV—who were poor, black, frequently unemployed, and bereft of formal education. However, while his access to medical schemes and antiretroviral medication distinguished him from most of South Africa's AIDS patients, Cameron was himself also HIV-positive and had a history working for progressive causes before 1994. Recalling what brought him to work on legal issues related to HIV/AIDS, Cameron mentions that the deportation of HIV-positive mineworkers left an impression because "I was a human rights lawyer doing trade-union work, that drew me into AIDS policy and litigation. Not my own condition, but a condition outside, graphically linked to apartheid injustice" (quoted in Moyle 2015, 17).

Since 1987, CALS had provided a space for lawyers to provide advice and work on litigation and policy related to AIDS, and Cameron served as its chair until 1996 (Moyle 2015, 23–24). Cameron was one of the few white lawyers who defended ANC guerillas (Power 2003). And in the final years of apartheid, working with other activists, Cameron sought to address the problem of stigma and discrimination against people with HIV/AIDS by founding the AIDS Consortium as a project within CALS in 1992 (Treatment Action Campaign 2010, 7). The consortium aimed to link organizations working on HIV/AIDS and promote a nondiscriminatory approach to the disease, guided by a human rights framework known as the AIDS Charter, which laid out the basic rights of people living with HIV and AIDS and served as the organization's founding document (AIDS Consortium 2015). The AIDS Consortium would grow to become its own independent NGO in 1998 and register as a network of more than one thousand AIDS Service Organizations in 2000 (AIDS Consortium 2015). Even more important than this, however, was Cameron's founding of the AIDS Law Project in 1993.

Cameron began raising money to start the ALP after serving as the lawyer for a man whose HIV status had been wrongfully disclosed by his doctor (Moyle 2015, 16). Just as he had with the AIDS Consortium, Cameron initially founded the ALP as a project within CALS, which provided it with resources and needed legitimacy with which to attract donors (Grebe 2011, 859). However, apart from size, what distinguished the ALP from the AIDS Consortium was that the ALP specifically focused on providing legal services to those who suffered from discrimination due to AIDS, effectively using "litigation and the courts to take the politics out of HIV/AIDS" (Moyle 2015, x, 17). As the first specialist AIDS legal organization in sub-Saharan Africa, the ALP drew on a wide range of strategies grounded in the law to address issues related to AIDS and social justice, from providing clients with legal advice to lobbying to helping companies adopt fair workplace policies to launching court cases and offering legal knowledge in high-profile cases (Moyle 2015, xii, 31). Over time, the ALP broadened its areas of focus to include public education and the promotion of legal awareness through publications and the media (Moyle 2015, 83). This approach led Mark Heywood—who would later become ALP's director—to remark that "Cameron pioneered the idea in South Africa of using the law to defend people with HIV and AIDS" (quoted in *Mail and Guardian* 1999).

After Cameron departed the ALP to become a High Court judge in 1994 (Moyle 2015, 17), Zackie Achmat became the director. While not a lawyer by training, Achmat was a gay HIV-positive intellectual who had received an initial grounding in the law through his time as an anti-apartheid activist and later as a gay rights activist. Achmat would himself leave the organization shortly after its founding to create and direct the National Coalition for Lesbian and Gay Equality in 1994, an organization that aimed to ensure that gay rights would be protected in the new South African constitution (Forbath 2011, 51; Power 2003). ALP's subsequent director, Mark Heywood, had worked with Achmat in the underground revolutionary socialist Marxist Workers' Tendency (MWT), a Trotskyite wing of the ANC, and the two developed an extraordinarily close relationship (Grebe 2011, 856). Drawing on the skills of professionals with training in the law, like Fatima Hassan and Adila Hassim, the ALP aimed to provide legal assistance to those who faced discrimination due to their HIV-positive status and would play an important role in upholding the rights of victims of AIDS (Cameron 2005, 32). As the only such organization providing these services, the ALP in 1994 set up a national referral system to help serve people seeking advice and assistance called the AIDS Legal Network and began to get involved in legal reform related to HIV/AIDS through the South African Law Commission (Moyle 2015, 32). While the leadership of the ALP has preferred that the story of the ALP be told as "the story of their clients and their cases" (Moyle 2015, x)—effectively extracting lawyers from the story and re-centering the history of ALP around citizen plaintiffs themselves—it has in fact been these legal activists who have taken up the cause of citizens and represented them in court.

Democratization and the Role of the Professional Movement in the Government's Changing Approach to HIV/AIDS

After the fall of apartheid, there was good reason for a sense of optimism that the incoming government's approach to HIV/AIDS would be much more aggressive than it had been under the apartheid government, which had for the most part neglected the epidemic entirely. However, pressure for the government to adopt a stronger stance on AIDS did not come from the masses: just 1 percent of citizens believed AIDS should be the government's top priority at the time of the elections in 1994, and that number would rise to just 13 percent in 2000 (Afrobarometer 2004, 4). AIDS was "not a central concern of voters" (Lieberman 2009, 132). In the absence of mass demands, pressure for the ANC to take a rights-based approach to the epidemic came from the professional movement.

The lead role played by the professional movement in fashioning the National AIDS Program and NACOSA before the fall of apartheid, in combatting stigma and discrimination through the creation of organizations like the AIDS Consortium, and in other related human rights work at CALS positioned the movement as a reliable source for advice and expertise related to policymaking on HIV/AIDS in the post-apartheid era. In this new environment, the ALP sought to monitor policy and legal developments and to inject the knowledge, expertise, and research into policy discussions that had been sorely lacking under the apartheid government and were largely absent in the first years of newly democratic South Africa (Moyle 2015, 45, 52). Although in some cases the transition from apartheid had led the movement to play a smaller role in health—NPPHCN's vaunted National AIDS Program, for example, was forced to wind down over lack of funding in 1995 as the democratically elected government took control (Pelser, Ngwena, and Summerton 2004, 304)—in other respects members of the movement now enjoyed greater access to the halls of power.

In spite of the lack of pressure from the general population, the government did immediately signal a higher profile approach to fighting AIDS when AIDS was granted status as a "Presidential Lead Project" (Sember 2008, 62). Members of the professional movement, including Manto Tshabalala-Msimang, a medical doctor who had been a member of NPHCCN and who would go on to become health minister in 1999, helped draft the country's new AIDS strategy; the strategy espoused human rights a central part of the government's approach to managing the epidemic (Fourie 2006, 107–8). In addition, the country's new constitution—widely recognized as one of the most progressive in the world—outlined a series of important new rights and granted citizens the power to take the state to court if it did not meet its obligations. In the area of health, Section 27 of the constitution stated that everyone should "have access to health care services, including reproductive health care," that no one "may be refused emergency treatment," and that the government must "take reasonable legislative and other measures, within its available resources, to achieve the progressive realisation" of the rights laid out in the constitution (Hassim et al. 2007, 33–34).

Almost immediately, however, the government committed a series of missteps related to its handling of HIV/AIDS. While NACOSA advanced a bold intersectoral plan for combating HIV/AIDS, the government decided to house NACOSA within the Department of Health rather than make it an autonomous organization that operated across social sectors, as had been recommended (Sember 2008, 62). It then proceeded to falter in executing NACOSA's plan (Pelser, Ngwena, and Summerton 2004, 305–6). And although Cameron, as the founding director of the AIDS Law Project, succeeded in obtaining a meeting with Mandela's deputy presidents, F. W. de Klerk and Thabo Mbeki, to discuss the government's AIDS policy in February of 1996 (Power 2003), Mandela's first significant public statement on AIDS would not come until February 1997, nearly three years after he took office (Cameron 2005, 124). Later that summer, the Health Minister announced that AIDS would be a notifiable disease (originally a policy of the apartheid government in 1987) (Fourie 2006, 131). Giving the disease notifiable status made quarantine of AIDS patients possible and threatened to drive carriers of the disease underground (Moyle 2015, 37), rather than according them confidentiality and respect for their rights as human beings.[2]

In the interim, more missteps followed. First, the government channeled a significant amount of money into a play aimed at raising AIDS awareness, called *Sarafina II* (Gevisser 2007, 732). Although the idea of using a play as a medium to increase public awareness of AIDS had its merits, AIDS experts had not been consulted to inform the production, underscoring the lack of connection between the government and the country's professional movement working on HIV/AIDS. The play was critically rebuked for being "confused and irrelevant" (Nattrass 2004, 45). The debacle "introduced and solidified a defensiveness in government" (Fourie 2006, 124), reinforcing a culture of closure within the ANC that was fueled by the party's unrivaled success at the polls.

Just one year later, the government played a leading role in raising false hopes around a South African antiretroviral treatment for AIDS that was being called virodene (Pieterse 2008, 367). But the academic team from the University of Pretoria that promoted it had not obtained proper ethical clearance for their research, and the government—which was supportive of the project—removed the chairperson and other members of the Medicines Control Council that had repeatedly rejected it as a viable therapy (Nattrass 2004, 45–46). The "therapy," it turns out, was made of toxic industrial chemicals. This debacle marked one of the government's first early dalliances with fringe science at the expense of the general public and a more informed and substantive connection with the country's professional movement working on HIV/AIDS. News outlets at the time also pointed to financial interests held by the ANC in the drug's development (Fourie 2006, 125). However, perhaps the greatest tragedy of the scandal, aside from marking the beginning of the government's alignment with dissident AIDS science, was the fact that the ability of combination antiretroviral therapy to effectively stop AIDS in its tracks had already been established one year earlier at the International AIDS Conference in Canada in 1996.

The remarkable political dynamics that led the ANC to claim such a wide margin of victory and to close ranks also led the health minister to insist on loyalty to the ANC's plan for transformation and to resist criticism, no matter the missteps. In this context, she deemed "any questioning of or negative comment on her department's actions of HIV and AIDS as either . . . disloyal or racist" (Fourie 2006, 119). Accusations of racism were also leveled against the opposition Democratic Alliance Party after it drew attention to the party's role in the scandals (Fourie 2006, 125).

If the government's actions to this point constituted a series of missteps, then in 1998 the administration's unorthodox approach to AIDS became dangerous when Health Minister Nkosazana Dlamini-Zuma announced that the government would not roll out a program to provide pregnant mothers with HIV with a therapy known to be effective in preventing transmission to unborn children in the womb (Nattrass 2004, 47). This program relied on administration of the drug zidovudine, or AZT, to prevent pregnant mother-to-child transmission (PMTCT) of HIV and stood to save some forty thousand infants from infection (Power 2003). Important international and local research had shown PMTCT to be cost-effective: A short course of AZT had been shown to cut transmission rates in half, although most mothers were too impoverished to be able to afford the cost of treatment, which cost roughly $75 (Gumede 2007, 195). The government (still under Mandela), however, refused to implement the program and attempted to justify its stance on the basis of cost and affordability (Nattrass 2004, 47) even though the cost amounted to less than 1 percent of the country's total health budget and the government had not succeeded in spending 40 percent of its budget for AIDS (Fourie 2006, 127–28; Gumede 2007, 200). At the same time, Deputy President Mbeki began arguing that Glaxo Wellcome was trying to use poor South Africans to test potentially dangerous medicines (Epstein 2001, 190). In the context of a new and democratic South Africa emerging from apartheid, these policies built upon Mbeki's view that an indigenous African remedy for AIDS was best, as the earlier virodene scandal also attested (Youde 2007, 80).

The Need for a Legal Response to the Growing Challenge Posed by Government

Most outsiders who are conversant about HIV/AIDS in South Africa have heard of the charismatic Zackie Achmat and the Treatment Action Campaign (TAC), often in that order. What they know of TAC usually comes in the form of stories of protest, picketing, and other traditional social movement activities. Where TAC's courtroom strategies are known, they are usually recognized as one important strategy that the organization has used among a wide range of others. Here I offer an alternative, historically informed account to the popular narrative advanced by TAC that emphasizes its mass base and traditional social movement activism.

Formed on December 10, 1998—International Human Rights Day—in response to the government's announcement that it would not roll out a program to prevent mother-to-child transmission of HIV, TAC sought to make access to treatment available and affordable for people living with HIV/AIDS (Fourie 2006, 130; Friedman and Mottiar 2005, 513). While the organization would eventually develop a mass membership, early on it was a child of the AIDS Law Project, and practice of the law was at the core of its work. Recognizing the growing problem posed by government and the need for "a more activist approach to the epidemic," members of the ALP helped to cofound the Treatment Action Campaign (Moyle 2015, xiv). As Fatima Hassan, a lawyer for TAC, recounts, "We practised activist lawyering, using every democratic institution and route—inspired by great lawyers of the anti-apartheid movement" (quoted in Treatment Action Campaign 2010, 29). Jonathan Berger, head of the ALP's Access Unit, stated, "TAC's work is deeply grounded in the Constitution—in the rights it recognises, in the obligations it imposes on the state and the private sector, and in its recognition of the importance of the rule of law to good governance, accountability and service delivery. This understanding of the Constitution has helped TAC to frame its demands in human rights language and use the law as a tool for progressive social change" (quoted in Treatment Action Campaign 2010, 29).

While Zackie Achmat's charisma and grassroots brand of activism have become synonymous with the organization, this popular understanding of the organization leaves out important pieces of its origin and evolution. TAC's founding members were actually a group of friends who had worked together in the anti-apartheid movement as part of the underground revolutionary socialist group MWT (Grebe 2011, 849, 853–54). As intellectuals, issues of class and the needs of the poor animated many of their concerns, and several of the group's members had worked together in the early 1990s at a community health project run by the Progressive Primary Health Care Network that provided them with early experience on the health-focused mobilization of local communities (Grebe 2011, 849, 853–34). Deena Bosch, who had been active in that project and saw great continuity between that work and the formation of TAC, suggested that "TAC is an extension of the work started in the Bellville Community Health Project" (quoted in Treatment Action Campaign 2010, 4). Others who were active in the movement drew lines between even earlier professional movement organizations involved in addressing issues of health equity and the formation of TAC.

William Pick, an honorary professor of public health and family medicine at the University of Cape Town, and his colleagues noted that the South African Health and Social Services Organization, as a formal organization, "no longer exists but its ideas live on in other organisations such as the Treatment Action Committee" (Pick et al. 2012, 405).

Sipho Mthathi, former general secretary of TAC, emphasizes that "TAC didn't begin as a grassroots movement. It started with a few middle-class people [who] had working-class roots. We knew we had to *become* a movement based in communities to have any integrity or we'd be just another NGO" (quoted in Treatment Action Campaign 2010, 30; emphasis added). Many of TAC's founding members and early activists—among them Mark Heywood (who would go on to serve as National Secretary), Jack Lewis, Deena Bosch, and Hermann Reuter—were neither poor nor black and did not reflect the broader demographics of South Africa's population of HIV-infected. As professionals with experience working in the medical and legal fields, they drew on expertise and resources that were largely unavailable to the vast majority of those in need. Zackie Achmat, who had previously served as director of the ALP and was HIV-positive, served as TAC's very visible first chairperson. An ethnic Cape Malay, he too though would develop formidable knowledge of the law through his work and eventually enroll in law school at the University of Cape Town with the aim (such as Edwin Cameron before him) of becoming a judge (Nolen 2008, 167, 180).

While the legal movement that would go on to challenge the government was therefore led by elite professionals who either had training in the law or developed competency in it, such as the HIV-positive lawyer and judge Edwin Cameron, and found a home in centers like CALS at the country's most elite universities, over time TAC's membership would grow to become comprised primarily of people with HIV/AIDS from the country's informal settlements and townships, and it would engage not just in challenges to government policy in the country's courts but also in community-level work to promote treatment literacy and education (Peacock, Budaza, and Greig 2008, 87–92). Transformation of TAC into a mass movement that was more reflective of the demographics of the nation was therefore a conscious effort (Treatment Action Campaign 2010, 8). But it did not start there. As one community member in a recent high-profile study of AIDS in South Africa said,

> I don't know where TAC is situated. But I think it is situated somewhere near the courts . . . because you'll see TAC whenever there is a court case. I think TAC's management is professional. They are intellectuals. . . . And their struggle is somewhere . . . up above. . . . It's not within the communities . . . it doesn't have an impact in and it doesn't represent communities. (quoted in Decoteau 2013, 119)

In confronting the challenges of the epidemic and the need for greater representativeness, Mark Heywood, former national secretary of TAC and director of ALP, argued, "I was acutely aware that it was not going to be possible to overcome HIV from little NGOs like the ALP. . . . Hence my decision in early 1999 to throw the ALP behind and literally into [TAC]. From 1999 to 2004 ALP was independent but in many ways subsumed in building TAC" (quoted in Moyle 2015, 110). Heywood continues, "TAC needed a leadership of black people who lived in the communities where TAC was organising, if possible people living with HIV, and we needed to go out and create that leadership" (quoted in Treatment Action Campaign 2010, 30).

Efforts to develop a mass base at the grassroots level eventually led the ranks of TAC to swell to between 8,000 and 9,500 volunteer members in 2005 (alongside forty paid staff members) (Friedman and Mottiar 2005, 514, 516, 540). TAC, however, has generally relied on a division of labor that includes a largely unemployed and poor and black base at the community level that turns out for mass actions and a small coterie of professionals who are skilled in the law to bring court challenges against pharmaceutical companies and the state. That has gradually changed with the replacement of Zackie Achmat by Nonkosi Khumalo as national chair (Decoteau 2013, 119). But the demographics of its non-dues-paying membership at the community level is more reflective of South Africa's AIDS epidemic than those who originally founded it and who carry out most of its legal advocacy; still, what bonds TAC members together is not a common HIV status but a desire to see those in need receive life-saving medicine (Friedman and Mottiar 2005, 3, 5). In this context, the activist lawyers who have played important roles in TAC and ALP's work have "marched with their clients, breaking down the distance the legal profession usually adopts" between clients and the lawyers who represent them (Moyle 2015, 111).

While TAC's high-profile legal actions relied on the expertise by legal professionals, it has used its base in the communities to demonstrate in large groups when needed and used other creative means to draw attention to the human rights dimensions of AIDS treatment. Zackie Achmat refused to take ARVs himself until they were available to all (Power 2003)—one of the world's first pharmaceutical strikes by someone in need of medication and a source of moral and political legitimacy for TAC's efforts (Overy 2011, 7). Following an attack on a woman who had announced her HIV status publicly, TAC confronted the problem of stigma and discrimination against those affected by AIDS head-on by printing bright T-shirts that read "HIV POSITIVE," suggesting that HIV had the potential to affect everyone (Power 2003). When the Mbeki administration refused to roll out access to ARVs, TAC put up "Wanted" posters of the health and trade ministers, accusing them of "culpable homicide" (Power 2003). These posters were accompanied by an actual filing of a docket at a police station, accusing them of failing to uphold their constitutional duties and negligence leading to the loss of life (Bond 2004, 68).

TAC also orchestrated a meeting between a group of renegade ANC officials who had begun distributing AZT in the township of Khayelitsha, just outside of Cape Town, and Doctors without Borders (MSF); TAC's role (as one of the leading professional movement organizations working on HIV/AIDS) proved crucial in convincing Médecins Sans Frontières to stay in the country and take over the program (using cheaper imported generic drugs from Brazil to save money) after being rebuffed by government officials (Power 2003). Until the government's hand was forced into providing treatment in 2003, just twenty thousand people in the whole country used ARVs out of an estimated five million in need (Gumede 2007, 188). The TAC-MSF program in Khayelitsha was therefore important as demonstration project, setting an example for how to accomplish treatment within communities for the rest of the country (von Soest and Weinel 2007, 218). The program began in 1999, four years before the announcement of the government's commitment to roll out antiretrovirals, and spawned TAC's Treatment Literacy Campaign, aimed at empowering HIV-positive patients (and sometimes clinic staff) with knowledge about care for HIV (Forbath 2011, 78, 82–84). So successful was the project that two years later, the TAC-MSF partnership initiated a new program to provide ARVs to a rural part of the Eastern Cape called Lusikisiki in a further demonstration of the viability of treatment in poor communities (Forbath 2011, 80). Against the backdrop of an intransigent government, these successes caused media to showcase the program's work with headlines like "It's So Easy to Save our AIDS Babies" (*Sunday Times* 2000 in von Soest and Weinel 2007, 218).

TAC's activist tendencies—and its close working relationship with the ALP—led ALP to become more of an "activist ally in the battle against discrimination and for the treatment of people living with HIV/AIDS" but also made the work of TAC and ALP at times hard to distinguish (Moyle 2015, xv). ALP lawyer Fatima Hassan remarks, "During the deadly period of AIDS denialism, we worked with the TAC on its legal cases and together won a number of victories" (quoted in Moyle 2015, 116). The ALP's expertise in law helped to "strengthen and empower a social movement" that was broader than the small group of lawyers working in ALP (Moyle 2015, xvii).

Advancing Legal Challenges to Expand Access to Medicine

The centrality of law in the expansion of access to antiretroviral medicines would become paramount in two court cases that TAC in which played a lead role.

Passed just one year after the announcement of the effectiveness of combination antiretroviral therapy at the 1996 International AIDS Conference, the country's 1997 Medicines and Related Substances Control Amendment Act enshrined in national law the country's right to import or produce generic medications at a greatly reduced price through compulsory licensing, including those that might be used to treat AIDS. The new law was explicitly born out of financial concerns related to the high cost of AIDS drugs (Fourie 2006, 163). However, the new law ran into tension with other international agreements to which South Africa was also a party. Much like Brazil, South Africa sought to deepen its commitment to the elimination of trade barriers even faster than the 1994 General Agreement on Tariffs and Trade (GATT) required (Bond 2004, 199). In particular, the Agreement on Trade-Related Aspects of Intellectual Property (TRIPS)—negotiated at the conclusion of the Uruguay Round of the GATT—was seen by many as a potential obstacle to expanding access to AIDS medicine, since it required developing countries to implement patent protections for intellectual property (including pharmaceuticals) by 2000 and least developed countries (LDCs) to implement protections by 2006—a provision that was later extended until 2016 (Cameron 2005, 166). A group of forty drug companies initiated a lawsuit aimed at preventing the government from implementing the law (Fourie 2006, 148; Hassim, Heywood, and Berger 2007, 174). Pressure from the pharmaceutical industry, which enjoyed the support of the U.S. government, laid bare some of the competing aims of the Clinton administration, which had publicly supported efforts to widen access to ARV medication in Africa (Gevisser 2007, 739).

The threat posed by big pharma temporarily led to an alliance between TAC and the government. For a government with a transformational mandate, the pursuit of price reductions (not just for AIDS drugs but medication more generally) had the potential of creating more fiscal space. So the government supported a TAC campaign that involved picketing Glaxo Wellcome's South Africa headquarters, which ultimately shamed the company into offering ARV drugs at a significantly reduced price (Power 2003).[3] And TAC participated in the lawsuit that the Pharmaceutical Manufacturers Association had brought against the government in 1998 as a friend of the court. The PMA argued that provisions of the 1997 Medicines and Related Substances Control Amendment Act that allowed for, among other things, parallel importation and generic production of medicine were unconstitutional; in a context of broader lack of capacity within the government, TAC supported the government's case by arguing that the act was neither unconstitutional nor a violation of international trade law (Heywood 2001, 135, 140, 144–49). During the case, TAC assembled large numbers of protesters, which caught the attention of the press and turned "a dry legal contest into a matter about human lives" (Heywood 2001, 147). After briefly withdrawing the lawsuit in late 1998 and then reinstating it in January 2001 when South

Africa was required to comply with TRIPS (von Soest and Weinel 2007, 215), the PMA ultimately dropped its case three months later, paving the way for the country to import generic medication from other countries or to use compulsory licenses to produce them locally (Pieterse 2008, 372).

However, this landmark victory—by Mandela's health minister, Nkosazana Dlamini-Zuma, with support from TAC—turned out to be hollow when the new health minister, Manto Tshabalala-Msimang, announced shortly afterwards that the drugs were too costly to import or produce locally (Fourie 2006, 149). In a political context that provided the ANC with the freedom to indulge in charlatan AIDS policy, the episode would underscore that initiatives to preserve fiscal space and policies to extend access to AIDS medicine to citizens were two different things. Zackie Achmat, TAC's founder, had been a strong proponent of the organization's loyalty to the ANC (Iliffe 2006, 145) but was taken aback by the government's response. He remarked, "We saw the government policy wouldn't change even with cheap drugs. . . . It was devastating" (quoted in Power 2003). This inaction would ultimately lead TAC to file a lawsuit against the government (Friedman and Mottiar 2004, 2).

TAC also opened another front in its campaign to expand access to medicines by launching a campaign against the pharmaceutical company Pfizer over the prices it was charging on fluconazole, a drug used to treat opportunistic infections. Working in cooperation with South Africa's Medicines Control Council, TAC went to Thailand and brought back a generic version of the drug manufactured in Thailand that cost just R2 ($0.32) per pill, some sixty times cheaper than the version available in South Africa (Cameron 2005, 163–64; Hassim, Heywood, and Berger 2007, 339). Pfizer, which had earned the equivalent of more than a billion U.S. dollars from the drug in 1999, bowed to the negative publicity that the campaign created and avoided a legal fight by creating the Diflucan Partnership Programme, which provided fluconazole at no charge to public hospitals in South Africa and other developing countries for use in the prevention and treatment of opportunistic infections (Cameron 2005, 164; Hassim, Heywood, and Berger 2007, 446). With the expiration of Pfizer's patent in 2002 and the introduction of generic versions of the drug, the price of the drug dropped by more than 50 percent from R120 ($10) per pill to R50–R60 ($4.15–$5) per pill in South Africa, and with the introduction of even more generics, the price dropped even further to R28 per pill ($4.17) by 2004 (Hassim, Heywood, and Berger 2007, 449).

While TAC enjoyed these successes in fighting pharmaceutical companies to make AIDS medicines more accessible, the government's disconnect with the professional movement on HIV/AIDS deepened as its views on the subject increasingly came into the open. In 1999, Thabo Mbeki, fresh from being elected president six months earlier, delivered his famous speech to Parliament that marked the beginning of the administration's association with "dissident science" on HIV/AIDS. In the speech, he expressed skepticism about the causes of AIDS and marked President Mbeki's first attempts to challenge the dominant paradigm related to the causes of AIDS (Cameron 2005, 103, 97–98; Gevisser 2007, 729). Responding to the president, Edwin Cameron wrote a letter to President Thabo Mbeki in 2000 defending the use of AZT, to which the president responded by "questioning the evidence" of the drug's efficacy (Power 2003). It was at this time that Mbeki invited dissident scientists to participate in an expert panel on HIV/AIDS alongside respected scientists and doctors who held accepted views on the causes of AIDS. While the credibility of the panel collapsed after the standard-bearers of mainstream science refused to participate, the AIDS dissidents' participation was something that the administration used to give further credence to its misguided policies (Gevisser 2007, 743).

Pressure began to mount against the government's unorthodox views on the causes of AIDS at the International AIDS Conference in Durban in July 2000. In his opening address, President Mbeki took the opportunity to advance his position that poverty and underdevelopment—not the HIV virus—causes AIDS (Gevisser 2007, 747). In an international show of condemnation of the administration's views just before the conference, five thousand people (including some prominent scientists) signed a statement known as the Durban Declaration affirming that HIV causes AIDS as a direct challenge of the Mbeki government's views (Cameron 2005, 108; Gevisser 2007, 747; Lieberman 2009, 193;). At this time, a document surfaced within the leadership circles of the ANC that attempted to offer broad support to the denialist views of the administration (Lieberman 2009, 194). As a rift between former President Mandela and current President Mbeki began to open up on the issue of AIDS—with Mandela increasingly taking a public leadership role on AIDS aligned with the views of TAC and mainstream science—Mbeki orchestrated a rotating cast of criticism of Mandela by attendees at the 2002 ANC leadership meeting at which Mandela was admonished for taking his concerns about the administration's AIDS policy public; he would leave the meeting "despondent about how the culture of debate and dissent had been stifled within the party" (Gevisser 2009, 290). With no real challenger and a willingness to admonish even the great Mandela, there was little real check to the government's increasingly preposterous policies.

While provincial governments that were not controlled by the ANC had announced their intention to provide PMTCT treatment to pregnant mothers as early as 1999, the national government led by the ANC continued to balk at providing ARVs for prevention of HIV/AIDS. The provincial government in the Western Cape announced that it would roll out PMTCT against the wishes of the national government in 1999 (Fourie 2006, 130); provincial leaders in

KwaZulu-Natal and Gauteng provinces followed suit in 2002, just as some of the ANC's closest partners in the Congress of South African Trade Unions (COSATU) and the South African Communist Party began to criticize the ANC for its AIDS policy (van der Vliet 2004, 71). At the same time, news became public that some ANC parliamentarians were taking ARVs, paid for by their state-sponsored medical schemes, even as the Mbeki government made repeated assertions about their toxicity (Gumede 2007, 207). While the actions of provincial governments and parliamentarians amounted to substantial cracks in the ANC's governing alliance, one set of voices, a corner from which the government would not tolerate dissent, came from the international community operating in its border. In 2002, Health Minister Manto Tshabalala-Msimang blocked a grant for $72 million from the Global Fund to Fight AIDS, Tuberculosis, and Malaria from going forward because it contained a component for antiretroviral treatment; the minister argued that the Global Fund had tried "to bypass the democratically elected government and put it (the money) in the hands of civil authorities" (quoted in SAPA 20 July 2002 in van der Vliet 2004, 76). During this period of denialism—when the government suspended and even fired doctors who secretly gave ARVs to their patients (Power 2003; Bateman 2008, 916)—organizations with access to medicines, such as the WHO, were reduced to channeling medication to those in need without government knowledge (Shasha interview 2008).

In 2001—the same year that AIDS had become the number one cause of death in the nation (Pelser, Ngwena, and Summerton 2004, 279)—TAC and the ALP launched another major legal campaign. Research had revealed nevirapine to be significantly cheaper and more effective than AZT, and once the drug had been cleared for use in South Africa by the Medicines Control Council, TAC decided that it had no choice but to take legal action against the state (Overy 2011, 3). With the support of more than 250 physicians, in August 2001 TAC filed a suit against the government in the Pretoria High Court to try to force the government to move forward with a PMTCT program (van der Vliet 2004, 69). Mark Heywood, director of the AIDS Law Project and a national chair of TAC, reflected at a news conference in 2001 that it was "regrettable that a government for which the people had struggled, had to be taken to court in pursuit of people's constitutional right to life, and to compel government to fulfill its obligations" (quoted in *Pulsetrack* November 22, 2001, in van der Vliet 2004, 69). Local researchers such as well-known health economist Nicoli Nattrass provided supportive affidavits to the suit, which demonstrated that a PMTCT program would actually save the government money (Overy 2011, 3). Just over three months later in December, TAC won the suit, requiring the government to provide nevirapine to pregnant mothers. When the government appealed to the country's constitutional court in *Minister of Health v. Treatment Action Campaign*, TAC filed a request that the order be executed while the appeal was being made. Illustrating its intransigence, the state then tried to prevent the execution order, which was eventually allowed to proceed in April 2002 (Gevisser 2007, 754; Hassim, Heywood, and Berger 2007, 40–41; Sember 2008, 64–65).

Following a cabinet session on AIDS in April 2002, the government, as it waited for its final appeal to be heard, began to shift course on the causes of AIDS and the efficacy of ARVs, coming more into line with the views of mainstream science and finally announcing its plan to commit to a universal rollout of PMTCT of nevirapine in 2003 (Gevisser 2007, 754, 757). On the appeal, the court again ruled in favor of TAC four months later (Sember 2008, 64–65; Hassim, Heywood, and Berger 2007, 40–41). The decision made clear that under South African law access to medicines were an essential part of the health care services to which South Africans were entitled. And to broader society and the international community, the decision amounted to a trenchant criticism of the government's handling of the HIV/AIDS epidemic and an indication that the court would not hold defenses based on dissident science as legitimate. As in the TAC case against the PMA, TAC—in partnership with the ALP—helped to draw local and international attention to the case and emboldened TAC's ongoing efforts to force the state to provide universal access to ARVs (Pieterse 2008, 384).

Another case brought to the South Africa Competition Commission in September 2002 by TAC, the AIDS Law Project, the AIDS Consortium, COSATU, and others charged two pharmaceutical companies, GlaxoSmithKline and Boehringer Ingelheim, with fixing prices of ARVs. When the case was referred to the Competition Tribunal, the complainants entered into settlement negotiations with the pharmaceutical companies. In December 2003, the complainants withdrew their complaints in exchange for the issuance of multiple licenses on the companies' patented ARVs for generic production and import; the settlement led to dramatic reductions in the cost of these medicines (Cameron 2005, 179–82; also Friedman and Mottiar 2005, 547).

In tandem with these high-profile legal tactics, TAC and the ALP mobilized grassroots pressure from below and helped turn out ten thousand protesters march on Parliament to press the government to adopt a treatment strategy (Fourie 2006, 166). The government's subsequent announcement that it would roll out a program of universal access to ARVs in November 2003 marked a decisive victory against dissident science and for the views of mainstream science held by the professional movement that advocated for expanded access to pharmaceuticals (Cameron 2005, 126). While the first treatment sites would not open until one year later, the advocacy of movement activists played an important role in bringing the cost of ARV combination down from over R4000 per month in 1997 to just R100 by 2004, paving the way for affordable access to treatment (Cameron 2005, 130, 155, 173–74).

A Slow Road to Victory, Marked by Delays

The government's reluctant leadership on the issue of treatment could again be seen in the slow rollout of the program: Although the plan to provide ARVs to the millions in need was announced in November 2003, the first ARVs did not reach patients until some five months later (Gumede 2007, 188). Shifting its focus from forcing the hand of government to adopt policy to ensuring its implementation, TAC again would mobilize as a watchdog that aimed to hold the government accountable in the context of a democratic South Africa (Peacock, Budaza, and Greig 2008, 86). Despite having set a goal of treating fifty-three thousand South Africans by March 2004, the government reached just fifteen thousand by October 2004, leading TAC to go to the courts to force government to make its treatment schedule public (Fourie 2006, 185). Three full years after the government's announcement, just over a fifth of people who needed ARVs in South Africa were receiving them (UNAIDS 2006 in Youde 2007, 8). TAC sent letters to government officials and staged open meetings to maintain pressure on government regarding targets and the timeline for rollout (Forbath 2011, 75).

Although continual delays marked the rollout, after the government announcement that it would agree to start a treatment program, international financial support for scaling up treatment that had been denied previously was now welcomed in. In 2004, PEPFAR donated $89.3 million to South Africa for prevention, treatment, and care, and by 2008, when nearly 550,000 people had gained access to treatment, this number had swelled to more than $590 million (PEPFAR 2008). Likewise, between 2004 and 2012, the Global Fund to Fight AIDS, Tuberculosis, and Malaria disbursed nearly $450 million to government, NGOs, and private organizations in South Africa to fund treatment programs, over three-quarters of which have been focused on HIV/AIDS (Global Fund to Fight AIDS, Tuberculosis, and Malaria 2012). Yet for all this support, responsibility for treatment over time was becoming more and more an obligation of government. By 2010, the South African government had taken responsibility for some 80 percent of funding for the country's AIDS treatment program, although it still relied on some R3 billion from the Global Fund to defray costs (Bodibe 2010).

Even though announcement of rollout of a treatment program officially marked the end of the government's policy of AIDS denialism, the fissures that had grown between the legal movement that had advocated for expanding access to treatment and government remained wide. In late 2006, the government prevented TAC and the ALP from being accredited to gain entrance to the UN General Assembly Special Sessions on AIDS, and it was only after protests that they were allowed in (Lieberman 2009, 157). The international community has continued to take the Mbeki administration to task for its policies: At the International AIDS Conference in Toronto in 2006, the UN Special Envoy on AIDS called the country's AIDS policies "wrong, immoral, and indefensible" and "more worthy of a lunatic fringe than of a concerned and compassionate state" (quoted in Gevisser 2007, 734–35, 743, 760). This, however, did not stop Mbeki from circulating a much longer version of the anonymously authored dissident manifesto that same year—three years after his government had finally committed to antiretroviral therapy (Gevisser 2009a, 294).

Ultimately, the tragic saga of AIDS under President Thabo Mbeki ended when four thousand delegates of the ruling ANC met at the 52nd National Conference of the ANC in Polokwane in 2007 and voted to remove the incumbent and replace him with his deputy, Jacob Zuma (Gevisser 2009a, 1). Following Mbeki's subsequent resignation from the presidency in 2008, new President Kgalema Motlanthe appointed ANC stalwart Barbara Hogan as minister of health. One of Hogan's first acts as health minister was to declare in no uncertain terms that HIV causes AIDS (Kapp 2009, 291). Under President Jacob Zuma, whose term began after national elections in 2009, the country's HIV/AIDS policies held a brighter future. While Zuma's personal actions left something to be desired in terms of modeling behavior for effective HIV prevention—while on trial for rape, Zuma admitted knowingly having unprotected sex with an HIV-infected woman and taking a shower afterwards to minimize the chance of infection—at the level of policy the government expanded access to PMTCT (Dugger 2009). More broadly, the government's efforts to expand access to treatment expanded significantly. In light of the new government's embrace of progressive treatment policy, the AIDS Law Project has since broadened its mandate, and TAC's efforts have shifted to putting pressure on international organizations to do more to expand access to treatment.

Conclusion

South Africa now boasts the largest antiretroviral treatment program in the world, with around 3.5 million people on combination therapy as of 2016 (Nordling 2016). The consequences of these life-saving drugs has been truly dramatic: Most strikingly, life expectancy in South Africa grew from just 54 years in 2005 to 60 in 2011 (Moyle 2015, ix). However, the country's recent gains are overshadowed by the government's descent into AIDS denialism and the estimated

330,000 preventable deaths that occurred on Thabo Mbeki's watch (Chigwe-dere et al. 2008). More broadly, for much of the time that the ANC has presided over government in South Africa, AIDS-related health measures have moved in the wrong direction: Between 1990 and 2005, the HIV prevalence of pregnant women from the ages of 15 to 49 soared from 0.8 percent to over 30 percent (Department of Health 2011c), and between 1996 and 2008, life expectancy in South Africa actually dropped from 57 to 50, while under-five child mortality increased from 60 to 69 deaths per 1,000 live births between 1990 and 2006 (Hassim, Heywood, and Berger 2007, 190). Near the peak of the epidemic in 2004, HIV prevalence rates of mothers attending antenatal clinics in KwaZulu-Natal—the country's hardest-hit province—stood at over 40 percent (SADOH 2006 in Youde 2007, 7). Close to two million people have died in South Africa since the epidemic began, and two-thirds of South Africa's 1.5 million maternal orphans have been orphaned due to AIDS (Gumede 2007, 214). More people now live with HIV in South Africa than in any other country in the world (Nattrass 2012, 77); by 2015, South Africa accounted for seven million of the world's 36.7 million infections (Nordling 2016).

As I have argued, the turning of the tide in South Africa's AIDS treatment story hinged on the mobilization of a small movement of professionals trained in the law. While some key figures in the movement are among those in need of treatment, by and large the demographics of the legal movement have not been reflective of the broader demographics of the population of HIV-positive people in the country. Although this small legal movement has over time grown into a broader mass movement more reflective of the country's race and class demographics—with estimates suggesting that between 50 percent and 70 percent of TAC's member-ship is HIV-positive (Friedman and Mottiar 2004, 3, 5)—the transition of the Treatment Action Campaign into a mass movement happened over time and was a conscious effort. This is not to say that some of the dramatic transformation in South Africa's AIDS policy could not have happened without the development of a mass movement. However, it is to suggest that a small legal movement of pro-fessionals has played a critical role in the transformation of the country's AIDS treatment policy.

When juxtaposed with Thailand and Brazil, South Africa's AIDS story lays bare the peculiar political dynamics that allowed an ascendant party of liberation to betray its own people. It begs us to interrogate the differences that led the ANC to embrace a denialist AIDS policy and ignore the entreaties of a well-organized and longstanding professional movement whose views were grounded in mainstream science and the law. I argue that the case illustrates the downside of citizens' unwavering commitment to a political party and highlights how uncompetitive political dynamics and a dominant party's unchecked success at the polls can translate into policy positions that reject science and cost the lives of hundreds of thousands of citizens. Given the sometimes slow and plodding path to legal victories, some leading members of the professional movement even opined that they did not challenge the ANC more forcefully and more quickly, "The tragedy for me is that we put our party loyalty ahead of people's lives" (Achmat quoted in Nolen 2008, 184). While the case shows that the luxury of being able to entertain dissident science and propagate charlatan AIDS policy can eventually be undone through Sisyphean legal struggles, the delay that such luxury entails is not indicative of success; it is a failure not only of policy but also of democracy.

Conclusion

The shift away from "aristocratic health care" and toward universal access to health care and life-saving medicine ("health universalism") stands as a remarkable moment in the history of the developing world. Countries with disparate laws, judicial systems, cultural and religious differences, demographic profiles, and resource bases are making efforts to move toward universal access to health care and medicine. In many ways, this sea change represents the actualization of some of the most cherished ideals of the professional movements surveyed here, namely, in the words of Dr. Sanguan Nitayarumphong, that "access to health care should be viewed as a right and not charity" (quoted in Sakboon 2000). Yet this watershed moment has largely been ignored by scholars and has only recently been acknowledged by international organizations involved in health issues. But as the comparison of Thailand, Brazil, and South Africa suggests, it is a moment that has not come to pass evenly around the world. It has touched some countries and neglected others. The very unevenness with which this pattern has unfolded demands scholarly attention to help illuminate how and why this is.

This book has explored this shift in two different but related policy areas (universal health coverage and access to AIDS medication) in three different countries. While the case studies affirm the larger theoretical point I seek to make about the surprising influence of professional movements in moments of democratic transition, consideration of case studies on AIDS medication alongside case studies on universal coverage serves an additional purpose: It illustrates that professional movement power rests on different mechanisms in the two different policy domains. Physician-led power in motivating universal health coverage largely rests on the privileged position of elites in the state apparatus, although the cases of Thailand and Brazil illustrate that professional movements sometimes use the state to advance reform in different ways. The power of professional movements to motivate access to ARVs, by contrast, rests largely on legal expertise.

In some other countries, reforms that have aimed to expand access to health care and medicine have come from other sources, among them mass movements, left-wing parties, and labor unions. While this book does not therefore claim to explain reform in all cases at this remarkable moment in history, it does use the cases of Thailand, Brazil, and South Africa to point to the highly influential role played by professional movements in the expansion of access to health care and medicine at times of democratic transition.

I have argued that professional movements constitute a category of collective action that occupies an important in-between space between social movements and the professions. Professional movements are distinct from mass movements due to their knowledge, networks, and privileged positions in the state. While these resources set them apart from ordinary citizens, movements of progressive elites exist as relatively marginal subdivisions of esteemed professions. However, these resources provide them with advantages relative to opposition forces we might typically imagine to be more powerful and enable them to push policy outcomes through agenda-setting, policy formulation and adoption, early implementation, and mechanisms aimed at holding governing political parties accountable to citizens for new policies.

In pointing to the influential role that elites from esteemed professions play in the institutionalization of policy, this research builds on foundational theoretical work in sociology (including contributions by Lenin and Gramsci), which has pressed us to think about the role of intellectuals in social change and has suggested that the beneficiaries of change are not always the purveyors. It also builds on more recent work that has sought to establish linkages between early experiences with grassroots activism and the entrance of radical liberation politics into historically conservative and exclusionary white collar professions (Bell 2014; Nam 2015). In drawing a distinction between the different kinds of resources available to mass movements and professional movements, this book implicitly underscores a classical sociological concern: the importance of class. In the cases I examine, class serves as an important (if relatively invisible) connective tissue underlying professional movements and distinguishing them from conventional mass movements. While shared social class is often an important part of the identity of professional movements, they are not reducible to it.

In Thailand, two elite professional movements, led by founding members of the Rural Doctors' Society and the Drug Study Group, advanced reforms that expanded access to health care and medicine. In Brazil, the *sanitarista* ("public health") movement worked with legal experts in civil society organizations to challenge the existing health care regime domestically and to promote a more supportive climate related to pharmaceutical access internationally. In South Africa, professional movements comprised of doctors and economists also advocated for national health insurance, while a legal movement led by the AIDS Law Project and the Treatment Action Campaign campaigned for antiretroviral therapy.

However, the outcome of reform campaigns in Thailand and Brazil diverged markedly from those taking place in South Africa. While in all cases democratic opening provided new opportunities for professional movements in medicine to use the organizational vehicle of the state to advance universal health coverage and the power of the law to deepen commitments to essential medicine, I have argued that differences in outcomes between Thailand and Brazil, on the one hand, and South Africa, on the other, hinged on dramatically different political dynamics. Whereas fierce political competition forced politicians to take the entreaties of elite professional movements seriously in Thailand and Brazil, in South Africa the African National Congress had no similar incentive. Although apartheid-era neglect had left policy on HIV/AIDS in disarray and allowed the public health care system to crumble in that country, the ANC did itself no favors in choosing to pursue policies that amounted to very little over more than twenty years on national health insurance and that actually resulted in harms to the population on HIV/AIDS.

The impact of the policies that were put in place in Thailand and Brazil has been unmistakable: Thailand's universal coverage program increased use of inpatient care by the poor between 8 and 12 percent and led to an estimated 6.5 fewer infant deaths per thousand births among the poor (Gruber et al. 2012). Financial protection increased dramatically, with the share of household spending devoted to health care (including catastrophic payments leading to impoverishment) declining dramatically, particularly among the poorest segments of society (Somkotra and Legrada 2008). Sir Michael Marmot has called the program "a model for other emerging economies in Asia, including India" (quoted in Corben 2016). And no less a figure than Amartya Sen has called attention to the program's contribution both to improved Thai life expectancy and to the correction of historical disparities in infant mortality in rich and poor regions of the country (Sen 2012).

As I have already recounted earlier in this book, we see a similar story in Brazil, which has achieved a greater rate of financial protection than the United States and seen catastrophic health spending plummet to some of the lowest levels in Latin America (Macinko in Khazan 2014). While it is imperative to remember that health is the product of many factors other than health care and medicine, the striking similarities between the Thai and Brazilian cases offer a sharp contrast with South Africa, where a fifteen-year-old girl in some parts of KwaZulu-Natal still has an 80 percent chance of contracting HIV in the course of her life (Nordling 2016). Primary care facilities are beset by problems ranging from lack of water and electricity to supplies (Bateman 2012), and barriers to accessing care at tertiary public hospitals has remained a problem (Ataguba and McIntyre 2013: 40–41). Table C.1 offers a direct comparison of the cases according to certain relevant measures.

The tactics used by professional movements in Thailand, Brazil, and South Africa differ markedly from those of traditional stakeholders, such as professional associations and pharmaceutical companies, whose primary strategies depend on the vast resources of money at their disposal. We have seen that a professional movement's strategies vis-à-vis the state may include embedding important principles and provisions in the constitution; financing and mobilizing grassroots petition campaigns to apply pressure from below; convening expert panels to apply pressure from above; embedding policy in the campaign platform of new political parties; drafting legislation from within the ministry; creating national strategies for implementation to bring health care to the masses; implementing policy as a national pilot project before it becomes law; and drawing on symbolic resources from friendly international organizations and civil society organizations to resist entrenchment and ensure implementation.

TABLE C.1 Comparison of health spending and outcomes

	THAILAND	BRAZIL	SOUTH AFRICA
Health spending per capita (Intl $, 2014)	$950	$1,318	$1,148
Health spending as percentage of GDP, 2014	6.5%	8.3%	8.8%
Life expectancy (m/f), 2015	72/78	71/79	59/66
Maternal mortality rate, 2013	26/100,000 live births	69/100,000 live births	140/100,000 live births
Under 5 mortality rate, 2013	13/1,000 live births	14/1,000 live births	44/1,000 live births
Percent of births attended by skilled health personnel, 2007	99%	99%	N/A
Measles Immunization, 2007	99%	99%	66%
Antenatal Care (4+ visits), 2007	80%	89%	N/A
Deaths due to HIV/AIDS, 2012	31/100,000	7.8/100,000	385.9/100,000
Probability of dying before age 70 (females), 2012	33%	36%	65%

Source: Latest data available from WHO Global Health Expenditure Database, Global Health Observatory.

Likewise, a professional movement's legal expertise has been used to ensure that new rights are embedded in emerging constitutions; to take advantage of these rights and to hold the state accountable for providing access to medicine; to challenge pharmaceutical companies' claims to patents; to empower the broader AIDS movement to engage in litigation with the state and pharmaceutical companies to expand access to medication; to build state capacity and confidence with respect to their rights regarding compulsory licensing; and to improve the international climate related to intellectual property and access to medicines.

While this is not intended to be an exhaustive list of all the actions that a professional movement may take, it does amount to an impressive and formidable array of strategies that are more or less uniquely accessible to professional movements. Mass movements, labor unions, left-wing parties, and medical associations simply do not enjoy the same comparative advantages, which helps to explain the remarkable impact professional movements can have on the policy process. Although they are not all powerful themselves and must frequently work in partnership with political parties in power, when taken into account their imprint on the policy process becomes nonetheless unmistakable.

This book has advanced a larger argument that turns the conventional wisdom related to democratization on its head. While it is true that democratization empowers the masses, this book argues that an unappreciated dynamic in democratic transitions is the extent to which elites are empowered and can have a progressive impact on politics. The striking influence of professional movements at times of democratic transition stems not only from the frequent disorganization and isolation of the masses but also from the relationship that elites from esteemed professions have with the state and the law, which they can use to outmaneuver an entrenched and powerful opposition. These findings challenge long-held notions within sociology and political science, including the primacy of the working class as "the most consistently pro-democratic force" (Rueschemeyer, Stephens, and Stephens 1992, 8). In many areas of social policy that contribute to the expansion of citizenship and the reduction of inequality, that sentiment may still be true, but not, I suggest, in the complex areas of health care and medicine.

For some, the notion that democratization empowers elites may be deeply troubling, as it threatens to spoil the very ideals that make democracy so palatable or, to quote Winston Churchill, that makes it "the worst form of government, except for those other forms that have been tried from time to time." Very simply, this is because it is not the great leveler that we thought it was. It empowers some among us who are already greatly advantaged much more than those who have almost nothing. Although I certainly understand the reasons for pessimism one may take from such an interpretation, I subscribe to an altogether different reading of the material. I believe the case studies offer great reasons for optimism, as they point to the existence of public-minded elites capable of delivering the promise of a better society to citizens in cases across two different domains on three different continents. Moreover, these movements have taken root in places where resources are tight, inequality is stark, and government corruption is commonplace. This suggests that this phenomenon may be much more widespread than is commonly acknowledged; it may serve as an important corrective to social science scholarship that all too often has cast a suspicious gaze on elites. While a critical gaze is always warranted, I would argue that scholarly interrogation must remain open to surprises if it is to retain its integrity. There are a multitude of different types of elites, and they can and sometimes do surprise us.

In Thailand and Brazil, we find some of the more unlikely policies we might imagine to find in resource-constrained countries. Amid historic levels of inequality, the countries' new universal health care and universal access programs might be thought of as "anti-elite" institutions in that they embody ideals that strive to make access to health care and medicine available to everyone. And yet, as I have shown, elites who frequently receive little or no benefit have played a prominent role in their creation. And while we might regard the implementation of universal health care and universal access to antiretroviral medication programs as big wins for citizens at large in developing countries (even if elites have played more of a role than we might expect), there are still some questions that need to be grappled with.

First, why don't mass movements coalesce around health care issues more often? Although I am not the only scholar to point this out, lack of organization frequently serves as an obstacle to the creation of mass movements. In developing countries, where many people live in rural areas, disconnected from the problems of the political center, these barriers are at times especially profound. Mass movements do sometimes take shape around other issues: While they were ultimately unsuccessful, more than a million joined popular protests in Brazil aimed at forcing the military dictatorship to hold direct elections for president (and more recently, as many as three million demonstrated against corruption). In Thailand, the Assembly for the Poor has forcefully represented concerns of rural farmers, particularly related to forest and land conflicts. These examples illustrate the regularity with which mass movements form in the industrializing world to represent citizen concerns.

For all this, health has somehow frequently remained a surprisingly small concern of mass movements, whether we measure this by the low ranking of health care access in polls conducted by Thai Rak Thai in Thailand, by the relatively small number of signatures in a petition campaign in Brazil,[1] or by the surveys of citizen priorities conducted when the ANC assumed power in South Africa.

I would argue (as others have) that this has much to do with the complexity that health care reform and intellectual property law entails. Next to the human brain, there are simply few things more complicated than the dynamics of health care systems. The daunting complexity of health care systems often lends itself to mystification, which can have the effect of blunting mobilization, no matter how great the need.

The cases point to the special role that trained professionals and technical experts have to play in issue advocacy and in empowering actors in the state and civil society through education and training. They also underscore the degree to which battles over reforms related to complex issues such as access to health care and medicine are primarily fought by stakeholders within the medical industry who understand the complexities involved in reform and have vested interests in the status quo—in particular, the medical profession and the medical associations that represent them, insurers, hospital groups, and pharmaceutical companies. Even in an advanced industrialized nation like the United States, health care reform rarely features as a central plank of grassroots movements. In the process, citizen interests—including those left unexpressed—become a casualty.

Second, how durable are professional movements? Can they be relied upon to protect and preserve the programs they put in place for the foreseeable future? In Thailand, the answer has thus far been yes. By instituting a regular meeting space like the Sampran Forum and recruiting members from younger generations to be mentored by and eventually replace those in an older one, Thailand's Rural Doctors' movement stands as an example of a sustainable professional movement that could be replicated in other countries. In Thailand, the Rural Doctors have actively sought to ensure that they maintain power over critical leadership posts in different ministerial positions, boards, and parastatal organizations. This foothold in powerful positions in the bureaucracy has not come without a challenge from business interests and politicians who are ever more keenly aware of the influence that members of the movement have wielded vis-à-vis these positions (Harris 2015, 18). However, they have also created new institutions, such as the National Health Assembly, to increase citizen participation in health care governance. From these longstanding forums and new institutions, we can expect a whole new generation of activists with shared policy goals to be born and join the ranks of the professional movement.

And even as they have been forced to confront domestic incursions that aim to erode their power base in the state, Thailand's professional movement has increasingly sought to project its power internationally. Members of the Rural Doctors' Movement have played an active role in sharing knowledge from the Thai experience and promoting universal coverage in dozens of countries around the world. And they have done so vis-à-vis ministerial appointments at the WHO and in parastatal organizations controlled by the movement, most notably the International Health Policy Program and the recently formed Capacity Building for Universal Health Coverage (CapUHC) organization. Similarly, members of the Drug Study Group have linked up with activists in other countries in Asia to monitor and mobilize against trade developments that threaten access to medicine. And Krisana Kraisintu, a former chief scientist and executive at Thailand's Government Pharmaceutical Office, has traveled to Africa and other countries around the world, seeking to help improve developing country capacity to produce generic medicine.

Recognizing some of the battles they had to fight against international organizations in their struggle for universal coverage in Thailand, members of Thailand's Rural Doctors' movement have sought to make the international climate more supportive of universal health care. In this, the Thais have been an exemplar of what it means to be entrepreneurial. A major public health conference in Thailand, called the Prince Mahidol Award Conference (mentioned in the introduction) has become a platform that the Rural Doctors have used to make sure that universal coverage—and the Thai experience—has a high place on the international political agenda. While the 2012 Prince Mahidol Award Conference (PMAC) led to the Bangkok Statement on Universal Coverage, which would lay the groundwork for the UN General Assembly resolution on universal coverage that would follow, the Rural Doctors used the 2015 PMAC to promote the inclusion of universal coverage in the development community's new Sustainable Development Goals, which will guide the direction of international aid through the year 2030. (They were successful.) The implications of this for reformers in other countries are staggering. Rather than confront an environment in which international organizations, like the World Bank and the Asian Development Bank, are critical of universal health care and promote policies that diminish access, they now seek to support it. The world has changed.

Brazil's *sanitarista* movement has taken a different tack altogether. While many important players in the public health sphere in Brazil still identify as *sanitaristas* today, their work in helping to enshrine important principles in the 1988 constitution remains an important reference point as the heyday of *sanitarista* activism and influence on the political process. As a more diffuse movement than Thailand's Rural Doctors, they have no similar Sampran Forum from which to reproduce the movement. Instead, they have pinned their hopes on the activism of citizens. By creating new participatory institutions, such as the state, local, and national health councils, and working in partnership with AIDS NGOs to monitor the accountability of local government provision, the *sanitaristas* have sought to invest citizens in the new health care system they have created.

While the improvements that have taken place in Brazil's universal ARV program and in the Unified Health System over the past twenty years offer some
suggestive evidence of the effectiveness of this strategy, it remains to be seen what
will come of the health system in the future when the *sanitaristas* are no longer
a durable and effective force on matters related to public health. With no formal
strategy for replacing an older generation of activist professionals with a younger
one, the future of public health in Brazil remains an open question. Depending
on one's interpretation, the movement has either been cavalier about its future
(and the future of public health in the country), or it has placed such an impressive faith in the country's citizens that it no longer believes that advocacy on
behalf of Brazil's citizens is necessary. Only time will tell what such an approach
will mean for public health in Brazil.

What does the current state of politics in Thailand, Brazil, and South Africa
mean for the health reforms in these countries? Until recently, prospects had
looked brightest in Thailand and Brazil while continuing to appear dim in South
Africa. However, recent developments in Thailand and Brazil have dampened
the success stories in those countries, while a new era of political competition
has altered the political landscape in South Africa and may have important consequences for reform there.

Thailand

A nearly fifteen-year break from military rule in Thailand (from 1992 to 2006)
and the electoral reforms and stronger political parties that arrived with the 1997
constitution led many to believe that democracy in Thailand was here to stay.
However, military coups in 2006 and 2014 put an end to the notion that dictatorship was a thing of the past. While the military government did away with the
30-baht co-payment in an effort to erase the memory of Thai Rak Thai's connection to the "30 baht to cure every disease" program following the first coup (*The
Nation* 2006), the second military government took a different approach entirely.
The idea of instituting a substantial new co-pay was raised just one week after
the second coup (Dawson 2014). In the context of a push by the junta to shore
up government coffers to purchase three submarines from China for 36 billion
baht (*Bangkok Post* 2016), the proposal amounted to a blatant effort to shrink the
government's fiscal responsibility for health and divert it to defense.

And while Thailand's Universal Coverage program would not only with-
stand repeal but also see its budget and benefit package grow following two
military coups and rule by six different prime ministers, serious tensions over
the program were mounting within the medical profession. Most notably, the
institutionalization of the 30-baht program led to a realignment within the
medical profession that would be most immediately visible in elections to

the country's Medical Council, which advocates for physicians and oversees medical curriculum, licensure, ethical standards, and medical complaints. As never before, the council's voice would be unified in representing the interests of physicians, particularly specialists and doctors working in large urban hospitals.

In the Medical Council's first election following passage of the act, the Doctors for the Medical Profession—the reform opponent famous for wearing all black in protest of the Universal Coverage policy—won eight of nineteen possible seats; nine other seats were won by medical school doctors and doctors from large private or public hospitals, institutions that stood to lose funding under a reform that sought to redirect financing to rural areas (Khwankhom and Shevajumroen 2003). The Private Hospital Association president was also elected to a seat, but just one Rural Doctor won a seat—giving the Rural Doctors their lowest level of representation on the Medical Council in decades (Khwankhom and Shevajumroen 2003).

Following the election, the head of the Doctors for the Medical Profession announced, "The council has never stood up for doctors . . . but from now on it will, I promise" (quoted in Khwankhom and Shevajumroen 2003). And despite the Medical Council's official role as investigator of medical complaints, a leading member flatly stated that the council wasn't a "consumer protection agency" and that "the council's objective is to work for the benefit of doctors" (Bhatiasevi 2003).

While the Rural Doctors' successful campaign for universal coverage enhanced the rights of patients, it also led to the doctors' marginalization within the profession. A decade after implementation of Universal Coverage in 2011, the Doctors for the Medical Profession—which was now led by the president of the Medical Council—would win 20 of 26 possible seats on the council (*Bangkok Post* 2011). Rural Doctors, now on the outside of the council looking in, would criticize the body for underrepresentation of rural interests and for oversight failures (Treerutkuarkul 2009).

The consequences of the program, however, would not only be confined to the makeup of the Medical Council. Tensions over the program would also simmer within the Ministry of Public Health. In 2014, the Permanent Secretary—the country's highest-ranking civil servant at the ministry—caused a stir when he proposed introducing a 30 to 50 percent co-pay and suggested that responsibility for the UC program's budget be returned to the ministry from the purchaser of services, the National Health Security Office, which the Rural Doctors controlled (*Bangkok Post* 2014). The proposed moves aimed to undercut key aspects of the reform that promised to ensure citizens' financial protection, to improve efficiency, and to stem corruption. This assault on the scheme ended when he was transferred to the Prime Minister's Office but not before one thousand ministry staff planned a gathering on his behalf as a show of support for his proposal (Wangkiat 2015). While the reform itself has so far remained intact, some leading members of the Rural Doctors' movement who occupy privileged positions in the state have recently come under attack (Phromkaew 2015; *Bangkok Post* 2016). Whether or not these attacks ultimately erode the base of the movement in the state over the long term, however, remains to be seen.

Brazil

While this book has focused primarily on the politics of health policy at the national level, important recent work has explored the reasons for the Unified Health System's slow and uneven implementation in Brazil at the subnational level (Gibson 2016). This research has again pointed to the critical role that *sanitaristas* have played in expanding Brazil's health workforce in places like Porto Alegre. However, it has also highlighted the limitations of municipal health councils as mechanisms for health policy decision-making relative to cabinet-level decision-making and pointed to the important role that political appointment of *sanitaristas* to head municipal health departments sometimes plays in this process. In a country whose governing arrangements are decentralized and state and local capacities varied and uneven, this work suggests the need not only to understand the politics of policymaking at the national level but also to be attentive to the politics of policymaking and implementation at the subnational level.

While subnational politics are extremely important, so too are macroeconomic and political issues. After the Unified Health System made steady gains during the 1990s and early 2000s, Brazil's economy has stumbled in recent years, and this has impacted government funding to the SUS. X-rays in São Paulo can now take months to receive (Khazan 2014). Pharmaceutical stockouts have left many families unable to get medication that is supposed to be free through the SUS, forcing them to pay out of pocket or purchase private health insurance (Gómez 2016). One public opinion poll in 2013 found that nearly 50 percent of respondents labeled health care as the country's greatest problem, ahead of other major issues, including corruption and violence (*Folha de S. Paulo* 2013 in Khazan 2014). In June 2013, protests over dissatisfaction with public services and corruption swept the federal capital of Brasilia as well as a dozen state capitals (*The Economist* 2013).

To help address some of these bottlenecks, the government made the decision to import some thirteen thousand doctors from Cuba in 2014 (Bevins 2014). And in 2015, the government would consider a few different means by which to shore up financing of the SUS, including revival of the CPMF tax on financial transactions (Santos, Delduque, and Alves 2016). However, in 2016, the Ministry of Health's budget was further slashed by another $631 million, almost 3 percent, at a time when the country was facing grave new challenges related to Zika and microencephaly (Worth 2016). And the country's new president proposed a constitutional amendment that would freeze public spending for twenty years (Soto and Marcello 2016). The resulting squeeze intensified regional disparities and left some public hospitals in a precarious position. Some hospitals in the state of Rio de Janeiro closed (*Folha de S. Paulo* 2015), and the number of hospital beds hovers at just two for every thousand Brazilians (Khazan 2014). As social worker Luzenir Ferreira noted of the conditions of the public hospital in her town of Goiana, which sometimes lacks places for people to sit in the waiting room at the emergency room, "Sometimes we take a plastic chair, set it in the hallway, and call it a hospital bed" (quoted in Worth 2016). Confronted with a lack of resources, the country's new health minister, Ricardo Barros, publicly suggested after the fall of Dilma Rousseff's leftist government that universal access to health care should be reconsidered (Collucci 2016), which prompted an outcry from public health professionals and citizens alike (ABRASCO 2016a, 2016b). Whether the new government succeeds in dismembering Brazil's health system in the coming months and years remains to be seen.

South Africa

In July 2016, on the eve of elections for mayors and councilors all over the country, the ANC's disdain for political competition and the "inconveniences" associated with democracy would grow increasingly transparent. The party's secretary-general, Gwede Mantashe, would publicly suggest that the ANC was "anointed by God to lead the country" (quoted in de Klerk 2016). And South Africa's sitting president Jacob Zuma opined in a media interview all the things he would get done in just six months as a dictator (Monama and Jordaan 2016).

While the public was not unaccustomed to inflammatory rhetoric from figures like departed ANC Youth League Chair Julius Malema, the surprising comments from some of the party's top leaders was significant news. Zuma's openness in decrying the inefficiency inherent in democracy, however, came at an unusual moment: An ANC activist who had been jailed alongside Mandela during apartheid had called for Zuma's resignation after the Constitutional Court found that he had ignored an order to repay millions of rand in state funds improperly used to renovate his private home (BBC 2016). The unabashed sense of entitlement voiced by leading members of the ANC stood in marked contrast to the growing frustration voiced both by citizens and activists in the country: Electoral participation had declined steadily (and protests increased) in the first two decades of democratic rule by the ANC (Schulz-Herzenberg and Southall 2014). And Mark Heywood (of AIDS Law Project fame) would flatly state that "the head of the state and parts of its body have been captured by people like President Zuma who appear to be subverting the state for personal enrichment" (quoted in *Alice News* 2014).

However, the unfortunate path taken by the ANC would have a silver lining: greater political competition. For the first time ever, on the eve of the 2016 local elections, the African National Congress stood to take home less than 60 percent of the vote nationally and to lose contests in some of the country's biggest cities (Burke 2016). In the lead-up to the election, sometimes violent protests over politicians' inability to deliver goods and services to communities were growing (Mapumulo 2016). The opposition Democratic Alliance, now led by a black South African, had even taken to evoking Mandela's name regularly throughout their campaign (*Gulf News* 2016). When all was said and done, the ANC took home just under 54 percent of the vote nationally, and for the first time, coalition governments would have to be formed in four of the country's eight largest cities (Vandome 2016).

Amid this increased political competition, the effectiveness of health care delivery was coming to play an increasingly important role in political campaigns. In the 2014 elections, both the Democratic Alliance and the ANC would tout their effectiveness in the building of hospitals in traditionally poor black communities like Khayelitsha and expanding treatment for HIV/AIDS (ANC Youth League 2014; Wilkinson 2014). Both issues would also feature in the State of the Western Cape address in 2015 by Democratic Alliance leader Helen Zille (Zille 2015), although the DA would respond to more transformative NHI proposals much more coolly. Despite the many unrealized hopes and dreams of citizens in the country's fledgling democracy, heightened political competition—now more than two decades removed from the country's democratic transition—paradoxically offered renewed prospects for incremental improvements to the country's health care system and ARV services, even if it meant that the window of opportunity for more transformative reform had passed.

Here again, the monumental and racialized nature of South Africa's democratic transition—relative to the other two cases—cannot be overstated. Black activists who stood outside the halls of power under apartheid for the first time had a chance to govern. In this context, the professional movement in South Africa confronted extraordinary challenges and sensitive racial dynamics. Many of the movement's leading black members were absorbed into the upper reaches of government, while many of its white members remained outside, leaving the movement less unified and less well incorporated into the state than it otherwise might have been. Some white members of the movement stayed in universities (like Max Price) while others either left the country or went into the private sector (such as Derek Yach and Johnny Broomberg). It therefore remains an open question as to whether a more cohesive and coordinated professional movement in South Africa could have succeeded in holding the government (and members of the movement inside it) accountable and altered the country's policy trajectory. However, the freedom to ignore outside voices afforded by the ANC's overwhelming electoral victories suggests that even if the professional movement had been stronger and more consolidated, it still would have faced a very difficult road.

As the conclusion to this book was being written, news articles continued to proclaim that South Africa's National Health Insurance program is imminent (Page 2015)—as has been the case often for most of the past twenty years. But in December 2015, four years after its scheduled release, South Africa's cabinet finally approved a "White Paper on National Health Insurance," nudging policy discussion on universal health care further, at least on paper. Among the key issues dealt with in the White Paper were the role that medical schemes would play under NHI (providing complementary benefits only and not benefits that duplicate what NHI offers) and the different possible sources of revenue that could be used to make up a projected R71.9 billion shortfall by 2025/26 needed to implement NHI (Department of Health 2015).

The paper pointedly spelled the end of private health insurance in South Africa as we had known it (Department of Health 2015, 82). It also acknowledged that such a massive transition would require legislative changes to existing laws such as the Medical Schemes Act (Department of Health 2015, 82). However, and somewhat tellingly, it put such hotly contested amendments off to the some unspecified date. One of the country's leading newspapers would look on these developments anxiously, suggesting that the NHI was at root about managing a large pool of money and that "how a government deals with corruption at a senior level is a good indicator of whether such a scheme will succeed or fail" (*Mail and Guardian* 2016).

While these recent developments may be read as the first meaningful developments on NHI in some time, a meandering approach—devoid of any real strategy—will continue to be the course the country takes, if history is any guide. In the meantime, only slow incremental changes are likely, though some may have meaningful consequences. While application of the means test that governs entrance in the country's public health system has frequently been weak, eliminating it and strengthening the system's financing and capacity would, on paper, give everyone universal access to health care, much as Brazil's National Health Service–type system offers.[2] However, without substantial efforts to improve the capacity of the public system, simply eliminating the means test will only make an already overburdened public system even more overburdened. As a major solution to South Africa's health care dilemmas will not happen overnight, this again points to the likelihood of slow (but again, not impossible) change in South Africa. And however plodding the pace of reform under the ANC, the recent relinquishing of government control by the ANC to parties less friendly to NHI suggests that transformative reform is not likely to happen any faster.

These developments also lead to a key question: Are human resource constraints a more parsimonious complementary explanation for the lack of movement on universal health care in South Africa over the past two decades than dynamics related to political competition? Certainly having appropriate human resources are fundamental pillars of any universal coverage program. And given the abysmal state of public health care that the ANC inherited in 1994, the lack of health care infrastructure and human resources in the former homelands meant that even had a universal health care program been put in place immediately at that time, it would have taken time to realize its potential.

A more serious approach to addressing South Africa's human resources needs in the health sector by the ANC earlier might have helped the public health system to achieve greater parity with the private system. While it cannot be emphasized enough that the distribution of health personnel matters a great deal, a comparison of the latest figures available on the number of doctors per thousand people in Thailand (.391), Brazil (1.891), and South Africa (.776) is instructive: South Africa falls squarely in the middle, and the country with the best outcomes has the lowest ratio (WHO Global Health Observatory 2016a).[3] This suggests that it might have been possible for South Africa to make great gains if a universal coverage policy had been put in place earlier, even if the full impact of the policy would not have been felt for some time.

What about cost? Is NHI in South Africa prohibitively expensive? How has cost contributed to the ANC's decision not to pursue NHI more vigorously at an earlier date? On this issue, the government's own estimates have varied wildly, ranging from "unaffordable," according to one estimate (Ministerial Task Team on Social Health Insurance 2005) to estimates in the more recent Green and White papers that suggest it is more tenable. Under any scenario, it is fair to say the cost is high. Here, though, the cases of Thailand and Brazil are both instructive in that they demonstrate that even if universal coverage programs are underfunded initially, they can still have dramatic impacts once in place. South Africa has had opportunities to make greater investments in health but has historically been content to place its bets on less complicated policy areas where the dividends to citizens are more direct. The country's social grant portfolio, for example—which includes grants for pensioners, child support, disability, caregivers, and veterans—has been growing over time and cost just over R121 billion in 2014/15, approximately 4 percent of GDP (Statistics South Africa 2016). If even some of this massive investment had been redirected toward financing national health insurance—and if the country's struggling public health care system could absorb it effectively—then perhaps different historical choices made earlier might have made a difference sooner. However, significant problems would need to be grappled with related to consumer preferences for private health insurance, how to build further parity among the public and private sectors, and how to involve the private sector in a way that would not lead to an exodus of capital and expertise.

If the role of professional movements loomed large in the stories of successful provision of antiretroviral medication in these countries, continued progress toward meeting the goal of providing access to all who need it in many other countries will likely hinge on developments at the global level and the role that legal movements play in them. The economic benefit of getting people on treatment as soon as possible is now well established, and studies have shown that the economic benefit of doing so in a country like South Africa would save the country some US$30 billion by 2050 (Granich et al. 2012). While international funding to support continued rollout of ARV provision in the world's poorest countries faced a squeeze following the 2008 recession, significant challenges also loom in industrializing countries like Thailand, Brazil, and South Africa, where the financing of AIDS treatment is largely provided for domestically. In Thailand and Brazil, those challenges largely relate to sustainability in the context of growing needs over time to rely on second- and third-line AIDS medication. In South Africa, they relate more grimly to the ability of continued substantial investments to slow down the pace of the epidemic: A 2010 report found that even if the country spends more than double what it already spends on treatment and prevention, five million more people will become infected by 2031 (Guthrie, Ndlovu, Muhib, Hecht, and Case 2010). While new technologies and an ever changing cost picture lead such estimates to be revised constantly, sometimes for the better, these projections are nonetheless sobering reminders of the gravity of South Africa's AIDS epidemic.

Although the cases have drawn out the ways in which compulsory licensing has enabled governments to produce AIDS drugs cheaply, the recent price hikes by pharmaceutical companies that produce generic drugs in the United States suggests that generics may no longer be the bastion of affordability that we thought they were. As private pharmaceutical companies become important suppliers of generic medications that patients need, like epinephrine injectors, so too may we see prices rise. This again points to the critical role that professional movements can play in helping to ensure that governments maintain leverage over pharmaceutical companies and that state pharmaceutical agencies are able to produce generics that meet their people's needs.

Whither Professional Movements in Other Places?

While this book has demonstrated the important role played by professional movements in expansionary reforms in health care and pharmaceuticals, some questions remain: Is the influence of professional movements limited to these two domains? In what other policy domains have professional movements left their mark? In other policy domains does holding a privileged position in the state figure so heavily into the pool of critical resources that professional movements use to gain advantage over entrenched political actors? If not, what other resources are critical?

In fact, the health domain is far from the only area in which professional movements play a substantial role that has yet to be accounted for theoretically. Scholars have pointed to a variety of other very different policy domains in which reform-minded professional movements have played an outsized role in policy-making, even if those scholars have not recognized the reformers as professional movements or understood their outsized contributions to the policymaking process as distinct from those of ordinary citizens, who lack knowledge, networks, or resources to make similar contributions.

Professional movements in the industrializing world have taken diverse forms and made varied and wide-ranging contributions to the betterment of societies to which they belong. In India, we find that the Lawyers Collective of Bombay has tried to play a similar role to South Africa's TAC and ALP on AIDS discrimination, access to medicine, and other important issues (d'Adesky 2004). When the lower classes and organized labor stood silent, progressive economists specializing in the labor market have promoted the institution of minimum income guarantees (Dowbor and Houtzager 2014). Labor lawyers have played key roles in the improvement and enforcement of new labor standards (Schrank 2013). Reformist engineers have contributed to improved water quality and sanitation policies that impact the health and lives of the poor (Gutiérrez 2010; Nance 2012). Social justice-minded tax professionals have championed financial reporting reforms globally to ensure that corporations pay their fair share of taxes (Seabrooke and Wigan 2015).

Although they have been less explored, professional movements have no doubt played a role in other complex policy areas related to social security, environmental policy, science and technology policy, and unemployment insurance. Scholarly contributions that help to draw out the unique contributions of professional movements to policy innovations in these areas, as well as the resources that professional movements have relied on to make them, are urgently needed.

Still, other important questions remain, such as whether or not we are more likely to see professional movements leave their mark on policy in the Global South than in the Global North. On this point, evidence from the case suggests that opportunities for professional movement influence may be greater in industrializing countries. For one, processes of democratic transition (typically already consolidated in the developed world) create unusual flux in the political system that well-positioned professional movements are poised to take advantage of. A general dearth of technical expertise in some industrializing nations may afford politically and technically savvy professional movements comparatively more opportunities relative to the rest of the political field to have an impact on complex issues such as health care and medicine. In addition, the foes they face in the medical profession (or other professions) may not be politically mobilized to the same extent as in the industrialized world. The types of resources and alliances professional movements have to draw on in reform battles (operating as coherent movements within the state and drawing on ties to international organizations, for example) are somewhat unique to the developing world. Finally, key strategies that would not be possible in the industrialized world, such as implementing a policy before it becomes law, seem to be available only in weakly institutionalized contexts. This is not to say that professional movements might not have a similar impact in the Global North, only that more research on the strategies they use and how they differ from their counterparts in the Global South is desperately needed.

What happens to professional movements in countries that transition away from democracy? If movements of progressive lawyers and doctors are especially empowered amid democratic opening, are they especially disadvantaged or disempowered when countries slide toward authoritarianism? More systematic research is needed, but if the recent cases of Hungary, Poland, or Turkey are any guide, then the answer is yes. In all three countries, democracy is gradually being hollowed out by parties that originally came to power through strong majorities. In Hungary, for example, this has meant not only that laws have been changed to favor the ruling party at the election box but also that the constitution itself has been rewritten and the very makeup of the Constitutional Court altered to ensure loyalty to Fidesz, the ruling party (Traynor 2014). In addition, a new secret police force, which exists outside of the police and armed forces, whose head is named by the prime minister, was recently set up (Scheppele 2012). This accumulation of power has led to a situation in which "the Hungarian state has been captured by powerful interest groups" (Transparency International 2012), instead of "developmental capture" of the state by professional movements, as in the cases explored in this book.

While these conditions have certainly done much to stifle dissent, professional movements have not been completely disempowered. Recently, two activist lawyers—Máté Szabó and Beatrix Vissy—working on behalf of the democracy watchdog organization, Eötvös Károly Közpolitikai Intézet, used the European Court of Human Rights to sue the government over mass surveillance and were successful (McCarthy 2016). However, it's worth noting that most industrializing countries don't have such supranational courts to which to appeal when transitions away from democracy occur. It is also worth noting that Fidesz owes its beginnings to political resistance in the 1980s to the communist Kadar regime by students at a law college at a time when no real mass movements existed (Sajo 1993, 142), implying not only that transitions away from democracy may do much to disempower progressive elites (movements of lawyers and doctors among them) but also that not all professional movements are necessarily progressive.[4]

Unlike the professional movements reviewed in this book, the strategies adopted by leading professional movements in the United States have been rather conventional, consisting of research, lobbying, petitions, protests, and op-eds. In other words, they have not as often adopted the same kinds of strategies outlined in this book that depend on the offices of the state or legal remedies. This is not to say that access to the state or litigation would necessarily be the magic remedy for physician-led movements in the United States, like Physicians for a National Health Program or other professional movements. Some strategies available to professional movements in the industrializing world are simply not available to professional movements in the industrialized world, where democracies are well established.

For example, in a two-party system such as the United States has, embedding a policy in an innovative new political party is a nonstarter. Drawing on the symbolic resources provided by supportive international organizations is likewise unlikely to sway the debates in the halls of Congress in ways that would benefit a professional movement's cause—and indeed, might even empower Republican opposition, given the contempt for international organizations in some portions of the U.S. political spectrum. And implementing the Patient Protection and Affordable Care Act as a national pilot project before it became law would be a laughable impossibility. While presidential administrations have been willing to test the bounds of authority in recent years in areas ranging from military intervention to immigration reform, the country's institutionalized system of checks and balances generally prevent such sweeping unilateral executive actions from taking place. And where congressional challenges to presidential powers do not halt executive overreach, the judiciary exists to apply further restraint.

Similarly, on the issue of expanding access to medicine, the U.S. context otherwise appears to offer few opportunities for legally minded professional movements to leverage. The U.S. Constitution contains no provisions related to the right to health care or medicine that a professional movement could use to hold the state accountable. And the relative availability of legal expertise in the industrialized world, compared to the developing world, makes the specialized skills that a professional movement represents less of an attractive, unique, and important resource for the state. While public-minded legal advocates might have both the government's interests (saving money) and citizen's interests (achieving access) in mind, in an electoral context that allows corporations to spend money and exercise tremendous power, the capture of U.S. government policy by large pharmaceutical companies presents a considerable challenge. In such contexts, legally minded professional movements have to contend with a vast pool of legal expertise that works for the profit-making entities that actively seek to bend government policy to serve the interests of pharmaceutical corporations.

Buoyed already by a great deal of legal expertise, the U.S. government knows that it has the right to issue compulsory licenses and has actually threatened to avail itself of that right in the past when needed. In the early 2000s, such threats led to an agreement with Bayer AG on a sharply reduced price for Ciprofloxacin following the anthrax scare. Similar actions have at times been taken to protect U.S. interests in other parts of the U.S. health care system. While a 2003 law forbids Medicare from negotiating with pharmaceutical companies over drug prices, the Veterans Administration is exempt from such non-negotiation clauses and has achieved lower prices through negotiation (Gellad et al. 2008; Pear 2007). Setting aside such rare moments of clarity, private health insurance and pharmaceutical interests have actually been preserved in the Affordable Care Act. This discussion would seem to paint a bleak picture of the opportunities available for professional movements in the United States to achieve transformative reform in the areas of health care and medicine. While the important contextual differences between the United States and the industrializing world must be fully acknowledged, there is one important area where a growing convergence of interests may lead to opportunities for transformative reform. Although the broader medical profession, represented by the American Medical Association, has not yet come around to the value of a single-payer health care system that provides universal coverage to everyone, there is growing frustration among physicians over issues such as the time that physicians and patients have to wait for insurance companies to approve procedures that doctors order and, later, for physicians to be reimbursed for those procedures. These tensions could be better exploited by professional movements in the United States.

Working from inside key offices in the government with partners on the outside, U.S.-based professional movements could do better to highlight the benefits that would come to physicians from substantive health care reform. Important reforms that could have meaningful impacts on the U.S. health care system might involve moving away from the fee-for-service payment system that dominates care in the United States and toward alternative arrangements that reward providers for quality rather than volume. Reforms of this variety have frequently been termed "value-based purchasing" and "alternative payment methods" by professionals. But the disconnect between how such clunky jargon can lead to meaningful changes in people's lives often makes mobilizing popular constituencies for these kinds of reforms incredibly difficult.

More sweeping reform aimed at reducing paperwork and making it easier for doctors to treat patients would involve eliminating third-party insurers altogether and making government the single payer of health care services. Support could be built by drawing on strategies that professional movements to expand access to health care have used in the developing world, such as convening expert panels and running small pilot projects that demonstrate the value of the program nationally.[5] Vermont's recent failed attempt at instituting a single-payer system, for example, would have amounted to quite a powerful demonstration project at the state level. (Some other states are weighing similar efforts.) Educational campaigns that emphasize the evidence-based benefits of a single-payer system could likewise make clear that such programs need not have a major impact on the salaries of physicians beyond those specialty fields constituting the top 5 percent of earners whose salaries are greatly increased through the ordering of medical procedures, such as gastroenterologists and interventional cardiologists.[6] While these highly compensated specialists would remain a powerful interest group opposing reform, such a strategy could fragment their opposition from the views of mainstream providers in the profession. And in a field whose battles are so frequently waged by people in the medical industry, this could be a meaningful intervention.

A final set of questions relates to whether or not the universal health care and universal access programs discussed in the book have fulfilled their promise or created unanticipated problems. Here I would offer the following: While expansionary reforms in the areas of health care and medicine have spelled relief for millions of people who lacked access previously, the existence of these programs has by no means led to disease-free utopias or eliminated all problems related to health care and medicine access in these countries. They too are subject to their own problems, challenges, and dilemmas. I will briefly review a few of the more challenging paradoxes of such expansionary commitments to public health by these nations.

First, it is important to reiterate that some of the most cost-effective interventions in public health are the simplest. Health promotion activities—embodied in programs that promote the importance of exercise and diet—and disease prevention activities—embodied in low-cost interventions, such as immunizations—often pay the biggest dividends for public health. Scholars, practitioners, and critics have expressed concern that universal access to health care and medicine may actually prevent citizens from doing the basic things necessary to maintain good health, leading to more expensive health interventions later. This is a serious concern and also one that is difficult to evaluate. At the very least, front-line physicians working in countries with universal health care systems must remain vigilant to these concerns. And the systems in which they work can and should provide proper incentives to monitor them. In other words, they would, like Brazil and Thailand's systems, ideally be universal health care systems that are, first and foremost, led by primary care physicians who are able to prevent problems that can be managed from becoming costly.

A larger problem that has accompanied one of the professional movement's primary tools to deliver medication to the people in Brazil—use of the right to health provisions in the constitution—is the explosion in litigation aimed at securing medication. Estimates suggest that there are more than forty thousand right to health cases in Brazil per year (Ferraz 2010, 1652). In the state of

Rio Grande do Sul alone, the number of right to health cases grew fifteen-fold between 2002 and 2009, from 1,126 cases to 17,025 cases (Biehl 2013, 426). Compared to other emerging democracies (including South Africa, where important health-related legal challenges have taken place), the use of litigation to protect and secure health rights has occurred at a rate thousands of times higher in Brazil than in four comparable countries (Gauri 2008, 1).

The frequency of the "judicialization of the right to health" in Brazil is in part a product of legal provisions related to the right to health in the constitution, but it is also a consequence of the fact that legal precedents set by courts in Brazil do not apply beyond individual cases (Ferraz 2010, 1656). In addition, the share of collective or class action cases in Brazil has been low relative to other comparable countries (Gauri 2008, 2), leading to a high rate of court cases being tried over and over again. One study found that 98 percent of lawsuits analyzed were put forward by individuals, only 2 percent by groups (Hoffman and Bentes 2008). This has led some to suggest that the very notion of public health in Brazil has changed from one that emphasizes primary care and prevention to one emphasizing pharmaceuticals (Biehl 2013, 425–26).

The degree to which courts have become an "alternative institutional voice for the poor" (as the professional movement and AIDS activists would hope) has also been a subject of debate (da Silva and Terrazas 2011). Research has begun to demonstrate that legal mobilization around economic and social rights has frequently benefited the wealthier socioeconomic strata more than the poor and has had important effects on the ability of the health ministry to prioritize resources effectively (Chieffi and Barata 2009). And indeed, more cases in Brazil have been brought forward in wealthier regions than poorer ones (Gauri 2008, 1), with over 93 percent of lawsuits generated by the ten states that rank highest on the UN's Human Development Index (Ferraz 2010, 1662). While important work has challenged these ideas and suggested that it is mostly the poor who rely on public assistance for both health care and legal assistance (Biehl et al. 2012; Biehl 2013), low-income filers have frequently requested low-cost medication, while those using private lawyers have more typically requested high-priced drugs (da Silva and Terrazas 2011, 847). Even more troubling is data that continues to point to problems in the basic operations of the Unified Health System: Not a small percentage of lawsuits have concerned medication that is supposed to be free and available through the Unified Health System (Macedo, Cruz Lopes, and Silvio Barberato-Filho 2011, 4–5). These dynamics have led some scholars to question openly whether the judicialization of the right to health that "excludes nothing from its scope" has worsened the country's "already pronounced health inequities" (Ferraz 2009b).

More broadly, the judicialization of public health in Brazil has led some prominent scholars to draw attention to the strange coterie of vested interests in making high-tech medicine available, a category that includes patient associations, industry advocates, physicians (both public and private), and researchers (Biehl 2013, 424). Pharmaceutical companies have realized the value of allying with victims of illness in need of medication as well as NGOs who can support them in litigation efforts; in some cases, they have actually gone so far as to sponsor NGO activities, publications, and awards (Scheffer, Salazar, and Grou 2005, 63–64). And in one case that generated a fair amount of public attention, pharmaceutical companies were found to have compensated lawyers and doctors in an effort to see that certain medications were provided vis-à-vis court orders (Ferraz 2009a, 25). Others have documented NGO sponsorship of lawsuits by pharmaceutical companies (Hoffman and Bentes 2008).

Legal mobilization around the right to health has not only made strange bedfellows of the actors involved, it has also perverted the priorities of the public health system. In 2005 in São Paulo state, an estimated $43 million—equal to 30 percent of the entire budget for high-cost pharmaceuticals and over 80 percent of the AIDS medication budget—was spent to comply with court-ordered injunctions to provide AIDS drugs that were not included in the benefit package covering only ten thousand people (Ferraz 2010, 1651). In Rio Grande do Sul state in 2008, the state spent over $30 million on court-ordered drugs, amounting to 22 percent of the total pharmaceutical expenditure by the state that year (Biehl 2013, 427). And a recent study of over twenty-three thousand active lawsuits in São Paulo found that imported drugs that were not otherwise used in the public health system due to lack of cost-effectiveness, with some not even available in Brazil more generally, amounted to 78.4 percent of the costs—drugs more likely to be demanded by the wealthy (Ferraz 2010, 1662–63).

While the new rights and principles embodied in the 1988 constitution clearly played an important role in helping the *sanitaristas* achieve their goals of expanding access to health care and medicine, it has also obviously led some to reassess the consequences of using the judiciary to expand access to medicine. From a utilitarian standpoint, protection of the ability of policymakers to set priorities for the general public seems paramount, and at the same time no person wants remedies that have the power to sustain their lives closed off to them.

Brazil offers an additional window into how universal health care systems interact with private health care providers. If South Africa is the case we want to avoid, in which universal access to health care does not exist, private health insurance benefits a privileged few, and a crumbling and overburdened public system is open to only some of those who need it, Brazil's health care system exists as a strange hybrid somewhere between Thailand and South Africa. For all of the impressive gains that the Unified Health System has made as a National Health Service designed to provide everyone with access to health care in the

British mold, use of the SUS remains highly stratified by income. One-fifth of Brazil's population (around 40 million people)—mostly those with incomes far above the minimum wage—use private health insurance, seeking to forego the long lines in public clinics and believing that higher-quality health care is in the private sector. Meanwhile, the vast majority of the population (150 million) rely on the SUS (Ferraz 2009a, 16–17).

This dual system means that the more than half of health spending that is private benefits a relatively small minority and that the SUS must serve the majority of the population using a resource base that is 2.26 times smaller than that which is in the private system (Ferraz 2009a, 16–17). Such deep divides and the inability of the government to address them calls into question the foundations of equity and universalism that are supposed to be embodied in Brazil's "anti-elite" universal health care system (for a further critique along these lines, see Ocké-Reis and Marmor 2010). This does not mean that Brazil's universal health care system is not a success, only that—set against other more clearly resounding successes, like that of Thailand's universal coverage program—it is a qualified and measured success, but also one that began more than a full decade before Thailand's program. The country's inability to discipline the private sector has meant that, rather than its health system as a whole, we might do well to emulate only some aspects of the country's approach to health care—most notably its Family Health Program, which has become an international model for universal health care. Some other industrialized countries with universal health care systems, such as France, have prevented this bifurcation of health care from happening by instituting regulation that allows for the purchase of private insurance only to cover user fees or services not included in the national benefit package (Commonwealth Fund 2015).

However, in Brazil, backwards public policies are leading the opposite to happen: Tax incentives effectively subsidize the purchase of private health insurance by those who can afford it, just as is the case in South Africa (and the United States). In other words, money that could otherwise be spent on a universal health care system designed to benefit everyone is effectively helping to fuel the growth of a private health insurance industry used by the well-to-do, which relies on private providers. And yet in cases involving high-cost complex care, those same people who buy private health insurance to forego the lines in simple office visits are choosing to rely on the Unified Health System for treatment, placing additional cost pressures on the state. While scholars in both Brazil (Ocké-Reis and Marmor 2010; Ocké-Reis 2012) and South Africa (Zwarenstein 1990) have argued for the need to undo the tax incentives that subsidize the purchase of private health insurance and channel those funds into the publicly maintained systems for some time, in opposition to a powerful and entrenched private health insurance industry that has had the ear of policymakers, these proposals have so far fallen on deaf ears. South Africa's recent white paper suggests that change along these lines may be coming, but only time will tell.

Finally, we must ask: Is the recent movement toward universal health coverage nothing more than the latest international development trend? To be sure, some have been critical of the movement toward universal coverage on the grounds that it is a neoliberal project that necessarily involves (1) getting the government out of the business of providing health care and into the business only of managing (financing) it, with a large role played by the private sector; and (2) maintaining low government spending on health care (see, for example, People's Health Movement et al. 2014, ch. B.1; also Birn, Nervi, and Siqueira 2016). Conversely, some have argued that resources spent on providing access for the well-to-do (who also benefit from the universal nature of the programs) would be better spent on programs for those who really need it through means-tested programs. Still others might suggest that the surprising about-face of former actors critical of universal health care, like former World Bank vice president David de Ferranti, is indicative not of a genuine turn toward universal health care but rather a recognition that universal coverage is simply the latest big development fad, and one which development contractors are eager to pursue.[7]

While these are certainly sobering, if not dispiriting, claims, even critics acknowledge that the shift from aristocratic to universal health care has achieved at least two things: international recognition of a role for the state in (1) correcting market failures resulting from private health care arrangements and (2) ensuring access to an important public good, even if the state is not the one providing it but only financing it (People's Health Movement et al. 2014, 81). The downsides of more limited, means-tested programs are well known: Aside from sometimes mistargeting populations in need, programs for the poor often gain reputations for providing second-class care, perpetuating narratives of the needy as somehow less deserving.[8] However, I would argue that the global movement toward universal health care has achieved more than just those two things. Even more substantive achievements that test critics' assertions can be found if we look inside Thailand's Universal Coverage program.

While private hospitals and clinics may contract with the program, Thailand's Universal Coverage program overwhelmingly relies on publicly provided services. By these critics' own measures, it is true that the country's health expenditure remains low relative to other low- and middle-income countries (People's Health Movement et al. 2014, 90). However, to stop at this fact is to ignore the way in which the program's budget and service package has grown substantially over time under markedly different political administrations. And it is also to ignore that government expenditures are at the same time a mark of strength and weakness of a country's health care system. If they are too high, they point to unsustainable spending. If they are too low, they point to weak government commitment.

In a world where controlling escalating costs will always be important if health care programs are to be sustainable, then perhaps a better measure of the success of a country's universal health care program would be the kinds of benefits citizens are actually receiving and the level of satisfaction people have with those services. In Thailand, this now includes a wide range of services, including heart surgery, chemotherapy for cancer, dialysis for kidney disease, and psychoactive drugs for mental illness. And while tensions there too must be managed between the country's universal coverage program and the elite private hospitals in Bangkok that have become a center for medical tourism,[9] that the Thais provide these services to their citizens at relatively low cost points to the possibilities that exist for universal health care elsewhere. However, the greater lessons, I would argue, are in the promise represented by professional movements themselves. Recognizing that complicated problems of health care and pharmaceutical access are above all political problems, the professionals who constitute these movements have deliberately sought to engage them on those terms, with specialized tools for doing so.

Notes

INTRODUCTION

1. Even world-society scholars, who give primacy to the global level, concede that local institutions give ultimate shape to national policies.

2. Haas (1992, 3) defines epistemic communities as "a network of professionals with recognized expertise and competence in a particular domain and an authoritative claim to policy-relevant knowledge within that domain or issue-area."

3. In other work (Harris 2015), I have used this term to refer to occupation of the state bureaucracy for the purposes of promoting inclusive developmental policies that enhance the welfare of the broader populace. I contrast this term with the notion of "regulatory capture," which refers to the takeover of state agencies by outside interest groups pursuing narrow agendas in the name of profit maximization.

4. The invocation of a compulsory license allows a country to produce or import a generic version of a drug without paying the full royalties normally required to the patent holder. While the practice is legal, it was hugely controversial. "Second-line" refers to drugs that are used after primary "first-line" treatments fail, normally when resistance to first-line drugs develops.

5. "Means-tested" social programs are not universally accessible to all but are open only to people who fall below a certain income threshold.

6. Primary health care, championed by the WHO in the 1970s, emphasized low-cost interventions, such as health prevention and promotion, child and maternal health, and essential drug lists, supported by volunteers working in the community (Green 2008, 155; Magnussen, Ehiri, and Jolly 2004).

7. Iliffe (2006, 43), for example, draws a contrast between an epidemic in Thailand that was concentrated among sex workers and infected drug users with an epidemic in South Africa that was not concentrated in a single group that could easily be targeted and which sat next to a much larger epidemic on its borders.

8. Related to concerns about dominant party rule and the quality of democracy in post-apartheid South Africa, see also Butler (2005), Giliomee (1998), Giliomee, Myburgh, and Schlemmer (2001), Habib and Taylor (1999), Mattes (2002), and Southall (2001).

9. This included consultation of primary and secondary sources at the Bangkok Post archives; the local UN and World Bank archives; the National Health Security Office library; the Health Systems Research Institute archive; the Chulalongkorn University, Mahidol University, and Chiang Mai University libraries; and attendance at local conferences of the Ministry of Public Health and the WHO in Thailand.

10. Informants included public health officials, officers at international organizations, members of civil society organizations, academics, doctors, nurses, and members of political parties. Interviews took place in organization offices, hospitals, and public meeting spaces in the Bangkok Metropolitan Area and Chiang Mai province.

11. Consulted libraries included the South African Historical Archives, the University of the Witwatersrand library, the archives of the AIDS Law Project, and the local UNDP and ILO archives.

12. Public health officials, officers at international organizations, members of civil society organizations, academics, doctors, nurses, and members of political parties were the subjects of interviews, which took place in organization offices, hospitals, and public meeting spaces.

1. DEMOCRATIZATION, ELITES, AND THE EXPANSION OF ACCESS TO HEALTH CARE AND MEDICINE

1. Economists (Chattopadhyay and Duflo 2004) have likewise pointed to the importance of representative institutions to the production of public goods.

2. Although these two explanations are the main ones against which I position my arguments, I do not mean to suggest that they are the only two explanations for the expansion of social policy. The logic of industrialism (Wilensky 1975) was, for example, a major focus of the literature for some time.

3. Kingdon points to "focusing events" as one prominent example of external events (or shocks) outside a policy that can ignite policy activity in an area (Kingdon 1984, 169).

2. THAILAND: CHASING THE DREAM OF FREE MEDICAL CARE FOR THE SICK

1. The two most famous projects of this ilk were the Saraphi project, which began in the late 1960s, and the Lampang project, started in 1974.

2. A senior member of the movement, Wichai Chokewiwat, described being run off the road after becoming known for his work on rural health problems (Chokewiwat interview 2009).

3. The Communist Party of Thailand had begun an armed struggle with the Thai military dictatorship in 1965. At its peak, some fourteen thousand insurgents operated in over 70% of the country's provinces, with historical ties to the northeast (Phatharathananunth 2006, 46–50).

4. Village drug cooperatives were especially popular, as access to pharmaceuticals was noticeably lacking in rural areas. One model cooperative expanded from an initial budget of 750 baht to 4,000 baht in two years, a significant increase at the time (Sirikanokvilai 1986, 25–26).

5. The doctor who would later become the chief economic architect of Thailand's universal health insurance program experimented with a school-based insurance program in the northeastern community where he worked at the time, while learning accounting at the hospital (Lertsuridej interview 2009; Thanprasertsuk interview 2009).

6. In rural areas, it is not uncommon for patients to bring doctors gifts as a token of gratitude. Many patients offer doctors a respectful *wai* (placing your hands together and bowing slightly) of thanks after a visit at a hospital.

7. Founded in the 1960s, the Thai Rural Reconstruction Movement has been recognized as the first development NGO in Thailand (Prasartset, Lele, and Tettey 1996, 62–63).

8. So great was the influence of Dr. Prawase that as early as 1989, he was involved in cabinet meetings of the government, seated next to the prime minister (*Thai Development Newsletter* 1989, 59).

9. So close were Sanguan's ties with Prawase that the director of LDI made a joke that the two were actually obstetricians who had delivered some NGOs together (Pinprateep interview 2009).

10. "Sampran" is the name of a district in Nakhon Pathom province that lies just outside of Bangkok. The group earned its name because it held regular monthly meetings at the Suan (Garden) Sampran Hotel (although it has been recently renamed). Members of the group also call it the Rose Garden Hotel Group.

11. These semiautonomous organizations included the Health Systems Research Institute, the Thai Health Promotion Foundation, the National Health Foundation, the Society and Health Institute, the International Health Policy Program, the National Health Security Office, and the National Health Assembly.

12. Prior to this, three military dictators had ruled Thailand from 1957 to 1973.

13. This is in no way to discount the roles that other leading figures played in the drafting of the constitution, including former prime minister Anand Panyarachun, lawyer Bowornsak Uwanno, or former speaker of the House Uthai Pimchaichon.

14. Somewhat ironically, these changes would end up costing the Democrat Party that had promoted reform in the first place.

15. The Rural Doctors' Society itself collected the second-highest number of signatures (Ford et al. 2009, 260).

16. The concrete benefits that universal coverage provided eventually proved to be of greater interest to politicians than the more sweeping but less concrete National Health Act bill. While serious discussions on that bill began under the Democrat government in 1999 and the Thai Rak Thai government had made a promise to deliver on it in 2002, it began to see universal coverage as a separate issue that could be separated from the other concerns promoted by the bill. By 2004 a civil society movement spearheaded by Dr. Amphon brought its own petition for the bill to Parliament after it became clear that the Thai Rak Thai government no longer saw the benefit of the bill (Charoenpo 2004). The bill languished in Parliament, and it would be another three years until it would be passed into law. Some close observers have suggested that Dr. Prawase was more supportive of Dr. Amphon's movement for a National Health Act than Dr. Sanguan's movement for Universal Coverage (Ungpakorn interview 2009).

17. Sanguan had originally envisioned that the country might achieve universal coverage by expanding this program (Pongpisut interview 2009).

18. Underscoring the party's fiscal conservatism, when universal health care began to be debated in Parliament in the summer of 2002, former prime minister Chuan Leekpai remarked, "I would like to remind [Thai Rak Thai] that the national budget is not only for the health sector" (Assavanonda 2002c).

19. Surapong had edited the Bulletin of the Rural Doctors' Society the year that Wichai Chokewiwat had been president decades earlier, and Sanguan had tried to recruit Surapong to come and work with him at Bua Yai Hospital in Korat province. Later Surapong worked with Sanguan on the Ayudhya Project (Suebwonglee interview 2009). Like Sanguan, Surapong was a devotee of Dr. Prawase Wasi.

20. After serving as a lecturer at Mahidol for twelve years, Dr. Surapong became the first doctor in Thailand to receive an MBA at Chulalongkorn University. From there, he served as director and assistant dean of the School of Hospital Administration at Ramathibodi Medical School before running for office with the Palang Tham party in 1996.

21. Thaksin also recognized the appeal of some of the Rural Doctors and asked Wichai Chokewiwat to join his party, which Wichai declined (Chokewiwat interview 2009).

22. Although his support of Thaksin would turn sour, Prawase initially supported Thaksin's Thai Rak Thai party (McCargo 2005, 513).

23. While the drug problem fell off the main tier of the party platform after the inclusion of the 30-baht program, it still featured prominently as an issue with Thai Rak Thai. The "drug war" under Thaksin is reputed to have claimed over two thousand lives.

24. One of the leading members of the professional movement would later note that he was able to push through five major policies championed by the Rural Doctors the year that Mongkol was health minister in 2006–2007 (Birmingham interview 2009).

25. This may in part be explained by the fact that, as a politician and not a doctor, the minister did not know much about health care. Deputy Minister Surapong Suebwonglee had been designated by Thaksin as the point person on the program.

26. While political pressures related to cost predisposed politicians to favor proposals with smaller cost estimates, a subsequent report by the Thailand Development Research Institute would call attention to a surprising mathematical error that led the initial budget that was accepted to be dramatically understated. Although it is impossible to say whether or not this mistake amounted to a deliberate attempt to make the cost of the program more palatable to politicians, it does underscore the important role of expertise in the story. Once in place, the program's budget would grow substantially in the years that followed.

27. The Thai legislative process involves first and second votes on a bill (called "readings") in the House of Representatives before a bill is sent to the Senate for consideration in a subcommittee and given a vote by the full Senate. If the bill passes these hurdles, it then returns to the House of Representatives for a final, third reading.

28. In his interview, Dr. Viroj described the stamp of approval as "*yan gan phii*" (protection from ghosts, which are a popular, if feared, aspect of Thai culture).

29. Years later, the World Bank's role in trying to stop Thailand's efforts at universal health care became public fodder for the Rural Doctors at international health conferences. Sitting next to a senior World Bank official at the International AIDS Conference in 2008, one Rural Doctor heaped shame on the World Bank, saying "When we started the universal health insurance, a World Bank consultant came into my office and asked me . . . to stop it. We are lucky we did not listen" (Wibulpolprasert 2008).

30. Sanguan was initially reluctant to head the NHSO over fear that doing so would create an opportunity for gossip. However, Dr. Ammar Siamwalla cited the positive role that Puey Ungpakorn had played in building a successful organizational culture at the Bank of Thailand after advocating for its creation. This ultimately helped convince Sanguan to take the post (Nitayarumphong 2008, 120–21).

3. BRAZIL: AGAINST ALL ODDS

1. For discussion of other important factors that contributed to the growth of political parties, see Mainwaring (1998, 539–40).

2. Hésio Cordeiro also had ties to international organizations such as the Pan-American Health Organization (PAHO), dating back to 1972 (*Cadernos de Saúde Pública* 1998).

3. "Fee-for-service" arrangements reimburse doctors for each billed service and offer providers few incentives to keep costs down, since providers can make more money by charging for additional services. This is the dominant provider-payment method in the United States and has been centrally implicated in the rise of costs in the United States and other countries.

4. Following the vetoing of automatic federal transfers, regulations known as the Basic Operating Guidelines (NOB) governed transfers and financing until the late 1990s (Melamed 2011, 64). After Collor was deposed, a new NOB was set up in an administration friendlier to the *sanitaristas* (Fleury 1997, 296). Other important mandates in the constitution, such as the requirement that 30 percent of the social security budget be allocated to the health sector, also failed to become reality.

5. As in the early years of Thailand's reform and South Africa's 1994 and 1996 free healthcare policies, the reform in Brazil was not accompanied by a budget increase that would account for the rise in patient demand (Lewis and Medici 1998, 280). Rather, in Brazil, amid a poor economic context, real health expenditures would go down in the programs' first years.

6. Pressure by the sanitaristas would lead to Guerra's resignation (Fleury 1997, 296).

7. The CPMF also played a role in funding other important Brazilian social programs, such as Bolsa Família. However, it would be abolished in 2007.

8. Sugiyama notes that due to an ingrained political culture in which patronage still matters a great deal, administrators report that personal requests for PSF jobs by politically connected individuals characterize hiring processes (2008, 92).

9. Sugiyama draws attention to the importance of the control of municipalities by left-wing parties more broadly for the programs' adoption (2008, 97).

10. While local health councils lack the constitutional mandate—and therefore veto power—that Municipal Health Councils enjoy, they have similar functions and aim to support local governments, health councils, and secretariats at the municipal level. Again, *sanitaristas* have been at the fore of promoting the creation and growth of these organizations as well, with thirty-one in operation in São Paulo alone as of 2007 (Coelho 2007, 34, 39, 41).

4. SOUTH AFRICA: EMBRACING NATIONAL HEALTH INSURANCE—IN NAME ONLY

1. Pieterse, however, notes that GEAR departed from the dominant neoliberal template in that it did allow for significant social spending (2008, 366).

2. It is important to note here that the government's own estimates on this have varied, though the percentage working in the private sector has generally been high. Some competing accounts suggest that the public sector holds a much greater share of the country's medical professionals than the government has acknowledged (Econex 2010; van den Heever 2011: 56–58).

3. Fourteen professional movement organizations signed a letter urging the World Medical Association not to readmit MASA as a result of its role in collaborating with the state in the death of Steve Biko and in maintaining an unequal apartheid healthcare system (Pick et al. 2012).

4. MASA held many of its meetings in facilities where blacks were barred from entry (Ncayiyana 1998).

5. Other professional movement organizations formed in the 1980s included the Organization for Appropriate Social Services (OASSA), which was formed by graduate students in psychology at the University of the Witwatersrand to develop a better vision for social services in South Africa. It stood in contrast to the more conservative Society of Psychiatrists of South Africa, which had represented psychiatric services to the international community as available to all South Africans, regardless of race, although a fact-finding team from the American Psychiatrists Association found this to be untrue (SAHWCO 1989a, 1–2).

6. The Mass Democratic Movement was a broad umbrella of "worker, civic, and student organizations," while the United Democratic Front was a "coalition of hundreds of community-based organizations built around day-to-day issues confronting people" (Coovadia 1999, 1505).

7. Hoosen Cooavdia advanced a similar proposal in 1988 (Coovadia 1988). Coovadia was a prominent physician who had been on the executive board of NAMDA and a member of the United Democratic Front who would go on to become head of Pediatrics and Child Health at the University of Natal in 1990. While in college in India, he had been active in the South African Students' Association, which invited members of the ANC in exile to speak (South African History Online 2014).

8. Similarly, scholars have drawn attention to the way in which activists seeking to address other issues, such as gender inequality and discrimination, were absorbed into government and changed the democratic discourse (Seidman 1999).

9. By 2009, more than 1,300 clinics had been built and more than 260 clinics upgraded (Coovadia et al. 2009, 828). While these are nontrivial achievements, they must also be read against the substantial *decline* of nurses per capita that occurred under the ANC, problems of staff competence and absenteeism notwithstanding (Coovadia et al. 2009, 830–31), as well as the abysmal condition of many of the country's public health facilities. As of 2012, nearly 170 clinics and 17 hospitals in the Eastern Cape did not have piped water, and 42 drew their electricity from generators; more than two-thirds lacked critical medical supplies (Bateman 2012).

10. While the tax subsidy to medical schemes amounted to approximately R7.8 billion in 2002, or about R1,000 per beneficiary (Hassim, Heywood, and Berger 2007, 167–69, 195), by 2008 the subsidy amounted to around R10 billion (Broomberg interview 2008).

11. To address poverty, the commission also recommended that a series of grants be set up as well. While these and other recommendations were important, I focus here only on the aspects of the policy that relate to health care.

12. The unofficial unemployment rate for South Africans under 25 was estimated at 50 percent in 2015 (McGroarty 2015).

13. The Medical Association of South Africa (MASA) was renamed SAMA in 1998 after apartheid fell and the former members of MASA had to reconcile with members of the professional movement.

14. Other researchers have found private general practitioners to be very critical of NHI (Surender et al. 2015). Fewer than 100 private sector doctors signed contracts to work in the government's NHI pilot projects in fiscal year 2013/14, well short of the government's goal of 600 (Kahn 2014).

15. While I focus on the racial dimensions, gendered dynamics have an impact on South African health care provision as well. Nurses on the public healthcare system's front lines are overwhelmingly female.

16. The GEMS program explicitly acknowledges increasing the number of medical scheme beneficiaries while reducing pressure on the public system (GEMS 2015).

17. Green Papers drafted by ministries in South Africa serve as discussion documents, which are intended to lead to public comment and subsequently the development of a more refined White Paper by the ministry, working in partnership with Parliament. White papers offer a broad statement of government policy (Parliament of the Republic of South Africa 2013).

18. One document surveying the development of NHI in other countries found that the transition time to achieve National Health Insurance took between 26 and 127 years (Ministerial Task Team on Social Health Insurance 2005, 16).

19. A 2013 policy of providing people who contribute to a medical scheme with an income tax credit rather than a deduction is an example (SAICA 2013).

5. THAILAND: FROM VILLAGE SAFETY TO UNIVERSAL ACCESS

1. Here it is worth noting that several NGOs make their homes at prestigious universities in Thailand. Focus on the Global South, for example, a vocal leftist anti-globalization NGO founded by Walden Bello, has maintained an office at Chulalongkorn University's Faculty of Political Science.

2. Process patents allowed Thai producers to produce the same drugs as patented medicine if they used a different process to do so (Limpananont interview 2009). As such, they were much weaker than product patents.

3. The original name of TCNA was the NGO against AIDS Consortium.

4. Due to patent protection, a monthly ddI regimen cost $136 in 1996, when office workers earned on average just $120 per month (Loos 2015, 219).

5. One informant suggested that Sanguan had made an agreement with the AIDS movement that AIDS medication would be included in the benefit package of the UC

program following its adoption by parliament but in return asked the movement not to agitate for its inclusion during sensitive parliamentary and budgetary discussions (Lamboray interview 2009). This tacit agreement could not be corroborated and, given the fractious nature of the broader movement, seems unlikely.

6. Somewhat ironically, this comment came from one of the core members of the RDS, Dr. Suwit Wibulpolprasert, who would go on to become vice chair of the Global Fund to Fight AIDS, Tuberculosis, and Malaria. While the nature of Dr. Suwit's objections may sound similar to statements that came out of the Mbeki government in South Africa around the same time, I would suggest that they essentially portray a concern with efficacy *in light of cost*, which was a major concern of the doctors who had taken great pains to found the program.

7. The funding financed coverage for approximately ten thousand people (Limpananont et al. 2009, 151).

8. Some involved in the deliberations have suggested that the founding of the Global Fund was due to the World Bank's lack of leadership on the issue of treatment.

9. In the longer term, he was actually promoted (Kijtiwatchakul interview 2009).

10. Others who were involved gave "due credit" to the Thai Network of People Living with HIV/AIDS and the academics involved while acknowledging that success hinged on Mongkol's work team (Kijtiwatchakul 2007, 59).

11. Zimbabwe had issued a blanket compulsory license on all AIDS medication in 2003 (WHO 2008, 38), but its lack of production capacity ensured that it would not gain the same notoriety as Thailand or Brazil.

6. BRAZIL: CONSTITUTING RIGHTS, SETTING PRECEDENTS, CHALLENGING NORMS

1. GAPA, the country's first AIDS service organization, was founded in 1985 in São Paolo (Larvie 1998, 284).

2. Led by HIV-positive activist Herbert de Souza (Betinho), ABIA was founded in 1986 by a diverse group of doctors, social scientists, and artists with a shared political intention of monitoring government policy related to HIV/AIDS (Larvie 1998: 284–85).

3. Founded by AIDS activist Herbert Daniel and an officer from ABIA in 1989, Grupo Pela VIDDA was the first AIDS organization founded by people living with HIV/AIDS and their friends and family (Parker 1994, 41). Rich notes that gay men formed the core of early AIDS activism (2013, 6).

4. Thailand's amended Patent Law took effect thirteen years before it was required to adopt minimum standards of protection. These agreements illustrate the strong desire of (and pressures faced by) industrializing nations hungry to capture the gains of free trade.

5. Some sixteen professionals from a range of relevant fields were selected to be part of the agency and went through a special training program in intellectual property (Cassier and Corrier 2003).

6. Former GTPI-REBRIP coordinator Carlos Passarelli would likewise later join UNAIDS as a senior expert.

7. Another *sanitarista* who played an influential role in Brazil's compulsory licensing decision was Reinaldo Guimarães, a professor of Social Medicine at the State University of Rio, who held the position of secretary of science, technology, and strategic procurement at the Ministry of Health.

7. SOUTH AFRICA: CONTESTING THE LUXURY OF AIDS DISSIDENCE

1. Gumede, for example, draws attention to the "combustible social mix" of "a large migrant population, people displaced because of apartheid, the breakdown of traditional

family bonds, a labor system that keeps men away from home for most of the year" (Gumede 2007; also Coovadia et al. 2009; Iliffe 2006).

2. The government would eventually backtrack on this decision in 2001 (Fourie 2006: 150–51).

3. By 2001, Boehringer Ingelheim would offer nevirapine for free to pregnant mothers (Gumede 2007, 196).

CONCLUSION

1. More recent petition campaigns on issues ranging from opposition to dam-building to anti-corruption to asylum for Edward Snowden have, by contrast, all garnered million-plus signatures.

2. And indeed, among other things, the White Paper on National Health Insurance calls for user fees at public hospitals to be abolished in the second phase of implementation (Department of Health 2015, 3).

3. A similar story plays out when we compare the latest data on the number of nursing and midwifery personnel per 1,000 people: Thailand (2.077), Brazil (7.601), and South Africa (5.114) (WHO Global Health Observatory 2016). As with the data on physicians, data are from 2010 for Thailand and from 2013 for Brazil and South Africa.

4. It is worth emphasizing the particular historical circumstances against which the students who formed Fidesz struggled, namely a communist dictator who ruled over Hungary for thirty-two years. Had the dictator against which the students struggled been fascist, the movement's ideology might well have been different.

5. Some have suggested that "direct primary care" could be used to challenge the primacy of the private insurance–based healthcare in the United States. Under direct primary care, patients pay doctors a monthly or annual fee to use their services but forego making insurance claims.

6. Gastroenterologists and cardiologists are two of the top three most highly compensated specialists in 2013 (Kane and Peckham 2014, 2).

7. De Ferranti is now head of a Washington, D.C.–based contractor of development and research projects that has made important contributions to work on universal coverage and AIDS treatment.

8. The much lower reimbursement rates of Medicaid compared to Medicare in the United States are one example.

9. Currently the mostly foreign users of these luxury health services are not taxed in any substantial way. Such taxes could help underwrite the sustainability and health of the country's Universal Coverage program, while at the same time helping to prevent the bifurcation of healthcare in Thailand.

References

Abbott, Andrew. 1988. *The System of Professions: An Essay on the Division of Expert Labor.* Chicago: University of Chicago Press.

Abdullah, F. 1987. *The Demand for a National Health Service.* University of Natal. July.

ABRASCO (Brazilian Post-Graduate Association for Public Health). 2016a. "Inaceitavel!" Last modified May 17. Available at http://www.abrasco.org.br/site/2016/05/inaceitavel/.

———. 2016b. "Trabalhadores e Movimentos Ocupam Quatro Sedes Estaduais do MS." Last modified June 9. Available at http://www.abrasco.org.br/site/2016/06/trabalhadores-e-movimentos-ocupam-quatro-sedes-estaduais-do-ms-e-reforcam-mobilizacao-desta-sexta.

Adler, Emanuel. 1986. "Ideological 'Guerrillas' and the Quest for Technological Autonomy: Brazil's Domestic Computer Industry." *International Organization* 40 (3): 673–705.

African National Congress (ANC). 1990. "Discussion Document for ANC Branches Towards Developing a Health Policy."

———. 1994. "A National Health Plan for South Africa. Johannesburg: ANC." Accessed June 27, 2007. Available at http://www.anc.org.za/show.php?id=257.

———. 2007. "52nd National Conference Resolutions." Accessed March 20, 2010. Available at http://www.anc.org.za/show.php?id=2536.

———. 2009. "National Elections Manifesto." Accessed May 25, 2012. Available at http://www.anc.org.za/docs/manifesto/2009/manifesto.pdf.

Afrobarometer. 2004. "Public Opinion and HIV/AIDS: Facing Up to the Future?" Afrobarometer Briefing Paper No. 12. April.

AIDS Consortium. 2015. "About AIDS Consortium." Accessed August 17, 2016. Available at http://www.aidsconsortium.org.za/About.htm.

Alice News. 2014. "South Africa Is at an Economic Impasse: An Interview with Mark Heywood." July 1.

AllAfrica.com. 2012a. "South Africa: National Health Insurance Is a Worldwide Trend—Motsoaledi." Last modified April 25. Available at http://allafrica.com/stories/201204250246.html.

———. 2012b. "South Africa: National Health Insurance Not a Panacea for All Ills." Last modified April 18. Available at http://allafrica.com/stories/201204240196.html.

———. 2012c. "South Africa: R1 Billion Pumped towards National Health Insurance." Last modified February 22. Available at http://allafrica.com/stories/201202221076.html.

Alvarez-Rivera, Manuel. 2014. "General Elections in the Republic of South Africa: April 26–29, 1994 General Election Results." Accessed January 24, 2015. Available at http://electionresources.org/za/provinces.php?election=1994.

Amenta, Edwin. 2003. "What We Know about the Development of Social Policy." In *Comparative Historical Analysis in the Social Sciences,* edited by James Mahoney and Dietrich Rueschemeyer, 91–130. Cambridge: Cambridge University Press.

Amenta, Edwin, Neal Caren, Elizabeth Chiarello, and Yang Su. 2010. "The Political Consequences of Social Movements." *Annual Review of Sociology* 36: 287–307.

Ames, Barry. 2002. *The Deadlock of Democracy in Brazil*. Ann Arbor: University of Michigan Press.

ANC Youth League. 2014. Twitter post. Accessed August 1, 2016. Available at https://twitter.com/ancylhq/status/437942147598139392.

Andersson, Neil, and Shula Marks. 1988. "Apartheid and Health in the 1980s." *Social Science and Medicine* 27(7): 667–81.

Arretche, Marta. 2003. "Financiamento Federal e Gestão Local de Políticas Sociais: O Difícil Equilíbrio Entre Regulação, Responsabilidade e Autonomia." *Ciencia and Saude Coletiva* 8(2): 331–45.

——. 2004. "Towards a Unified and More Equitable System: Health Reform in Brazil." In *Crucial Needs, Weak Incentives*, edited by Robert Kaufman and Joan Nelson, 155–88. Washington, D.C.: Woodrow Wilson Center Press and Johns Hopkins University Press.

Assavanonda, Anjira. 2001a. "30-Baht Scheme Extended to Cover Anti-Retroviral Drugs." *Bangkok Post*, December 1.

——. 2001b. "Care Suffers as Hospitals Slash Costs." *Bangkok Post*, November 22.

——. 2001c. "Including New AIDS Drugs Could Prove Too Costly." *Bangkok Post*, November 15.

——. 2002a. "Amendments Prescribed by Health Sector." *Bangkok Post*, August 5.

——. 2002b. "Civic Groups Back Reform Measure." *Bangkok Post*, July 13.

——. 2002c. "Govt Urged to Heed Criticism of Scheme." *Bangkok Post*, July 19.

——. 2002d. "ILO Specialist Backs Universal Coverage." *Bangkok Post*, July 26.

——. 2002e. "Strong Lobbying as Bill Heads for Final Scrutiny by Senate." *Bangkok Post*, August 1.

——. 2002f. "Top Doctor Slams 30-Baht Scheme." *Bangkok Post*, July 17.

Ataguba, John, and Di McIntyre. 2013. "Who Benefits from Health Services in South Africa?" *Health Economics, Policy and Law* 8(1): 21–46.

AusAid. 1983. "PHC in Thailand: Current Status and Potential for Australian Involvement." Consulting Mission Report. February.

Avritzer, Leonardo. 2000. "Democratization and Changes in the Pattern of Association in Brazil." *Journal of Interamerican Studies and World Affairs* 42(3): 59–76.

——. 2009. *Participatory Institutions in Democratic Brazil*. Washington, D.C.: Woodrow Wilson Center Press.

Bachmann, Max. 1994. "Would Social Health Insurance Improve South African Health Care? What Other Middle Income Countries Can Teach Us." *Transformations* 24: 26–39.

Bacon, Oliver, Maria Lúcia Pecoraro, Jane Galvão, and Kimberly Page-Shafer. 2004. "HIV/AIDS in Brazil." AIDS Policy Research Center, University of California San Francisco.

Baiocchi, Gianpaolo. 2005. *Militants and Citizens: The Politics of Participatory Democracy in Port Alegre*. Palo Alto: Stanford University Press.

Balzer, Harley D., ed. 1996. *Russia's Missing Middle Class: The Professions in Russian History*. Armonk, NY: M.E. Sharpe.

Bamber, Scott. 1997. "The Thai Medical Profession and Political Activism." In *Political Change in Thailand*, edited by Kevin Hewison, 233–50. London: Routledge.

Bangkok Post. 1995. "AIDS Drug Bill in Question." Reprinted in 1996, *Thai Development Newsletter* no. 31: 43–44.

——. 2001. "Cover Limited to Opportunistic Infections." March 22.

——. 2002. "Doubts over Insurance Bill Raised." July 14.

——. 2006. "Leap in Lawsuits Against Doctors." January 9.

——. 2011. "Govt Gets No Respite from Council Poll." January 21.

——. 2014. "30-baht Healthcare Under Attack." December 7.

——. 2016. "7 Thai Health Executives Suspended." January 6.

Bateman, Chris. 2008. "Manana's Costly Machinations: Naude Vindicated." *South African Medical Journal* 98(12): 916–18.

——. 2009. "'Loose-Cannon' Letlape Says He Was 'Misinterpreted.'" *South African Medical Journal* 99(3): 132–36.

——. 2012. "Will our Public Health Sector Fail the NHI?" *South African Medical Journal* 102(11): 817–18.

Baumgartner, Frank R., and Christine Mahoney. 2005. "Social Movements, the Rise of New Issues, and the Public Agenda." In *Routing the Opposition: Social Movements, Public Policy, and Democracy,* edited by David Meyer, Valerie Jenness, and Helen M. Ingram, 65–86. Minneapolis: University of Minnesota Press.

BBC. 2011. "South Africa Unveils Universal Health Care Scheme." August 12.

——. 2016. "Anti-Apartheid Veteran Kathrada Calls for Zuma to Resign." April 2.

Bell, Joyce M. 2014. *The Black Power Movement and American Social Work.* New York: Columbia University Press.

Benatar, Solomon. 1985. "Letter to the Editor." *South African Medical Journal* 68: 839.

Benjamin, Ruha. 2013. *People's Science: Bodies and Rights on the Stem Cell Frontier.* Palo Alto: Stanford University Press.

Berger, Sebastian. 2008. "ANC Party Dominance Hurts South Africa, Says Experts." *The Telegraph,* October 6. Accessed September 15, 2014. Available at http://www.telegraph.co.uk/news/worldnews/africaandindianocean/southafrica/3147033/ANC-party-dominance-hurts-South-Africa-say-experts.html.

Besley, Timothy, and Masayuki Kudamatsu. 2006. "Health and Democracy." *American Economic Review* 96 (2): 313–18.

Bevins, Vincent. 2014. "Brazil's President Imports Cuban Doctors to Ease Shortage." *Los Angeles Times,* January 6.

Bhatiasevi, Aphaluck. 2001a. "Generic Aids Pills Get Push for Care Plan." *Bangkok Post,* March 21.

——. 2001b. "Hospitals Could Crack from Strain." *Bangkok Post,* March 17.

——. 2002. *People's Participation towards Health Reform in Thailand.* Master's Thesis. University of Leeds.

——. 2003. "New Line-Up Worries Consumer Advocates." *Bangkok Post.* January 18.

Biehl, João. 2004. "The Activist State: Global Pharmaceuticals, AIDS, and Brazil." *Social Text* 22(3): 105–32.

——. 2007. *Will to Live: AIDS Therapies and the Politics of Survival.* Princeton, NJ: Princeton University Press.

——. 2008. "Drugs for All: The Future of Global AIDS Treatment." *Medical Anthropology* 27(2): 1–7.

——. 2013. "The Judicialization of Biopolitics: Claiming the Right to Pharmaceuticals in Brazilian Courts." *American Ethnologist* 40(3): 419–36.

Biehl, João, Joseph J. Amon, Mariana P. Socal, and Adriana Petryna. 2012. "Between the Court and the Clinic: Lawsuits for Medicines and the Right to Health in Brazil." *Health and Human Rights* 14(1): E36–E52.

Birmingham, Maureen. 2009. WHO country representative. Interview by author, May 26.

Birn, Anne-Emanuelle, Laura Nervi, and Eduardo Siqueira. 2016. "Neoliberalism Redux: The Global Health Policy Agenda and the Politics of Cooptation in Latin America and Beyond." *Development and Change* 47: 734–59.

Bisseker, Claire. 2001. "Work It Out or Watch It Die." *Financial Mail,* June 29.

Bodibe, Khopotso. 2010. "South Africa: Govt's Responsibility in AIDS Funding." Last modified October 28. Available at http://allafrica.com/stories/201010280549.html.

Boix, Carles. 2001. "Democracy, Development, and the Public Sector." *American Journal of Political Science* 45(1): 1–17.

Bond, Patrick. 2000. *Elite Transition: From Apartheid to Neoliberalism in South Africa.* Sterling, VA: Pluto Press.

———. 2004. *Talk Left, Walk Right: South Africa's Frustrated Global Reforms.* Scottsville, South Africa: University of KwaZulu-Natal Press.

Bor, Jacob. 2007. "The Political Economy of AIDS Leadership in Developing Countries: An Exploratory Analysis." *Social Science and Medicine* 64(8): 1585–99.

Brenny, Patrick. 2009. UNAIDS country director. Interview by author, July 5.

Brint, Steven. 1994. *In an Age of Experts.* Princeton, NJ: Princeton University Press.

Broomberg, Jonathan. 1991. "The Future of Medical Schemes in South Africa: Towards National Insurance or the American Nightmare?" *South African Medical Journal* 79: 2–5.

———. 2008. Executive, Discovery Health. Interview by author, November 18.

Brown, Lawrence D. 1984. "Health Reform, Italian-Style." *Health Affairs* 3(3): 75–101.

Brown, Mark. 2009. *Science in Democracy: Expertise, Institutions, and Representation.* Cambridge: MIT Press.

Brown, Phil. 1992. "Popular Epidemiology and Toxic Waste Contamination: Lay and Professional Ways of Knowing." *Journal of Health and Social Behavior* 33(3): 267–81.

Brown, Phil, and Stephen Zavestoski, eds. 2005. *Social Movements in Health.* Malden, MA: Blackwell Publishing.

Brown, Phil, Stephen Zavestoski, Sabrina McCormick, Brian Mayer, Rachel Morello-Frosch, and Rebecca Gasior Altman. 2004. "Embodied Health Movements: New Approaches to Social Movements in Health." *Sociology of Health and Illness* 26(1): 50–80.

Brown, Tim, and Wiwat Peerapatanapokin. 2004. "The Asian Epidemic Model: A Process Model for Exploring HIV Policy and Programme Alternatives in Asia." *Sexually Transmitted Infections* 80(Supplement 1): i19–i24.

Brulliard, Karin. 2009. "Predicted Win Has Some Asking: Is South Africa Becoming a One-Party State?" *Washington Post,* April 22.

BuaNews. 2012. "South Africa Gears Up for National Health." *BuaNews,* February 22.

Bucher, Rue. 1962. "Pathology: A Study of Social Movements within a Profession." *Social Problems* 10(1): 40–51.

Bucher, Rue, and Anselm Strauss. 1961. "Professions in Process." *American Journal of Sociology* 66(4): 325–34.

Bunpanya, Bamrung. 1982. "A Commentary on Development in Thailand." *Thai Development Newsletter,* Issue 1, Last Quarter.

Burke, Jason. 2016. "Breaking the Mould? South Africa at a Crossroads as Country Goes to Polls." *The Guardian.* August 1.

Burns, Monica. 2002. *Thailand: Extension of Social Protection for the Formal and Informal Sectors.* Bangkok: ILO.

———. 2009. ILO technical expert. Interview by author, May 20.

Burstein, Paul, and Sarah Sausner. 2005. "The Incidence and Impact of Policy-Oriented Collective Action: Competing Views." *Sociological Forum* 20: 403–19.

Buss, Paolo, and Paolo Gadelha. 1996. "Healthcare Systems in Transition: Brazil Part 1: An Outline of Brazil's Health Care Reforms." *Journal of Public Health Medicine* 18(3): 289–95.

Butler, Anthony. 2005. "How Democratic Is the African National Congress?" *Journal of Southern African Studies* 31(4): 719–36.

Cameron, Edwin. 2005. *Witness to AIDS*. New York: I.B. Taurus.

Campbell, John. 2014. "Election Outcome: South Africa Is Moving Away from a One-Party State." *Christian Science Monitor*. Last modified May 12. Available at http://www.csmonitor.com/World/Africa/Africa-Monitor/2014/0512/Election-outcome-South-Africa-is-moving-away-from-a-one-party-state.

Capoccia, Giovanni, and R. Daniel Kelemen. 2007. "The Study of Critical Junctures: Theory, Narrative, and Counterfactuals in Historical Institutionalism." *World Politics* 59(3): 341–69.

Carbone, Giovanni. 2001. "Democratic Demands and Social Policies: The Politics of Health Reform in Ghana." *Journal of Modern African Studies* 49(3): 381–408.

Carpenter, Daniel. 2001. *The Forging of Bureaucratic Autonomy: Reputations, Networks, and Policy Innovation in Executive Agencies, 1862–1928*. Princeton, NJ: Princeton University Press.

Cassier, Maurice, and Marilena Correa. 2003. "Patents, Innovation and Public Health: Brazilian Public-Sector Laboratories' Experience in Copying AIDS Drugs." In *Economics of AIDS and Access in Developing Countries: Issues and Challenges*, edited by Jean-Paul Moatti, Benjamin Coriat, Yves Souteyrand, Tony Barnett, Jérôme Dumoulin, and Yves-Antoine Flori, 89–107. Paris: Agence Nationale de Recherche sur le SIDA.

———. 2007. "Intellectual Property and Public Health: Copying of HIV/AIDS Drugs by Brazilian Public and Private Pharmaceutical Laboratories." *RECIIS* (1): 83–90.

Castro-Leal, Florencia. 1996. *The Impact of Public Health Spending on Poverty and Inequality in South Africa*. Poverty and Social Policy Department, Human Capital Development, Washington, D.C.: World Bank.

Cawthorne, Paul. 2009. Access campaign coordinator, MSF. Interview by author, April 24.

Chaitrong, Wichit. 2002. "'We Cannot Afford This.'" *The Nation,* July 29.

Chan, Jennifer. 2015. *Politics in the Corridor of Dying*. Baltimore: Johns Hopkins University Press.

Chan, Margaret. 2012. "Universal Coverage Is the Ultimate Expression of Fairness." Speech, May 23. Available at http://www.who.int/dg/speeches/2012/wha_20120523/en/.

———. 2016. "Making Fair Choices on the Path to Universal Health Coverage." *Health Systems and Reform* 2(1): 5–7, doi: 10.1080/23288604.2015.1111288.

Charoenpo, Anucha. 2004. "Petition Urges Action on Stalled Legislation." *Bangkok Post,* May 28.

Chattopadhyay, Raghabendra, and Esther Duflo. 2004. "Women as Policy Makers: Evidence from a Randomized Policy Experiment in India." *Econometrica* 72(5): 1409–43.

Chaves, Gabriela Costa, Marchell Fogaca Vieira, and Renata Reis. 2008. "Access to Medicines and Intellectual Property in Brazil: Reflections and Strategies of Civil Society." *SUR-International Journal on Human Rights* 5(8): 163–89.

Chieffi, Ana Luiza, and Rita Barradas Barata. 2009. "Judicialização Da Política Pública de Assistência Farmacêutica e Eqüidade" (Judicialization of public health policy for distribution of medicines). *Cadernos de Saúde Pública* 25(8): 1839–49.

Chigwedere, Pride, George R. Seage III, Sofia Gruskin, Tun-Hou Lee, and Max Essex. 2008. "Estimating the Lost Benefits of Antiretroviral Drug Use in South Africa." *JAIDS: Journal of Acquired Immune Deficiency Syndromes* 49(4): 410–15.

Childs, Katharine. 2011. "Motsoaledi Unveils 'Radical' NHI Plan." *Mail and Guardian,* August 11.

Chokewiwat, Wichai. 2009. Former chair, Government Pharmaceutical Office. Interview by author, April 19.

Chorev, Nitsan. 2012a. *The World Health Organization between North and South.* Ithaca, NY: Cornell University Press.

——. 2012b. "Changing Global Norms through Reactive Diffusion: The Case of Intellectual Property Protection of AIDS Drugs." *American Sociological Review* 77(5): 831–53.

Chunharas, Somsak. 2009. Director, National Health Foundation. Interview by author, March 25.

——. 2013. Personal communication, December 23.

Codato, Adriano. 2006. "A Political History of the Brazilian Transition from Military Dictatorship to Democracy." *Revista de Sociologia e Política* (2): 1–33.

Coelho, Vera. 2004. "Brazil's Health Councils: The Challenge of Building Participatory Political Institutions." *IDS Bulletin* 35(2): 33–39.

——. 2007. "Brazil's Health Councils: Including the Excluded?" in *Spaces for Change? The Politics of Citizen Participation in New Democratic Arenas,* edited by Andrea Cornwall and Vera Coelho, 33–54. New York: Zed Books.

Coelho, Vera, P. Schattan, Ilza Araújo L. de Andrade, and Mariana Cifuentes Montoya. 2002. "Deliberative Fora and the Democratisation of Social Policies in Brazil." *IDS Bulletin* 33(2): 1–16.

Cohen, Jillian, and Kristina Lybecker. 2005. "AIDS Policy and Pharmaceutical Patents: Brazil's Strategy to Safeguard Public Health." *The World Economy* 28(2): 211–30.

Cohen, Paul. 1989. "The Politics of Primary Health Care in Thailand, with Special Reference to Non-Governmental Organizations." In *The Political Economy of Primary Health Care in Southeast Asia,* edited by Paul Cohen and John Purcal, 159–76. Canberra: Australian Development Studies Network, ASEAN Training Center for Primary Health Care Development.

——. 2007. "Public Health in Thailand: Changing Medical Paradigms and Disease Patterns in Political and Economic Context." In *Public Health in Asia and the Pacific,* edited by Milton Lewis and Kerrie MacPherson, 106–21. London: Routledge.

Collucci, Claudia. 2016. "Universal Access to Healthcare Should Be Reconsidered, Says Brazil's New Health Minister." *Folha de S. Paulo,* May 17.

Committee Submission on the Report of Inquiry into a NHS System. 1995. "Submission from the National Assembly Portfolio Committee on Health in Respect of the Report of the Committee of Inquiry into a National Health Insurance System." June 9.

Commonwealth Fund. 2015. "France." Accessed August 17, 2016. Available at http://www.commonwealthfund.org/topics/international-health-policy/countries/france.

Conrad, Peter. 2008. *The Medicalization of Society: On the Transformation of Human Conditions into Treatable Disorders.* Baltimore: Johns Hopkins University Press.

Coovadia, Hoosen. 1988. "The Case for a National Health Service: A Framework for Discussion." In *Towards a National Health Service,* edited by C. P. Owen, 11–21. Cape Town: NAMDA Publishers.

———. 1999. "Sanctions and the Struggle for Health in South Africa." *American Journal of Public Health* 89(10): 1505–8.

Coovadia, Hoosen, Rachel Jewkes, Peter Barron, David Sanders, and Diane McIntyre. 2009. "The Health and Health System of South Africa: Historical Roots of Current Public Health Challenges." *The Lancet* 374: 817–34.

Corben, Ron. 2016. "Thai Health Policy Seen as Model for Emerging Economies." *Voice of America News,* February 9.

Cornwall, Andrea. 2006. "Democratizing the Governance of Health Services: Experiences from Brazil." In *Spaces for Change? The Politics of Citizen Participation in New Democratic Arenas,* edited by Andrea Cornwall and Sera V. Coelho, 155–79. London: Zed Books.

———. 2008. "Deliberating Democracy: Scenes from a Brazilian Municipal Health Council." *Politics and Society* 36(4): 508–31.

Cornwall, Andrea, Silvia Cordeiro, and Nelson Delgado. 2006. "Rights to Health and Struggles for Accountability in a Brazilian Municipal Health Council." In *Rights, Resources, and the Politics of Accountability,* edited by Peter Newell and Joanna Wheeler, 144–59. London: Zed Books.

Cornwall, Andrea, Jorge Romano, and Alex Shankland. 2008. "Brazilian Experiences of Citizenship and Participation: A Critical Look." *Institute of Development Studies Discussion Paper* 389.

Cornwall, Andrea, and Alex Shankland. 2008. "Engaging Citizens: Lessons from Building Brazil's National Health System." *Social Science and Medicine* 66(10): 2173–84.

Crewe, Mary. 1992. *AIDS in South Africa: The Myth and the Reality*. London: Penguin Books.

Critical Health. 1983. "A Chronology of Women's Health Struggles." *Critical Health*. May.

———. 1990. "Editorial." August.

D'Adesky, Anne-Christine. 2004. *Moving Mountains: The Race to Treat Global AIDS*. London: Verso.

Da Silva, Virgílio, and Fernanda Terrazas. 2011. "Claiming the Right to Health in Brazilian Courts: The Exclusion of the Already Excluded?" *Law and Social Inquiry* 36(4): 825–53.

Dal Poz, Mario Roberto, and Roseni Pinheiro. 1998. "A Participação Dos Usuários Nos Conselhos Municipais de Saúde e Seus Determinantes." *Ciência & Saúde Coletiva* 3(1): 28–30.

Damrongplasit, Kannika, and Glenn A. Melnick. 2009. "Early Results from Thailand's 30 Baht Health Reform: Something to Smile About." *Health Affairs* 28(3): w457–w466.

Daniel, Herbert, and Richard Parker. 1993. *Sexuality, Politics, and AIDS in Brazil*. London: Falmer Press.

Dargent, Eduardo. 2014. *Technocracy and Democracy in Latin America*. Cambridge: Cambridge University Press.

Dawson, Alan. 2014. "The Big Issue: If Not 30 Baht, How Much?" *Bangkok Post,* July 20.

De Beer, Cedric, and J. Broomberg. 1990. "Financing Health Care for All—Is National Health Insurance a First Step?" *South African Medical Journal* 78(4): 144–47.

De Ferranti, David, and Julio Frenk. 2012. "Toward Universal Health Coverage." *New York Times*, April 5. Accessed June 2, 2013. Available at http://www.nytimes.com/2012/04/06/opinion/toward-universal-health-coverage.html.

de Klerk, Aphiwe. 2016. "'God Chose ANC to Lead.'" *Times Live,* July 18.

De Mattos, Ruben Araujo, Veriano Terto, and Richard Parker. 2003. "World Bank Strategies and the Response to AIDS in Brazil." *Divulgação em Saúde para Debate* 27(4): 215–27.

De Souza, Maria do Carmo Campello. 1989. "The Brazilian 'New Republic': Under the Sword of Damocles." In *Democratizing Brazil: Problems of Transition and Consolidation,* edited by A. C. Stepan, 351–94. Oxford: Oxford University Press.

Decoteau, Claire. 2013. *Ancestors and Antiretrovirals: The Biopolitics of HIV/AIDS in Post-Apartheid South Africa.* Chicago: University of Chicago Press.

Department of Health. 2011a. *National Health Insurance in South Africa: Policy Paper.* Pretoria: Government of South Africa. Accessed January 22, 2013. Available at http://www.gov.za/sites/www.gov.za/files/nationalhealthinsurance.pdf.

——. 2011b. *National Health Insurance: Healthcare for all South Africans.* Pretoria: Government of South Africa.

——. 2011c. National Antenatal HIV and Syphilis Prevalence Survey. Pretoria: Government of South Africa.

——. 2015. "White Paper on National Health Insurance." Pretoria: Government of South Africa.

Dobbin, Frank, Beth Simmons, and Geoffrey Garrett. 2007. "The Global Diffusion of Public Policies: Social Construction, Coercion, Competition, or Learning?" *American Review of Sociology* 33: 449–72.

Dorrington, R., and L. Johnson. 2002. "Epidemiological and Demographic." In *Impacts and Interventions,* edited by J. Gow and C. Desmond. Pietermaritzburg, South Africa: University of Natal Press.

Dowbor, Monika. 2007. "Origins of Successful Health Sector Reform: Public Health Professionals and Institutional Opportunities in Brazil." *IDS Bulletin* 38(6): 73–80.

——. 2009. "Origins of Successful Health Sector Reform: Public Health Professionals and Institutional Opportunities in Brazil." Paper presented at IPSA's 21st World Congress of Political Science, Santiago, Chile.

——. 2011. "Institutional Dimensions of Social Movements: Case Study of the Sanitario Movement and its Fight for Universal Access to Health in Brazil." Queen Elizabeth House Working Paper Series. Oxford Department of International Development.

Dowbor, Monika, and Peter Houtzager. 2014. "The Role of Professionals in Policy Reform: Cases from the City Level, São Paulo." *Latin American Politics and Society* 56(3): 141–62.

Dreze, Jean, and Amartya Sen. 1989. *Public Action for Social Security: Foundations and Strategy.* Development Economics Research Programme, Suntory-Toyota International Centre for Economics and Related Disciplines.

Drug Study Group. 1984. "The Pharmaceutical Situation in Thailand." *Thai Development Newsletter* 3(2).

Dugger, Celia. 2009. "Breaking with Past, South Africa Issues Broad AIDS Policy." *New York Times.* Accessed May 10, 2013. Available at http://www.nytimes.com/2009/12/02/world/africa/02safrica.html.

Duncan, Felicity. 2014. "Cosatu Feud Could Crack ANC Ruling Alliance." BizNews.com. November 11.

Econex. 2010. *Updated GP and Specialist Numbers for SA.* Health Reform Note 7. October.

Eimer, Thomas, and Suzanne Lütz. 2010. "Developmental States, Civil Society, and Public Health: Patent Regulation for HIV/AIDS Pharmaceuticals in India and Brazil." *Regulation and Governance* 4(2): 135–53.

Eisenstein, Hester. 1996. *Inside Agitators: Australian Femocrats and the State.* Philadelphia: Temple University Press.

Eksaengsri, Achara. 2009. Director, Research and Development Institute, Government Pharmaceutical Organization. Interview by the author. May 25.

Elias, Paulo Eduardo, and Amelia Cohn. 2003. "Health Reform in Brazil: Lessons to Consider." *American Journal of Public Health* 93(1): 44–48.

Ellis, Stephen. 2015. "Introduction." In *Movements in Times of Democratic Transition,* edited by B. Klandermans and Cornelis van Stralen, 209–15. Philadelphia: Temple University Press.

Encarnacion-Tadem, Teresa. 2001. "The Thai Social Movements and the Democratisation Process: Challenging the State through the Anti-Asian Development Bank Campaigns." *Asian Studies* 37(1–2): 35–53.

Epstein, Helen. 2001. *AIDS in South Africa: The Invisible Cure.* New York: Picador.

Epstein, Steven. 1996. *Impure Science: AIDS, Activism, and the Politics of Knowledge.* Berkeley: University of California Press.

Escorel, Sarah. 1999. *Reviravolta na Saúde: Origem e Articulação do Movimento Sanitário.* Rio de Janeiro: Editoria FIOCRUZ.

Esping-Andersen, Gosta. 1990. *Three Worlds of Welfare Capitalism.* Princeton, NJ: Princeton University Press.

European AIDS Treatment Group (EATG). 2008. "Bangkok Declaration on Compulsory Licensing, Innovation, and Access to Medicines For All." Accessed April 20, 2009. Available at http://www.eatg.org/news/164246/ Bangkok_Declaration_on_compulsory_licensing,_innovation,_and_access_to_ medicines_for_all.

Evans, Peter. 1995. *Embedded Autonomy: States and Industrial Transformation.* Princeton, NJ: Princeton University Press.

Evans, Peter, and Patrick Heller. 2015. "Human Development, State Transformation and the Politics of the Developmental State." In *The Oxford Handbook of Transformations of the State,* edited by Stephan Leibfried, Frank Nullmeier, Evelyne Huber, Matthew Lange, Jonah Levy, and John D. Stephens, 691–713. Oxford: Oxford University Press.

Evans, Peter, Dietrich Rueschemeyer, and Theda Skocpol. 1985. *Bringing the State Back In.* New York: Cambridge University Press.

Ewig, Christina. 2010. *Second-Wave Neoliberalism.* College Park: Pennsylvania State Press.

Fah Diaw Kan. 2009. "Investigative Article on the 'Public Participation Development for Social Well-Being.'" Proposal by Pipob Thongchai, *Fah Diaw Kan,* July–September.

Falleti, Tulia. 2010. "Infiltrating the State: The Evolution of Health Care Reforms in Brazil, 1964–1988." In *Explaining Institutional Change: Ambiguity, Agency, and Power,* edited by James Mahoney and Kathleen Thelen, 38–62. New York: Cambridge University Press.

Fassin, Didier. 2007. *When Bodies Remember: Experiences and Politics of AIDS in South Africa.* Berkeley: University of California Press.

Ferraz, Ocatvio. 2009a. "Right to Health Litigation in Brazil: An Overview of the Research." Accessed May 15. Available at http://ssrn.com/abstract=1426011.

——. 2009b. "The Right to Health in the Courts of Brazil: Worsening Health Inequities?" *Health and Human Rights* 1(2): 33–45.

——. 2010. "Harming the Poor through Social Rights Litigation: Lessons From Brazil." *Texas Law Review* 89: 1643–68.

Financial Mail. 2009. "Will NHI Draft Be Good for Health?" October 5.

Fishlow, Albert. 1989. "A Tale of Two Presidents: The Political Economy of Crisis Management." In *Democratizing Brazil: Problems of Transition and Consolidation,* edited by A.C. Stepan, 83–119. Oxford: Oxford University Press.

Fleury, Sonia. 1997. "A Questão Democrática Na Saúde." In *Saúde e Democracia: A Luta do Cebes,* edited by Sonia Fleury, 25–44. São Paulo: Lemos Editorial.

Flynn, Matthew. 2013. "Origins and Limitations of State-Based Advocacy: Brazil's AIDS Treatment Program and Global Power Dynamics." *Politics and Society* 41(1): 3–28.

——. 2014. *Pharmaceutical Autonomy and Public Health in Latin America: State, Society, and Industry in Brazil's AIDS Program.* New York: Routledge.

Folha de S. Paulo. 2013. "Para Quase 50%, Saúde é o Maior Problema do País." June 30.

——. 2015. "Rio: Financial Crisis Leads to Chaos in the State's Health System." December 25.

Font, Mauricio. 2003. *Transforming Brazil: A Reform Era in Perspective.* Lanham, MD: Rowman and Littlefield.

Forbath, Peter (with assistance from Zackie Achmat, Geoff Budlender, and Mark Heywood). 2011. "Cultural Transformation, Deep Institutional Reform, and ESR Practice." In *Stones of Hope: How African Activists Reclaim Human Rights to Challenge Global Poverty,* edited by Lucie White and Jeremy Perelman, 51–90. Palo Alto: Stanford University Press.

Ford, Nathan, David Wilson, Onanong Bunjumnong, and Tido von Schoen Angerer. 2004. "The Role of Civil Society in Protecting Public Health over Commercial Interests: Lessons From Thailand." *The Lancet* 363: 560–63.

Ford, Nathan, David Wilson, Paul Cawthorne, Aree Kumphitak, Siriras Kasi-Sedapan, Suntharaporn Kaetkaew, Saengsri Teemanka, Boripat Donmon, and Chalerm Preuanbuapan. 2009. "Challenge and Co-operation: Civil Society Activism for Access to HIV Treatment in Thailand." *Tropical Medicine and International Health* 14(3): 258–66.

Foundation for Consumers. 2004. *FFC and the Thai Universal Healthcare Coverage Scheme: The Fight for a Security of Health Care System in Thailand.* Bangkok: FFC.

Fourie, Pieter. 2006. *The Political Management of HIV and AIDS in South Africa: One Burden Too Many?* New York: Palgrave Macmillan.

Freidson, Eliot. 1970. *Profession of Medicine.* New York: Harper and Row.

——. 1986. *Professional Powers.* Chicago: University of Chicago Press.

Frenk, Julio, Octavio Gómez-Dantés, and Felicia Marie Knaul. 2009. "The Democratization of Health in Mexico: Financial Innovations for Universal Coverage." *Bulletin of the World Health Organization* 87(7): 542–48.

Frickel, Scott, and Neil Gross. 2005. "A General Theory of Scientific/Intellectual Movements." *American Sociological Review* 70(2): 204–32.

Friedman, Elisabeth Jay, and Kathryn Hochstetler. 2002. "Assessing the Third Transition in Latin American Democratization: Representational Regimes and Civil Society in Argentina and Brazil." *Comparative Politics* 35(1): 21–42.

Friedman, Irwin. 2008. Director of Research, Health Systems Trust. Interview by author, November 28.

Friedman, Stephen, and Shauna Mottiar. 2004. "A Moral to the Tale: The Treatment Action Campaign and the Politics of HIV/AIDS." Globalisation, Marginalisation and New Social Movements in Post-Apartheid South Africa project. Centre for Policy Studies. Durban: University of KwaZulu-Natal.

——. 2005. "A Rewarding Engagement? The Treatment Action Campaign and the Politics of HIV/AIDS." *Politics and Society* 33(4): 511–65.

Fung, Archon, and Erik Olin Wright. 2003. *Deepening Democracy: Institutional Innovations in Empowered Participatory Governance,* vol. 4. New York: Verso.

Galvão, Jane. 2002. "Access to Antiretroviral Drugs in Brazil." *The Lancet* 360(9348): 1862–65.

——. 2005. "Brazil and Access to HIV/AIDS Drugs: A Question of Human Rights and Public Health." *American Journal of Public Health* 95(7): 1110–16.

Gamson, William. 1990. *The Strategy of Social Protest.* Homewood, IL: Dorsey.

Gantsho, Monwabisi. 2008. "SAMA and NHI Debate." *SAMA Insider,* November.

Garrett, Geoffrey, and Deborah Mitchell. 2001. "Globalization, Government Spending, and Taxation in the OECD." *European Journal of Political Research* 39(2): 145–77.

Gauri, Varun. 2008. *Courting Social Justice in Health and Education.* Research at the World Bank: Human Development and Public Services Research, May.

Gauri, Varun, and Peyvand Khaleghian. 2002. "Immunization in Developing Countries: Its Political and Organizational Determinants." *World Development* 30(12): 2109–32.

Gauri, Varun, and Evan Lieberman. 2006. "Boundary Institutions and HIV/AIDS Policies in Brazil and South Africa." *Studies in Comparative International Development* 41(3): 47–73.

Geddes, Barbara. 1994. *Politician's Dilemma: Building State Capacity in Latin America.* Berkeley: University of California Press.

Gellad, Walid F., Sebastian Schneeweiss, Phyllis Brawarsky, Stuart Lipsitz, and Jennifer S. Haas. 2008. "What If the Federal Government Negotiated Pharmaceutical Prices for Seniors? An Estimate of National Savings." *Journal of General Internal Medicine* 23(9): 1435–40.

Gentle, Leonard. 2009. "South Africa: The Debate on National Health Insurance." *Third World Resurgence* 231(2).

Gerring, John, Strom Thacker, and Rodrigo Alfaro. 2012. "Democracy and Human Development." *Journal of Politics* 74(1): 1–17.

Gevisser, Mark. 2007. *Thabo Mbeki: The Dream Deferred.* Johannesburg: Jonathan Ball.

——. 2009a. *A Legacy of Liberation: Thabo Mbeki and the Future of the South Africa.* New York: St. Martin's Griffin.

——. 2009b. "South Africa: Beyond a One-Party State." *The Guardian.* Accessed April 19, 2009. Available at http://www.theguardian.com/commentisfree/2009/apr/20/south-africa-anc-election-democracy.Gibson, Christopher. 2012. "Making Redistributive Direct Democracy Matter: Development and Women's Participation in the Gram Sabhas of Kerala, India." *American Sociological Review* 77(3): 409–34.

——. 2016. "*Sanitaristas, Petistas,* and the Post-Neoliberal Public Health State in Porto Alegre." *Latin American Perspectives* 43(2): 153–71.

Gilbert, Jess, and Carolyn Howe. 1991. "Beyond 'State vs. Society': Theories of the State and New Deal Agricultural Policies." *American Sociological Review* 56(2): 204–20.

Giliomee, Hermann. 1995. "Democratization in South Africa." *Political Science Quarterly* 110(1): 83–104.

——. 1998. "South Africa's Emerging Dominant-Party Regime." *Journal of Democracy* 9(4): 128–42.

Giliomee, Hermann, James Myburgh, and Lawrence Schlemmer. 2001. "Dominant Party Rule, Opposition Parties, and Minorities in South Africa." *Democratization* 8(1): 161–82.

Glaser, Mishka, and Ann Marie Murphy. 2010. "Patients Versus Patents: Thailand and the Politics of Access to Pharmaceutical Products." *Journal of Third World Studies* 27(1): 215–34.

Global Fund to Fight AIDS, Tuberculosis, and Malaria. 2012. "Fact Sheet." April 30.

Gomes, Fábio. 2011. *Interações Entre o Legislativo e o Executivo Federal do Brasil na Definição de Políticas de Interesse Amplo: uma abordagem sistêmica, com aplicação na saúde.* PhD diss., Universidade do Estado do Rio de Janeiro, Instituto de Estudos Sociais e Políticos.

Gómez, Eduardo. 2016. "Brazil's Health System Suffers as Recession Bites." BBC News, June 5.

Gómez, Eduardo, and Joseph Harris. 2015. "Political Repression, Civil Society, and the Politics of Responding to AIDS in the BRICS Nations." *Health Policy and Planning* 31(1): 56–66.

Gough, Ian, and Geoffrey Wood, eds. 2004. *Insecurity and Welfare Regimes in Asia, Africa, and Latin America.* New York: Cambridge University Press.

Gourevitch, Peter. 1986. *Politics in Hard Times: Comparative Responses to International Economic Crises.* Ithaca, NY: Cornell University Press.

Government Employees Medical Scheme (GEMS). 2015. "Background." Accessed February 4, 2015. Available at http://www.gems.gov.za/default.aspx?vBR48Vf9K NL7jeeIJMpLEXLCY7A8Hh2rirUmN/aKb7k=.

Government of the Republic of South Africa. 1996. Constitution.

Granich, Reuben, et al. 2012. "Expanding ART for Treatment and Prevention of HIV in South Africa: Estimated Cost and Cost-Effectiveness 2011–2050." *PLoS ONE* 7(2): e30206.

Grebe, Eduard. 2011. "The Treatment Action Campaign's Struggle for AIDS Treatment in South Africa: Coalition-Building through Networks." *Journal of Southern African Studies* 37(4): 849–68.

Green, Andrew. 2008. "Reflections on Alma Ata." *Global Social Policy* 8(2): 155–57.

Gruber, Jonathan, Nathaniel Hendren, and Robert Townsend. 2012. "Demand and Reimbursement Effects of Healthcare Reform: Health Care Utilization and Infant Mortality in Thailand." Working Paper 17739. National Bureau of Economic Research.

Grzymala-Busse, Anna. 2007. *Rebuilding Leviathan: Party Competition and State Exploitation in Post-Communist Democracies.* Cambridge: Cambridge University Press.

Gulf News. 2016. "ANC Faces Tough Test in South Africa Local Elections." August 1.

Gumede, William. 2007. *Thabo Mbeki and the Battle for the Soul of the ANC.* New York: Zed Books.

Guthrie, Teresa, Nhlanhla Ndlovu, Farzana Muhib, Robert Hecht, and Kelsey Case. 2010. *The Long Run Costs and Financing of HIV/AIDS in South Africa.* Washington, DC: Results for Development Institute.

Gutiérrez, Ricardo A. 2010. "When Experts Do Politics: Introducing Water Policy Reform in Brazil." *Governance* 23(1): 59–88.

Haas, Peter. 1992. "Epistemic Communities and International Policy Coordination." *International Organization* 46(1): 1–35.

Habib, Adam, and Rupert Taylor. 1999. "South Africa: Anti-Apartheid NGOs in Transition." *Voluntas: International Journal of Voluntary and Nonprofit Organizations* 10(1): 73–82.

Hacker, Jacob. 1998. "The Historical Logic of National Health Insurance." *Studies in American Political Development* 12: 57–130.

———. 2002. *The Divided Welfare State.* Cambridge: Cambridge University Press.

Hafferty, Fred, and John B. McKinlay. 1993. *The Changing Medical Profession: An International Perspective.* Oxford: Oxford University Press.

Haggard, Stephen, and Robert Kaufman. 2008. *Development, Democracy, and Welfare States*. Princeton, NJ: Princeton University Press.

Hagopian, Frances. 1990. "'Democracy by Undemocratic Means'? Elites, Political Pacts, and Regime Transition in Brazil." *Comparative Political Studies* 23(2): 147–70. Harris, Joseph. 2014. "Who Governs? Autonomous Political Networks as a Challenge to Power in Thailand." *Journal of Contemporary Asia* 45(1): 3–25.

——. 2015. "'Developmental Capture' of the State: Explaining Thailand's Universal Coverage Policy." *Journal of Health Politics, Policy, and Law* 40(1): 165–93.

Hassim, Adila. 2008. Head of litigation and legal services, AIDS Law Project. Interview by author, November 16.

Hassim, Adila, Mark Heywood, and J. Berger. 2007. *Health and Democracy: A Guide to Human Rights, Health Law, and Policy in Post-Apartheid South Africa*. West Lake, South Africa: Siber Ink.

Health Policy Coordinating Unit (HPCU). 1995. *Report of a Meeting with Health Policy Groups*. January 19.

Health Policy Sub-Committee. 1991. "Eric Buch, Manto Tshabalala, Mawethu Bam, Hugh Gosnell, and Joan Muller Attending." Minutes. East London, September 21.

Health Systems Trust. 1995. *South African Health Review*. Durban, South Africa: HST.

——. Undated. *Health Care in Other Countries—A Brief Glimpse*.

Health Workers' Organization (HWO). 1988. *Hospital Tariffs Go Up Again!* Health Workers' News.

Hein, Wolfgang, Sonja Bartsch, and Lars Kohlmorgen. 2007. *Global Health Governances and the Fight against HIV/AIDS*. New York: Palgrave Macmillan.

Heller, Patrick. 1999. *The Labor of Development: Workers and the Transformation of Capitalism in Kerala, India*. Ithaca, NY: Cornell University Press.

Hess, David. 2005. "Medical Modernization, Scientific Research Fields, and the Epistemic Politics of Health Social Movements." In *Social Movements in Health*, edited by Phil Brown and Stephen Zavestoski, 17–30. Malden, MA: Blackwell Publishing.

Hewison, Kevin. 1997. *Political Change in Thailand: Democracy and Participation*. New York: Psychology Press.

——. 2010. "Thaksin Shinawatra and the Reshaping of Thai Politics." *Contemporary Politics* 16(2): 119–33.

Heywood, Mark. 2001. "Debunking 'Conglomo-talk': A Case Study of the Amicus Curiae as an Instrument for Advocacy, Investigation and Mobilisation." In *Law, Democracy and Development*. 5(2): 133–62.

——. 2008. Director, AIDS Law Project. October 14. Interview with author.

Hicken, Allen. 2006. "Party Fabrication: Constitutional Reform and the Rise of Thai Rak Thai." *Journal of East Asian Studies* 6(3): 381–408.

Hirschman, Dan, and Elizabeth Berman. 2014. "Do Economists Make Policies? On the Political Effects of Economics." *Socio-Economic Review* 12(4): 779–811.

Hochstetler, Kathryn. 2000. "Democratizing Pressures From Below? Social Movements in the New Brazilian Democracy." In *Democratic Brazil: Actors, Institutions, and Processes,* edited by Peter R. Kingston and Timothy Joseph Power, 157–84. Pittsburgh: University of Pittsburgh Press.

Hoffman, Florian, and Fernando Bentes. 2008. "Accountability for Economic and Social Rights in Brazil." In *Courting Social Justice: Judicial Enforcement of Social and Economic Rights in the Developing World,* edited by Varun Gauri and Daniel M. Brinks, 100–145. Cambridge: Cambridge University Press.

Hoffman, Lily. 1989. *The Politics of Knowledge: Activist Movements in Medicine and Planning*. New York: SUNY Press.

Huber, Evelyn, and John Stephens. 2001. *Development and Crisis of the Welfare State: Parties and Policies in Global Markets*. Chicago: University of Chicago Press.

——. 2012. *Democracy and the Left: Social Policy and Inequality in Latin America*. Chicago: University of Chicago Press.

Hunter, Qaannitah. 2015. "ANC Squirms over Voter Discontent." *Mail and Guardian*, July 31. Accessed August 6, 2015. Available at http://mg.co.za/article/2015-0 7-30-anc-squirms-over-voter-discontent/.

Hunter, Wendy. 2011. "Brazil: The PT in Power." In *The Resurgence of the Latin American Left*, edited by Steven Levitsky and Kenneth M. Roberts, 306–24. Baltimore: Johns Hopkins University Press.

Hunter, Wendy, and Natasha Borges Sugiyama. 2009. "Democracy and Social Policy in Brazil: Advancing Basic Needs, Preserving Privileged Interests." *Latin American Politics and Society* 51(2): 29–58.

Iliffe, John. 2006. *A History of the African AIDS Epidemic*. Oxford: James Currey Ltd.

Immergut, Ellen. 1992. *Health Politics: Interests and Institutions in Western Europe*. Cambridge: Cambridge University Press.

Innovative Medicines South Africa. 2011. "Myths About Medical Schemes." National Health Insurance Policy Brief 21.

Jinabhal, Noddy. 1989. "Development of a Strategy for Primary Health Care in South Africa." *Proceedings from Second National Consultation*, September.

Joffey, Carole, Tracy Weitz, and Claire Stacey. 2005. "Uneasy Allies: Pro-Choice Physicians, Feminist Health Activists, and the Struggle for Abortion Rights." In *Social Movements in Health*, edited by Phil Brown and Stephen Zavestoski, 94–114. Malden, MA: Blackwell Publishing.

Johnson, R. W. 2009. "The ANC's Health Lesson for Obama." *Standpoint Magazine*, September 9. Available at http://www.standpointmag.co.uk/node/2061.

Joint United Nations Programme on HIV/AIDS (UNAIDS). 2016. *Fact Sheet 2016*. Geneva: UNAIDS.

Joint Working Group for Health Policy. 1991. *Proposal for a Joint Policy Program*, December 10.

Jongudomsuk, Pongpisut. 2009. Director, Health Systems Research Institute. Interview by author, March 4.

Kahn, Tamar. 2014. "Doctors too Greedy for NHI, Says Motsoaledi." *Business Day*, March 6.

Kane, Leslie, and Carol Peckham. 2014. *Medscape Physician Compensation Report 2014*. Presentation. Accessed April 15. Available at http://www.medscape.com/ features/slideshow/compensation/2014/public/overview.

Kaplan, Karyn, and Paisan Suwannawong. 2009. Thai Treatment Action Group officials. Interview by author, April 10.

Kapp, Claire. 2009. "Barbara Hogan: South Africa's Minister of Health." *The Lancet* (373): 291.

Kapstein, Ethan, and Busby, Joshua. 2013. *AIDS Drugs for All: Social Movements and Market Transformations*. New York: Cambridge University Press.

Kasza, Gregory. 2006. *One World of Welfare*. Ithaca, NY: Cornell University Press.

Kaufman, Robert, and Joan Nelson. 2004. *Crucial Needs, Weak Incentives: Social Sector Reform, Democratization, and Globalization in Latin America*. Washington, D.C.: Woodrow Wilson Center Press.

Kaufman, Robert, and Alex Segura-Ubiergo. 2001. "Globalization, Domestic Politics, and Social Spending in Latin America: A Time-Series Cross-Section Analysis, 1973–97." *World Politics* 53(4): 553–87.

Keck, Margaret. 1992. *The Workers' Party and Democratization in Brazil*. New Haven: Yale University Press.

Keck, Margaret, and Kathryn Sikkink. 1998. *Activists Beyond Borders*. Ithaca, NY: Cornell University Press.

Kepp, Michael. 2008. "Cracks Appear in Brazil's Primary Health-Care Programme." *The Lancet* 372: 877.

Khazan, Olga. 2014. "What the U.S. Can Learn from Brazil's Healthcare Mess." *The Atlantic*, May 8.

Khumalo, Gene. 2012. "South Africa Pilots National Health." *BuaNews*, March 23.

Khwankhom, Arthit, and Nerisa Noeykhiew. 2002. "Doctors Give Two Months." *The Nation*, November 10.

Khwankhom, Arthit and Usa Shevajumroen. 2003. "Doctors revolt." *The Nation.* January 17.

Kiatyingungsulee, Niyada. 2009. Professor, Faculty of Pharmacy, Chulalongkorn University. Interview by the author. May 11.

Kijtiwatchakul, Kannikar. 2007. *The Rights to Life*. Bangkok: Médecins Sans Frontières-Belgium; Pharmacy Network for Health Promotion; Thai Health Promotion Foundation; Third World Network.

——. 2009. Access Campaigner, Médecins Sans Frontières. June 5. Interview with author.

Kijtiwatchakul, Kannikar, and Uayporn Daechutragun. 2007. *Iik Gaaw Thii Glaa Khong Mor Khii Maa Klap* (The biography of Dr. Mongkol na Songkhla). In Thai. Bangkok: Penthai Publishing.

Kingdon, John. 1984. *Agendas, Alternatives, and Public Policies*. Boston: Little, Brown.

Kitschelt, Herbert P. 1986. "Political Opportunity Structures and Political Protest: Anti-Nuclear Movements in Four Democracies." *British Journal of Political Science* 16(1): 57–85.

Klandermans, Bert. 2015. "Movement Politics and Party Politics in Times of Democratic Transition: South Africa, 1994–2000." In *Movements in Times of Democratic Transitions*, edited by Bert Klandermans and Cornelis van Stralen, 241–58. Philadelphia: Temple University Press.

Klopper, J. M. 1986. "Towards a National Health Service for South Africa." *South African Medical Journal* 70(5): 293–95.

Klug, Heinz. 2008. "Law, Politics, and Access to Essential Medicines in Developing Countries." *Politics and Society* 36(2): 207–46.

Korpi, Walter. 1983. *The Democratic Class Struggle*. London: Routledge.

Krasner, Stephen D., Eric Nordlinger, Clifford Geertz, Stephen Skowronek, Charles Tilly, Raymond Grew, and Ellen Kay Trimberger. 1984. "Approaches to the State: Alternative Conceptions and Historical Dynamics." *Comparative Politics* 16(2): 223–46.

Krücken, Georg, and Gili Drorik, ed. 2009. *World Society: The Writings of John W. Meyer*. Oxford: Oxford University Press.

Kuanpoth, Jakkrit, Jiraporn Limpananont, Kingkorn Narintarakul, Benja Silarak, Supanee Taneewuth, Witoon Lianchamroon, Jacques-chai Chomthongdi, Saree Aongsomwang, and Niramon Yuwanaboon. 2005. *Free Trade Agreements: Impact in Thailand*. Nonthaburi, Thailand: FTA Watch.

Kudamatsu, Masayuki. 2012. "Has Democratization Reduced Infant Mortality in Sub-Saharan Africa? Evidence from Micro Data." *Journal of the European Economic Association* 10(6): 1294–1317.

Kuhonta, Erik. 2008. "The Paradox of Thailand's 1997 'People's Constitution': Be Careful What You Wish For." *Asian Survey* 48(3): 373–92.

Kwon, Oh-Jung. 2011. "The Logic of Social Policy Expansion in a Neoliberal Context: Health Insurance Reform in Korea After the 1997 Economic Crisis." *Theory and Society* 40: 645–67.

Lamboray, Jean-Louis. 2009. Co-Founder of UNAIDS. Interview by the author. October 2.

Larson, Magali. 1977. *The Rise of Professionalism: A Sociological Analysis*. Berkeley: University of California Press.

Larvie, Sean Patrick. 1998. *Managing Desire: Sexuality, Citizenship, and AIDS in Contemporary Brazil*. PhD diss., University of Chicago.

Leechanavanichaphan, Rakawin. 2009. Civil society activist and ILO officer. Interview by author, October 27.

Lenski, Gerhard E. 1966. *Power and Privilege: A Theory of Social Stratification*. Chapel Hill: University of North Carolina Press.

Lertsuridej, Prommin. 2009. Former Thai Rak Thai executive. Interview by author, May 7.

Lewis, Maureen, and Andre Medici. 1998. "Health Care Reform in Brazil." In *Do Options Exist? The Reform of Pension and Health Care Systems in Latin America*, edited by Maria Amparo Cruz-Saco and Carmelo Mesa-Lago, 267–92. Pittsburgh: University of Pittsburgh Press.

Lieberman, Evan. 2009. *Boundaries of Contagion: How Ethnic Politics Have Shaped Government Responses to AIDS*. Princeton, NJ: Princeton University Press.

Light, Donald. 2010. "Health-Care Professions, Markets and Countervailing Powers." In *Handbook of Medical Sociology*, edited by Chloe E. Bird, Peter Conrad, Allen M. Fremont, and Stefan Timmermans, 270–89. Nashville: Vanderbilt University Press.

Limpananont, Jiraporn. 2005. "EFTA-Thailand FTA: Access to Medicines and TRIPS." Presentation at 1st Technical Advisory Group for Improving Access to Essential Medicines in the Western Pacific Region 2005–2010, November 14–15.

——. 2009. Associate professor, Faculty of Social Pharmacy, Chulangkorn University. Interview by author, April 7.

Limpananont, Jiraporn, Achara Eksaengsri, Kannikar Kijtiwatchakul, and Noah Metheny. 2009. "Access to AIDS Treatment and Intellectual Property Rights' Protection in Thailand." In *Intellectual Property Rights and Access to ARV Medicines: Civil Society Resistance in the Global South: Brazil, Colombia, China, India, and Thailand*, edited by Renata Reis, Veriano Terto Jr., and Maria Cristina Pimenta, 137–63. Rio de Janeiro: ABIA.

Lipset, Seymour. 1959. "Some Social Requisites of Democracy: Economic Development and Political Legitimacy." *American Political Science Review* 53(1): 69–105.

Lo, Ming-Cheng. 2005. "The Professions: Prodigal Daughters of Modernity." *Remaking Modernity: Politics, History, and Sociology*. Durham, NC: Duke University Press.

Lodge, Tom. 2004. "The ANC and the Development of Party Politics in Modern South Africa." *Journal of Modern African Studies* 42(2): 189–219.

Lohmann, Larry. 1986. "Primary Health Care and People's Movements." *Thai Development Newsletter* 4(2).

Loos, Tamara. 2009. "Introduction." In *Cocktail*, edited by Vince LiCata and Ping Chong. Chiang Mai, Thailand: Silkworm Books.

——. 2015. "Dilemmas of Development: Dr. Krisana Kraisintu's Praxis in Asia and Africa." In *Modernities: Sites, Concepts, and Temporalities in Asia and Europe*, edited by Arif Dirlik, 215–57. New York: SUNY Press.

Macedo, Eloisa Israel de, Luciane Cruz Lopes, and Silvio Barberato-Filho. 2011. "A Technical Analysis of Medicines Request-Related Decision Making in Brazilian Courts." *Revista de Saúde Pública* 45(4): 706–13.

Macinko, James, Frederico C. Guanais, and Maria De Fátima Marinho De Souza. 2006. "Evaluation of the Impact of the Family Health Program on Infant Mortality in Brazil, 1990–2002." *Journal of Epidemiology and Community Health* 60(1): 13–19.

Macinko, James, Inês Dourado, Rosana Aquino, Palmira de Fátima Bonolo, Maria Fernanda Lima-Costa, Maria Guadalupe Medina, Eduardo Mota, Veneza Berenice de Oliveira, and Maria Aparecida Turci. 2010. "Major Expansion of Primary Care in Brazil Linked to Decline in Unnecessary Hospitalization." *Health Affairs* 29(12): 2149–60.

Macinko, James, and Matthew Harris. 2015. "Brazil's Family Health Strategy—Delivering Community-Based Primary Care in a Universal Health System." *New England Journal of Medicine* 372(23): 2177–81.

Magnussen, Lesley, John Ehiri, and Pauline Jolly. 2004. "Comprehensive Versus Selective Primary Health Care: Lessons for Global Health." *Health Affairs* 23(3): 167–76.

Mail and Guardian. 1999. "The Judge Who Lives with AIDS." Last modified April 23. Available at http://mg.co.za/article/1999-04-23-the-judge-who-lives-with-aids.

———. 2010a. "SAIRR Warns against National Health Insurance." June 28.

———. 2010b. "Union Says Foreign Doctors Needed for NHI." September 29.

———. 2011a. "Budget Takes First Steps in Establishing NHI." February 23.

———. 2011b. "Mandatory NHI payments on cards." August 12.

———. 2011c. "NHI to be Passed in 2012, Says Health Minister." February 22.

———. 2014. "Zuma Promises to Go Ahead with Free Health Delivery. Accessed June 14, 2015. Available at http://africajournalismtheworld.com/tag/south-africa-health-service/.

———. 2016. "Editorial: Disarray Bodes Ill for NHI." January 22.

Mainwaring, Scott. 1986. "The Transition to Democracy in Brazil." Working Paper No. 66. Helen Kellogg Institute for International Studies. March.

———. 1987. "Urban Popular Movements, Identity, and Democratization in Brazil." *Comparative Political Studies* 20(2): 131–59.

———. 1988. "Political Parties and Democratization in Brazil and the Southern Cone." *Comparative Politics* 21(1): 91–120.

———. 1989. "Grass-Roots Catholic Groups and Politics in Brazil." In *The Progressive Church in Latin America,* edited by Scott Mainwaring, 151–92. Terre Haute, IN: Notre Dame Press.

———. 1998. "Electoral Volatility in Brazil." *Party Politics* 4(4): 523–45.

Makgetla, Neva. 2008. Lead economist, Development Bank of South Africa. Interview by author, October 20.

Malan, Mia. 2011. "NHI: Behind the Proposals." *Mail and Guardian,* July 22.

Malloy, James. 1979. *The Politics of Social Security in Brazil.* Pittsburgh: University of Pittsburgh Press.

Mandela, Nelson. 1998. Speech by President Nelson Mandela at the Opening of the Sangoni Clinic. Accessed January 24, 2015. Available at http://www.anc.org.za/show.php?id=2982.

Mapumulo, Zinhle. 2016. "Service Delivery Protests Intensifying in Run-Up to the Election." *City Press,* June 3.

Mares, Isabela. 2003. *The Politics of Social Risk: Business and Welfare State Development.* Cambridge: Cambridge University Press.

Marks, Sheila. 1988. "The Historical Origins of National Health Services." In *Towards a National Health Service: Proceedings of the 1987 NAMDA Conference*, edited by Peter Owen. Cape Town: NAMDA.

Marrian, Natasha. 2014. "NUM and ANC: The Price of Loyalty." *Financial Mail*, July 3. Accessed August 10, 2014. Available at http://www.financialmail.co.za/coverstory/2014/07/03/num-anc-the-price-of-loyalty.

Marshall, Thomas H. 1950. *Citizenship and Social Class*. Cambridge: Cambridge University Press.

Martel-García, Fernando. 2014. "Democracy Is Good for the Poor: A Procedural Replication of Ross (2006)." *Research and Politics* 1(3): 1–10.

Massard da Fonseca, Elize. 2015. *The Politics of Pharmaceutical Policy Reform: A Study of Generic Drug Regulation in Brazil*. Cham, Switzerland: Springer International Publishing.

Matsoso, Precious. 2013. "National Health Insurance: The First 18 Months." *South African Medical Journal* 103(3). Accessed November 15, 2014. Available at http://www.samj.org.za/index.php/samj/article/view/6601/4920.

Mattes, Robert. 2002. "South Africa: Democracy Without the People?" *Journal of Democracy* 13(1): 22–36.

Maxwell, William. 1975. "Modernization and Mobility into the Patrimonial Medical Elite in Thailand." *American Journal of Sociology* 81(3): 465–90.

McAdam, Douglas, John McCarthy, and Mayer Zald. 1996. *Comparative Perspectives on Social Movements: Political Opportunities, Mobilizing Structures, and Cultural Framings*. Cambridge: Cambridge University Press.

McCann, M. 2006. "Law and Social Movements: Contemporary Perspectives." *Annual Review of Law and Social Science* 2: 17–38.

McCargo, Duncan. 1997. "Thailand's Political Parties: Real, Authentic, Actual?" in *Political Change in Thailand: Democracy and Participation*, edited by Kevin Hewison, 114–31. New York: Psychology Press.

——. 2001. "Populism and Reformism in Contemporary Thailand." *South East Asia Research* 9(1): 89–107.

——. 2002. *Reforming Thai Politics*, edited by Duncan McCargo, 183–89. Copenhagen: Nordic Institute of Asian Studies.

——. 2003. "Balancing the Checks: Thailand's Paralyzed Politics Post-1997." *Journal of East Asian Studies* 3(1): 129–52.

——. 2005. "Network Monarchy and Legitimacy Crises in Thailand." *Pacific Review* 18(4): 499–519.

McCargo, Duncan, and Ukrist Pathmanand. 2005. *Thaksinization of Thailand*. Copenhagen: NIAS Press.

McCarthy, Kieren. 2016. "European Human Rights Court Rules Mass Surveillance Illegal." *The Register*, January 20.

McCoy, David, and Solani Khosa. 1996. "'Free Health Care' Policies." In *South African Health Review 1996*, edited by David Harrison. Durban: Health Systems Trust.

McGroarty, Patrick. 2015. "South Africa Unemployment Hits 11-Year High." *Wall Street Journal*, May 26. Accessed on August 1, 2015. Available at http://www.wsj.com/articles/south-africa-unemployment-hits-11-year-high-1432640795.

McGuire, James. 2010. *Wealth, Health, and Democracy in East Asia and Latin America*. New York: Cambridge University.

——. 2013. "Political Regime and Social Performance." *Contemporary Politics*. 19(1): 55–75.

McIntyre, Di, Jane Doherty, and Lucy Gilson. 2003. "A Tale of Two Visions: The Changing Fortunes of Social Health Insurance in South Africa." *Health Policy and Planning* 18(1): 47–58.

McIntyre, Di, and Alex van den Heever. 2007. "Social or National Health Insurance." In *South African Health Review 2007,* edited by Stephen Harrison, Rakshika Bhana, Antoinette Ntuli, J. Roma-Reardon, J. Day, and P. Barron. Durban: Health Systems Trust.

McKinley, Dale. 2001. "Democracy, Power, and Patronage: Debate and Opposition within the African National Congress and the Tripartite Alliance since 1994." *Democratization* (8)1: 183–206.

Melamed, Clarice. 2011. "Regulamentação, Produção de Serviços e Financiamento Federal do Sistema Único de Saúde: Dos Años 90 aos 2000." In *Políticas Públicas e Financiamento Federal do Sistema Único de Saúde,* edited by Clarice Melamed and Sérgio Piola, 59–84. S. F. Brasília: IPEA.

Melo, Marcus. 1993. "Anatomia do Fracasso: Intermediacao de Interesses e a Reforma das Políticas Sociais na Nova Republica." *Dados e Revista de Ciencias Sociais* 36(1): 119–63.

Messeder, Ana Marcia, Claudia Garcia Serpa Osorio-de-Castro, and Vera Lucia Luiza. 2005. "Mandados Judiciais Como Ferramenta Para Garantia do Acesso a Medicamentos No Setor Público: A Experiencia do Estado do Rio de Janeiro, Brasil." *Cadernos de Saude Pública* 21(2): 525–34.

Ministerial Task Team on Social Health Insurance. 2005. *Social Health Insurance Options: Financial and Fiscal Impact Assessment.* Pretoria: Government of South Africa.

Ministry of Health. 2006. "IDB 2006 – Brasil – Indicadores e Dados Basicos para a Saude." *annual:* MS, RIPSA.

Ministry of Public Health and National Health Security Office. 2008. *The Ten Burning Questions on the Government Use of Patents on the Four Anti-Cancer Drugs in Thailand.* Nonthaburi, Thailand: MOPH and NHSO.

Missingham, Bruce. 2003. *The Assembly of the Poor in Thailand: From Local Struggles to National Protest Movement.* Chiang Mai, Thailand: Silkworm Books.

Mitchell, Timothy. 1991. "The Limits of the State: Beyond Statist Approaches and Their Critics." *American Political Science Review* 85(1): 77–96.

Mji, D., K. S. Chetty, H. M. Coovadia, and C. P. Owen. 1989. "NAMDA Responds." Letter to the Editor. *Canadian Medical Association Journal* 140(2): 115.

Monama, Tebogo, and Jennifer Jordaan. 2016. "Zuma Wants Six Months as a Dictator." *IOL,* July 21.

Monamodi, Isaac Seboko. 1996. *Medical Doctors under Segregation and Apartheid: A Sociological Analysis of Professionalization among Doctors in South Africa, 1900–1980.* PhD diss., Indiana University.

Moodley, Keymanthri, and Sharon Kling. 2015. "Dual Loyalties, Human Rights Violations, and Physician Complicity in Apartheid South Africa." *AMA Journal of Ethics* 17(10): 966–72.

Moore, Barrington. 1966. *Social Origins of Dictatorship and Democracy: Lord and Peasant in the Making of the Modern World.* Boston: Beacon Press.

Moyle, Didi. 2015. *Speaking Truth to Power: The Story of the AIDS Law Project.* Johannesburg: Jacana Media.

Mustago, Bernard. 2008. "National Health Insurance (NHI) for South Africa: Beyond Definitions." *SAMA Insider,* October.

Nance, Earthea. 2013. *Engineers and Communities: Transforming Sanitation in Contemporary Brazil.* Lanham: Rowman & Littlefield.

Na Songkhla, Mongkol. 2009. Former Permanent Secretary and Minister of Public Health. Interview by author, May 12.

Nam, Illan. 2015. *Democratizing Health Care: Welfare State Building in Korea and Thailand.* New York: Palgrave Macmillan.

National Medical and Dental Association (NAMDA). 1990. Summary of Details for the Maputo Conference.

National News Bureau of Thailand. 2008. "Rural Doctors Society Chairman Challenges Public Health Minister for Televised Debate on CL Changes." March.

National Progressive Primary Health Care Network (NPPHCN). 1989. *Second National Conference Document*. Durban, South Africa, January 27–28.

——. 1991. Summary Report to Organizations on the Workshop Held to Prepare Progressive Health Organizations' Views on Funding Matters and Other Matters Related to the IDT, June 22–23.

——. Undated a. Brochure. Johannesburg: NPPHCN.

——. Undated b. Brochure. Johannesburg: NPPHCN.

National Statistical Office. 1979. *Report of the Socio-Economic Survey 1975/6*. Bangkok, Thailand.

Nattrass, Nicoli. 2004. *The Moral Economy of AIDS in South Africa*. New York: Cambridge University Press.

——. 2012. *The AIDS Conspiracy: Science Fights Back*. New York: Columbia University Press.

Ncayiyana, Daniel. 1998. "MASA Is Dead—Long Live the South African Medical Association!" *South African Medical Journal* 88(7).

Nelson, Joan. 2001. "The Politics of Pension and Health-Care Reforms in Poland and Hungary." In *Reforming the State*, edited by Janos Kornai and Stephan Haggard. Cambridge: Cambridge University Press.

Nelson, Joan, and Robert Kaufman. 2004. *Crucial Needs, Weak Incentives*. Baltimore: Johns Hopkins University Press.

Nelson Mandela Foundation. 2015. "Biography of Nelson Mandela." Accessed January 26, 2015. Available at http://www.nelsonmandela.org/content/page/biography.

Neser, Christian. 1989. "Should Canadians Support NAMDA or MASA?" *Canadian Medical Association Journal* (140)2: 115.

Niedzwiecki, Sara. 2014. "The Effect of Unions and Organized Civil Society on Social Policy: Pension and Health Reforms in Argentina and Brazil, 1988–2008." *Latin American Politics and Society* 56(4): 22–48.

Nitayarumphong, Sanguan. 2006. *Struggling Along the Path to Universal Health Care for All*. Bangkok: National Health Security Office.

——. 2008. *Ngaan Gap Udomgaankoti Khong Chiwit* (My work and ideology in life). In Thai. Bangkok: National Health Security Office.

Nolen, Stephanie. 2008. *Twenty-Eight Stories of AIDS in Africa*. New York: Walker Publishing Company, Inc.

Nontharit, Wut. 2002. "Rally Planned after Senate Passes Health Bill." *Bangkok Post*, September 1.

Nordling, Linda. 2016. "South Africa Ushers in a New Era for HIV." *Nature*, July 14.

North, Douglass. 1990. *Institutions, Institutional Change, and Economic Performance*. Cambridge: Cambridge University Press.

Nunn, Amy. 2009. *The Politics and History of AIDS Treatment in Brazil*. New York: Springer.

Nunn, Amy, E. Da Fonseca, and Sofia Gruskin. 2009. "Changing Global Essential Medicines Norms to Improve Access to AIDS Treatment: Lessons from Brazil." *Global Public Health* (4)2: 131–49.

O'Brien, Kevin, and Lianjiang Li. 2006. *Rightful Resistance in Rural China*. Cambridge: Cambridge University Press.

Ocké-Reis, Carlos Octávio. 2012. *SUS: o Desafio de Ser Único*. Rio de Janeiro: FIOCRUZ.

Ocké-Reis, Carlos Octávio, and Theodore R. Marmor. 2010. "The Brazilian National Health System: An Unfulfilled Promise?" *International Journal of Health Planning and Management* 25(4): 318–29.

Ockey, James. 2004. *Making Democracy*. Honolulu: University of Hawaii Press.

O'Donnell, Guillermo. 1988. "Challenges to Democratization in Brazil." *World Policy Journal* 5(2): 281–300.

Okie, Susan. "Fighting HIV – Lessons from Brazil." *New England Journal of Medicine* 354(19): 1977–81.

Olsen, Tricia D., and Aseema Sinha. 2013. "Linkage Politics and the Persistence of National Policy Autonomy in Emerging Powers: Patents, Profits, and Patients in the Context of TRIPS Compliance." *Business and Politics* 15(3): 323–56.

Ondam, Bantorn. 2004. "The Thai NGO Movement on Health." In *The NGO Way: Perspectives and Experiences from Thailand,* edited by Shin'ichi Shigetomi and Kasīan Tēchaphīra. Chiba, Japan: IDES-JETRO.

Ongsomwang, Saree. 2009. Secretary-General, Foundation for Consumers. Interview by author, June 11.

Onishi, Norimitsu. 2014. "In South Africa, A.N.C. is Counting on the Past." *New York Times,* May 5.

Overy, Neil. 2011. *In the Face of Crisis: The Treatment Action Campaign Fights Government Inertia with Budget Advocacy and Litigation.* International Budget Partnership Study No. 7, August.

Page, Thomas. 2015. "After a 70 Year Wait, Is Universal Healthcare Finally Coming to South Africa?" *CNN,* September 22. Available at http://www.cnn.com/2015/09/21/africa/south-africa-nhi-universal-health-care/.

Paim, Jairnilson, Claudia Travassos, Celia Almeida, Ligia Bahia, and James Macinko. 2011. "The Brazilian Health System: History, Advances, and Challenges." *The Lancet* 377:1778–97.

Pannarunothai, Supasit. 2009. Dean, Naresuan School of Medicine. Interview by author, April 30.

Parker, Faranaaz. 2010. "NHI Will Cost Same as Current Healthcare." *Mail and Guardian,* September 10.

Parker, Richard. 1994. "Public Policy, Political Activism, and AIDS in Brazil." In *Global AIDS Policy,* edited by Douglas Feldman. Westport, CT: Greenwood Publishing.

——. 2003. "Building the Foundations for the Response to HIV/AIDS in Brazil: The Development of HIV/AIDS Policy, 1982–1996." *Divulgação em Saúde para Debate,* August 27, 143–83.

——. 2007. "From the Ground Up: Solidarity, Citizenship, and the Response to HIV and AIDS in Brazil." Paper presented at the Conference on Values and Experience in Global Health. May. Harvard University.

Parker, Richard, and Veriano Terto, eds. 2001. *Solidariedade: A ABIA na Virada do Milênio.* ABIA: Rio de Janeiro.

Parliament of the Republic of South Africa. 2013. "How a Law is Made." Accessed February 10, 2012. Available at http://www.parliament.gov.za/live/content.php?Item_ID=1843.

Paton, Carol. 2009. "Left-Hand Drive." *Financial Mail,* July 2009.

Peacock, Dean, Thokozile Budaza, and Alan Greig. 2008. "The Treatment Action Campaign's Activism." In *HIV/AIDS and Society in South Africa,* edited by Angela Ndinga-Muvumba and Robyn Pharaoh, 85–102. Scottsville: University of KwaZulu-Natal Press.

Pear, Robert. 2007. "Bill to Let Medicare Negotiate Drug Prices Is Blocked." *New York Times,* April 18.

Pelser, A. J., C. G. Ngwena, and J. V. Summerton. 2004. "The HIV/AIDS Epidemic in South Africa: Trends, Impacts and Policy Responses." In *Health and Health Care in South Africa,* edited by H. C. J. van Rensburg, 276–315. Hatfield, South Africa: Van Schaik.

People's Health Movement, Medact, Medicao International, Third World Network, Health Action International, and ALAMES. 2014. *Global Health Watch Vol. 4.* London: Zed Books.

Phatharathananunth, Somchai. 2006. *Civil Society and Democratization: Social Movements and Northeast Thailand.* Copenhagen: NIAS Press.

Phongpaichit, Pasuk, and Chris Baker. 2004. *Thaksin: The Business of Politics in Thailand.* Chiang Mai, Thailand: Silkworm Books.

Phromkaew, Natthapat. 2015. "Rajata and Deputy Face Probe over 'Power Abuse.'" *The Sunday Nation,* June 28.

Pick, W., J. W. B. Claassen, C. A. Le Grange, and G. D. Hussey. 2012. "Health Activism in Cape Town: A Case Study of the Health Workers Society." *South African Medical Journal* 102(6): 403–5.

Picq, Manuela Lavinas. 2004. *The Politics of Human Rights in Brazil: Imposition of Norms from Without or Innovation from Within?* PhD diss., University of Miami.

Pieterse, Marius. 2008. "Health, Social Movements, and Rights-Based Litigation in South Africa." *Journal of Law and Society* 35(3): 364–88.

Pinprateep, Poldej. 2009. Secretary-General, Local Development Institute. Interview by author, March 27.

Pitayarangsarit, Siriwan. 2004. "The Introduction of the Universal Coverage of Health Care Policy in Thailand: Policy Responses." PhD diss., University of London.

Piven, Frances Fox. 2006. *Challenging Authority: How Ordinary People Change America.* Lanham, MD: Rowman and Littlefield.

Politics Web. 2009. "ANC Must End Secrecy Over NHI—DA." Accessed September 15, 2013. Available at http://www.politicsweb.co.za/news-and-analysis/anc-must-end-secrecy-over-nhi--da.

Pongsuphap, Yongyuth. 2007. "Introducing a Human Dimension to Thai Health Care." PhD diss., University of Brussels.

Power, Samantha. 2003. "The AIDS Rebel." *The New Yorker,* May 19.

Prasartset, Suthy, J. Lele, and W. Tettey. 1996. "The Rise of NGOs as Critical Social Movements in Thailand." In *Asia: Who Pays for Growth? Women, Environment and Popular Movements,* edited by Jayant Lele and Wisdom Tettey, 62–75. Brookfield, VT: Dartmouth Publishing Company.

President's Emergency Plan For AIDS Relief (PEPFAR). 2008. "South Africa Country Profile. Available at http://www.pepfar.gov/documents/organization/81668.pdf.

Price, Max. 1989. "Explaining Trends in the Privatization of Health Services in South Africa." *Health Policy and Planning* 4(2): 121–30.

Quadagno, Jill. 2004. "Why the United States Has No National Health Insurance: Stakeholder Mobilization against the Welfare State, 1945–1996." *Journal of Health and Social Behavior* 45: 25–44.

——. 2005. *One Nation, Uninsured: Why the U.S. Has No National Health Insurance.* Oxford: Oxford University Press.

Quinn, Rapin. 1997. *NGOs, Peasants, and the State: Transformation and Intervention in Rural Thailand, 1970–1990.* PhD diss., Australian National University.

Rao, Hayagreeva, Philippe Monin, and Rodolphe Durand. 2003. "Institutional Change in Toque Ville: Nouvelle Cuisine as an Identity Movement in French Gastronomy." *American Journal of Sociology* 108(4): 795–843.

Reich, Michael. 1994. "The Political Economy of Health Transitions in the Third World." In *Health and Social Change in International Perspective,* edited by

Lincoln C. Chen, Arthur Kleinman, and Norma C. Ware, 413–51. Cambridge: Harvard University Press.

Reis, Renata, Marcela Foçaça Vieira, and Gabriela Chaves. 2009. "Access to Medicines and Intellectual Property in Brazil: Reflections and Strategies of Civil Society." In *Intellectual Property Rights and Access to ARV Medicines: Civil Society Resistance in the Global South: Brazil, Colombia, China, India, and Thailand,* edited by Veriano Terto Jr., Renata Reis, and Maria Cristina Pimenta, 12–54. Rio de Janeiro: ABIA.

Report of the Committee of Inquiry into a Comprehensive System of Social Security for South Africa. 2002. *Transforming the Present-Protecting the Future.* Pretoria: Government of South Africa. Accessed March 10, 2008. Available at http://www.cdhaarmann.com/Publications/Taylor%20report.pdf.

Rich, Jessica. 2013. "Grassroots Bureaucracy Intergovernmental Relations and Popular Mobilization around AIDS Policy in Brazil." *Latin American Politics and Society* 55(2): 1–25.

Rich, Jessica, and Eduardo Gómez. 2012. "Centralizing Decentralized Governance in Brazil." *Publius: The Journal of Federalism* 42(4): 636–61.

Robins, Steven, and Christopher Colvin. 2015. "Social Movements after Apartheid: Rethinking Strategies and Tactics in a Time of Democratic Transition." In *Movements in Times of Democratic Transition,* edited by Bert Klandermans and Cornelis van Stralen, 259–80. Philadelphia: Temple University Press.

Rocha, Romero, and Rodrigo Soares. 2010. "Evaluating the Impact of Community-Based Health Interventions: Evidence from Brazil's Family Health Program." *Health Economics* 19(S1): 126–58.

Rodrik, Dani. 1998. "Has Globalization Gone Too Far?" *Challenge* 41(2): 81–94.

Ross, M. 2006. "Is Democracy Good for the Poor?" *American Journal of Political Science* 50(4): 860–74.

Ruangdit, Pradit, and Apiradee Treerutkuerkul. 2008. "Senators Sign Petition over Chaiya." *Bangkok Post,* April 17.

Rudra, Nita. 2002. "Globalization and the Decline of the Welfare State in Less-Developed Countries." *International Organization* 56(2): 411–45.

Rudra, Nita, and Stephen Haggard. 2005. "Globalization, Democracy, and Effective Welfare Spending in the Developing World." *Comparative Political Studies* 38(9): 1015–49.

Rueschemeyer, Dietrich, Evelyne Huber Stephens, and John D. Stephens. 1992. *Capitalist Development and Democracy.* Chicago: University of Chicago Press.

Safreed-Harmon, Kelly. 2008. "Human Rights and HIV/AIDS in Brazil." *GMHC Treatment Issues,* April.

Sajo, Andras. 1993. "The Role of Lawyers in Social Change: Hungary." *Case Western Reserve Journal of International Law* 25(2): 137–46.

Sakboon, Mudawan. 1992. "Campaigning in the Wards." *The Nation,* September.

——. 1999. "The AIDS Battle Takes a Turn for the Worse." *The Nation,* December 1. Reprinted in *Thai Development Newsletter* 37: 13.

——. 2002. "Problems Are 'Decades Old.'" *Bangkok Post,* March 27.

Sakunphanit, Thaworn. 2009. Senior Expert, National Health Security Office. Interview by author, September 28.

Sandbrook, Richard, Marc Edelman, Patrick Heller, and Judith Teichman. 2007. *Social Democracy in the Global Periphery: Origins, Challenges, Prospects.* Cambridge: Cambridge University Press.

Santimataneedol, Ampa. 2003. "Medical Council Calls for Pay Increase for Doctors." *Bangkok Post,* November 12.

Santoro, Wayne A., and Gail M. McGuire. 1997. "Social Movement Insiders: The Impact of Institutional Activists on Affirmative Action and Comparable Worth Policies." *Social Problems* 44: 503–19.

Santos, Alethele Oliveira, Maria Celia Delduque, and Sandra Mara Campos Alves. 2016. "The Three Branches of Government and Financing of the Brazilian Unified National Health System: 2015 in Review." *Cadernos de Saude Publica* 32(1): 1–3.

Sarat, Austin, and Stuart Scheingold. 2006. *Cause Lawyers and Social Movements*. Palo Alto: Stanford University Press.

Scheffer, Mário, Andrea L. Salazar, and Karina B. Grou. 2005. *O Remédio via Justiça: Um Estudo Sobre o Acesso a Novos Medicamentos e Exames em HIV/AIDS no Brasil Por Meio de Ações Judiciais*. Brasília, DF: Ministério da Saúde, Secretaria de Vigilaˆncia em Saúde, Programa Nacional de DST e AIDS.

Scheppele, Kim. 2012. "The New Hungarian Secret Police." *New York Times*, April 19.

Schneider, Helen. 2002. "On the Fault-Line: The Politics of AIDS Policy in Contemporary South Africa." *African Studies* 61(1): 145–67.

Schneider, Helen, and Lucy Gilson. 1999. "The Impact of Free Maternal Health Care in South Africa." In *Safe Motherhood Initiatives: Critical Issues*, edited by Marge Berer and T. K. Sundari Ravindran, 93–101. Oxford: Blackwell Science.

Schönleitner, Günther. 2004. "Can Public Deliberation Democratise State Action? Municipal Health Councils and Local Democracy in Brazil." In *Politicising Democracy: Local Politics and Democratisation in Developing Countries*, edited by John Harriss, Kristian Stokke, and Olle Törnquist. Basingstoke, U.K.: Palgrave Macmillan.

Schrire, Robert. 2001. "The Realities of Opposition in South Africa: Legitimacy, Strategies, and Consequences." *Democratization* 8(1): 135–48.

Schulz-Herzenberg, Collette. 2007. *A Lethal Cocktail: Exploring the Impact of Corruption on HIV/AIDS Prevention and Treatment Efforts in South Africa*. Pretoria: Institute for Security Studies.

Schulz-Herzenberg, Collette, and Roger Southall. 2014. *Election 2014 South Africa: The Campaign, Results, and Future Prospects*. Johannesburg: Jacana Media.

Scott, Richard. 2008. "Lords of the Dance: Professionals as Institutional Agents." *Organization Studies* 29: 219–38.

Seabrooke, Leonard and Wigan, Duncan. 2015. "Powering Ideas through Expertise: Professionals in Global Tax Battles." *Journal of European Public Policy*, 1–18.

Seekings, Jeremy, and Nicoli Nattrass. 2005. *Class, Race, and Inequality in South Africa*. New Haven: Yale University Press.

Seidman, Gay. 1999. "Gendered Citizenship: South Africa's Democratic Transition and the Construction of a Gendered State." *Gender & Society* 13(3): 287–307.

Selway, Joel. 2011. "Electoral Reforms and Public Policy Outcomes in Thailand." *World Politics* 63(1): 165–202.

———. 2015. *Coalitions of the Well-Being: How Electoral Rules and Ethnic Politics Shape Health Policy in Developing Countries*. Cambridge: Cambridge University Press.

Sember, R. 2008. "The Social Construction of ARVs in South Africa." *Global Public Health* 3(S2): 58–75.

Sen, Amartya. 1999. *Development as Freedom*. New York: Alfred A. Knopf.

———. 2015. "Universal Healthcare: The Affordable Dream." *The Guardian*, January 6.

Shadlen, Kenneth. 2009. "The Politics of Patents and Drugs in Brazil and Mexico: The Industrial Bases of Health Policies." *Comparative Politics* 42(1): 41–58.

Shandra, John M., Jenna Nobles, Bruce London, and John B. Williamson. 2004. "Dependency, Democracy, and Infant Mortality: A Quantitative, Cross-National Analysis of Less Developed Countries." *Social Science and Medicine* 59(2): 321–33.

Shankland, Alex, and Andrea Cornwall. 2007. "Realizing Health Rights in Brazil: The Micropolitics of Sustaining Health System Reform." In *Development Success:*

Statecraft in the South, edited by W. McCourt. Basingstoke, U.K.: Palgrave Macmillan.

Shasha, Welile. 2008. Former Country Director, WHO South Africa. Interview by author, October 27.

Shevajumroen, Usa. 2002a. "Bt30 Health Plan Makes Hospitals Miserly." *The Nation,* October 29.

———. 2002b. "Doctors Relent on Defensive Medicine." *The Nation,* September 28.

Shim, Janet. 2014. *Heart-Sick: The Politics of Risk, Inequality, and Heart Disease.* New York: NYU Press.

Siamwalla, Ammar. 2009. Former Director, Thailand Development Research Institute. Interview by author, June 9.

Sidley, Pat. 1994. "Radical Option for Healthcare for All." *Weekly Mail and Guardian,* December 15–23.

Sirikanokvilai, Somjai. 1986. "Primary Health Care and Community Participation: A Case Study of Noan Kui Village." *Thai Development Newsletter* 4(2): 21–26.

Sirisinsuk, Yupadee. 2009. Assistant professor, Social Pharmacy Research Unit, Chulalongkorn University. Interview by author, March 12.

Skidmore, T. E. 1989. "Brazil's Slow Road to Democratization: 1974–1985." In *Democratizing Brazil: Problems of Transition and Consolidation,* edited by Alfred C. Stepan, 5–42. Oxford: Oxford University Press.

Skocpol, Theda. 1979. *States and Social Revolutions.* Cambridge: Cambridge University Press.

———. 1992. *Protecting Soldiers and Mothers.* Cambridge: Belknap Press.

———. 1997. *Boomerang: Health Care Reform and the Turn Against Government.* New York: W. W. Norton.

———. 2003. *Diminished Democracy: From Membership to Management in American Civic Life.* Norman: University of Oklahoma Press.

Skocpol, Theda, and Margaret Somers. 1980. "The Uses of Comparative History in Macrosocial Inquiry." *Comparative Studies in Society and History* 22(2): 174–97.

Somkotra, Tewarit, and Leizel Lagrada. 2008. "Payments for Health Care and Its Effect on Catastrophe and Impoverishment." *Social Science and Medicine* 67(12): 2027–35.

Somsin, Benjawan. 2002. "Senators Unleash 'Monster.'" *The Nation,* September 2.

Soto, Alonso, and Maria Marcello. 2016. "Brazil Seeks 20-Year Spending Cap to Curb National Debt." Reuters. Accessed September 12, 2016. Available at http://www. reuters.com/article/us-brazil-politics-idUSKCN0Z120S.

South African Department of Health. 2006. *National HIV and Syphilis Antenatal Sero-Prevalence Survey in South Africa 2005.* Pretoria: Department of Health.

South African Health and Social Services Organisation (SAHSSO). Undated. *Health for All Brochure.*

South African Health Workers Congress (SAHWCO). 1989a. *The Case for the Expulsion of South Africa from International Psychiatry.* August 4.

———. 1989b. *The Constitutional Guidelines and the Right to Health.*

———. 1990a. *Health and the Constitutional Guidelines,* April.

———. 1990b. *Proposal for Unity in the Health Sector.* Discussion paper.

———. 1991. *Suggested POA for TVL Unity Forum,* May.

South African History Online. 2014. "Professor Hoosen 'Jerry' Mahomed Coovadia." Available at http://www.sahistory.org.za/people/ professor-hoosen-jerry-mahomed-coovadia.

South African Institute of Chartered Accountants (SAICA). 2013. "Medical Tax Credit in Force by SARS." Accessed July 7, 2014. Available at http://www.saica.co.za/

News/NewsArticlesandPressmediareleases/tabid/695/itemid/4215/language/
en-ZA/Default.aspx.

South African Private Practitioners Forum (SAPPF). 2010. "SAPPF Position Statement
Regarding the Re-Establishment of the Specialist Private Practice Committee of
SAMA (SPPC)." SAPPF website.

——. 2011. "Exco." South African Private Practitioners Forum (SAPPF) website. Last
modified August 22, 2011.

Southall, Roger. 2001. "Opposition in South Africa: Issues and Problems."
Democratization 8(1): 1–24.

Starr, Paul. 1982. *Social Transformation of American Medicine*. New York: Basic Books.

Statistics South Africa. 2016. "Facts You Might Not Know about Social Grants."
Accessed August 10, 2016. Available at http://www.statssa.gov.za/?p=7756.

Steinbrook, Robert. 2007. "Thailand and the Compulsory Licensing of Efavirenz." *New
England Journal of Medicine* 356: 544–46.

Steinhoff, Patricia, ed. 2014. *Going to Court to Change Japan: Social Movements and the
Law in Contemporary Japan*. Ann Arbor: Center for Japanese Studies, University
of Michigan.

Stephens, John. 1979. *The Transition from Socialism to Capitalism*. Urbana: University
of Illinois Press.

Suebwonglee, Surapong. 2009. Former deputy minister of public health. Interview by
author, March 13.

Sugiyama, Natasha. 2007. *Ideology and Social Networks: The Politics of Social Policy
Diffusion in Brazil*. PhD diss., University of Texas-Austin.

——. 2008. "Ideology and Networks: The Politics of Social Policy Diffusion in Brazil."
Latin American Research Review 43(3): 82–108.

Supachutikul, Anuwat, and Petchsri Sirinirund. 1993. *A Report on the German-Thai
Health Card Project*. Nonthaburi, Thailand: Ministry of Public Health.

Supakankunti, Siripen, Witanee Phetnoi, and Keiko Tsunekaw. 2004. *Costing of the
National Access to Antiretroviral Program for People Living with HIV and AIDS in
Thailand*. Bangkok: Chulalongkorn University.

Surender, Rebecca, Robert Van Niekerk, Bridget Hannah, Lucie Allan, and Maylene
Shung-King. 2015. "The Drive for Universal Healthcare in South Africa: Views
from Private General Practitioners." *Health Policy and Planning* 30(6): 759–67.

Susanpoolthong, Suwadee. 2001. "House Backs Health Insurance Fund Bill." *Bangkok
Post,* November 23.

Suwanphattana, Niwat, et al. 2008. *From People of Number Zero to a Leader in the
People's Sector: Lessons Learned and the Struggle of PLWHA Networks*. Bangkok:
PLAN Printing.

Swenson, Peter. 2002. *Capitalists against Markets: The Making of Labor Markets and
Welfare States in the United States and Sweden*. Oxford: Oxford University Press.

Tangcharoensathien, Viroj. 2009. Director of International Health Policy Program.
Interview by author, April 8.

Tangcharoensathien, Viroj, Supachutikul Anuwat, and Lertiendumrong Jongkol. 1999.
"The Social Security Scheme in Thailand: What Lessons Can Be Drawn?" *Social
Science and Medicine* 48(7): 913–23.

Tantivess, Sripen, and Gill Walt. 2008. "The Role of State and Non-State Actors in
the Policy Process: The Contribution of Policy Networks to the Scale-Up of
Anti-Retroviral Therapy in Thailand." *Health Policy and Planning* 23: 328–38.

Tarrow, Sidney. 1996. "States and Opportunities: The Political Structuring of Social Move-
ments." *In Comparative Perspectives on Social Movements: Political Opportunities,
Mobilizing Structures, and Cultural Framings,* edited by Doug McAdam, John D.
McCarthy, and Mayer N. Zald, 41–61. New York: Cambridge University Press.

Teixeira, Paulo. 2003. "Universal Access to AIDS Medicines: The Brazilian Experience." *Divulgação em Saúde para Debate* 27: 184–91.

Tendler, Judith. 1997. *Good Government in the Tropics.* Baltimore: Johns Hopkins University Press.

Thabchumpon, Naruemon. 2002. "NGOs and Grassroots Participation in the Political Reform Process." In *Reforming Thai Politics,* edited by Duncan McCargo, 183–89. Copenhagen: Nordic Institute of Asian Studies.

Thai Development Newsletter. 1986a. "The Co-operation between Governmental and Non-Governmental Organizations: An Interview with Dr. Sanguern Nittayaramphong." 4(2).

——. 1986b. "Pharmaceutical Patent Law: Whose Profit?" 3(4): 9.

——. 1987. "Drug Patent and Thai People." 15.

Thai Development Support Committee Staff. 1989. "Thais Meet the Cabinet." *Thai Development Newsletter* 17: 59–62.

——. 1987. "News from the NGOs (Drug Patent and Thai People)." *Thai Development Newsletter* 15: 36.

——. 1993. "Drug Patent Demands From the U.S. 'Unacceptable.'" *Thai Development Newsletter* 22: 69.

——. 1995. "AIDS Group to Petition House Panel on Rights." *Thai Development Newsletter* 29: 67.

——. 1996. "Mystery 'Or' Group Steps Out of the Shadows." *Thai Development Newsletter* 31: 50–52.

Thaiprayoon, Suriwan, and Richard Smith. 2015. "Capacity Building for Global Health Diplomacy: Thailand's Experience of Trade and Health." *Health Policy and Planning* 30(9): 1118–28.

Thanprasertsuk, Sombat. 2009. Former director of Thai AIDS Bureau. Interview by author, September 28.

Thanprasertsuk, S., C. Lertpiriyaswat, and S. Chasombat. 2004. "Developing a National Antiretroviral Programme for People with HIV/AIDS: The Experience of Thailand." In *AIDS in Asia: The Challenge Ahead,* edited by J. P. Narain. New Delhi: WHO,: Regional Office for South-East Asia.

The Economist. 2013. "The Streets Erupt." June 18.

The Nation. 2001. "HIV Drugs Included." December 1.

——. 2002a. "Head-Count Row." May 9.

——. 2002b. "The Two Architects Who Shaped the Low Cost Scheme." April 17.

——. 2006. "Bt30 Health Fee May Scrapped." October 12.

Thomas, Stephen, and Lucy Gilson. 2004. "Actor Management in the Development of Health Financing Reform: Health Insurance in South Africa, 1994–1999." *Health Policy and Planning* 19(5): 279–91.

Thompson, Leonard Monteat. 1995. *A History of South Africa.* New Haven: Yale University Press.

Thulare, Aquina. 2008. Secretary-general, South African Medical Association. Interview by author, December 1.

Timmermans, Stefan, and Hyeyoung Oh. 2010. "The Continued Social Transformation of the Medical Profession." *Journal of Health and Social Behavior* 51(1 Suppl.): S94–S106.

Toms, Ivan. 1990. "AIDS in South Africa: Potential Decimation on the Eve of Liberation." *Progress,* Fall/Winter: 13–16.

Transparency International. 2012. *National Integrity Study 2011.* Accessed August 10, 2016. Available at http://transparency.hu/National_integrtity_study.

Traynor, Ian. 2014. "Budapest Autumn: Hollowing Out Democracy on the Edge of Europe." *The Guardian,* October 29.

Treatment Action Campaign. 2010. *Fighting for Our Lives: The History of the Treatment Action Campaign 1998–2010.* Cape Town: TAC.

Treerutkuarkul, Apiradee. 2008a. "Kidney Patients, NHSO in Subsidy Row." *Bangkok Post,* September 12.

———. 2008b. "The Pursuit of Happiness." *Bangkok Post,* February 2.

———. 2008c. "FDA Chief Removed in Health Shake-Up." *Bangkok Post,* February 27.

———. 2009. "Somsak Leads Team to Keep Grip on Board." *Bangkok Post,* January 22.

Trirat, Nualnoi. 2000. "Two Case Studies of Corruption in Medicine and Medical Supplies Procurement in the Ministry of Public Health (Thailand)." Civil Society and Governance Programme, IDS.

Ubon Ratchathani University. 2015. "Biography Krisana Kraisintu, Ph.D." Available at http://www.ubu.ac.th/krisana_h/bio_en%20_update_.pdf.

Ungpakorn, Jon. 1994. "Human Rights of People with HIV/AIDS Still Violated." *Thai Development Newsletter:* 25.

———. 2009. Founder, TVS and AIDS Access. Interview by author, August 27.

UNAIDS. 2006. South Africa. Available at http://www.unaids.org/en/in+focus/hiv_aids_human_rights.asp

———. 2015. AIDS. Info Online Database. http://www.aidsinfoonline.org/devinfo/libraries/aspx/Home.aspx, accessed 9 January 2015.

United Nations Department of Economic and Social Affairs. 2015. *World Population Prospects.* Interactive Data: Thailand. Available at https://esa.un.org/unpd/wpp/DataQuery/.

United Nations Development Programme (UNDP) et al. 2006. *Free Trade Agreements and Intellectual Property Rights: Implications for Access to Medicine.* Bangkok: UNDP.

Van den Heever, Alex. 2008. Health economist and consultant. Interview by author, November 24.

———. 2011. Evaluation of the Green Paper on National Health Insurance.

———. 2016. "South Africa's Universal Health Coverage Reforms in the Post-Apartheid Period." *Health Policy:* 1–9.

Van der Linde, Ivan. 1995. "Mandates for Mandatory Health Insurance." *South African Medical Journal* 85(8): 722–24.

Van der Vliet, Virginia. 1994. "Apartheid and the Politics of AIDS." In *Global AIDS Policy,* edited by Douglas Feldman, 107–28. Westport, CT: Greenwood Publishing.

———. 2004. "South Africa Divided against AIDS: A Crisis of Leadership." In *AIDS and South Africa: The Social Expression of a Pandemic,* edited by D. L. Lindauer, 48–96. London: Palgrave Macmillan UK.

Van Gunten, Tod. 2015. "Cycles of Polarization and Settlement: Diffusion and Transformation in the Macroeconomic Policy Field." *Theory and Society* 44(4): 321–54.

Van Rensburg, H. C. J., ed. 2004. *Health and Health Care in South Africa.* Hatfield, South Africa: Van Schaik.

Vandome, Christopher. 2016. "South Africa Left in Limbo by Landmark Election Results." *Newsweek,* August 9.

Vathesatogkit, Prakit. 2005. "Funding of the Health Promotion Foundation by Earmarked Taxation: Thailand's Experience." Presentation at the Health Promotion and Tobacco Control Meeting, Taipei, Taiwan, March 30.

Ventura, Miriam. 2003. "Strategies to Promote and Guarantee the Rights of People Living with HIV/AIDS." *Divulgação em Saúde para Debate* 27: 239–46.

Victora, Cesar G., et al. 2011. "Health Conditions and Health-Policy Innovations in Brazil: The Way Forward." *The Lancet* 377(9782): 2042–53.

Vitória, Marco Antônio de Ávila. 2003. "The Experience of Providing Universal Access to ARV Soest Drugs in Brazil." *Divulgação em Saúde para Debate* 27: 247–51.

Von Soest, Christian, and Martin Weinel. 2007. "The Treatment Controversy: Global Health Governance and South Africa's Fight Against HIV/AIDS." In *Global Health Governance and the Fight against HIV/AIDS,* edited by Wolfgang Hein, Sonja Bartsch, and Lars Kohlmorgen, 202–25. New York: Palgrave Macmillan.

Wallee-ittikul, Suradej. 2009. Director, NHSO Bangkok. Interview by author, September 12.

Wampler, Brian, and Leonardo Avritzer. 2004. "Civil Society and New Institutions in Democratic Brazil." *Comparative Politics* 36(3): 291–312.

Wangkiat, Paritta. 2015. "Prayut Shunts Narong to Inactive Post." *Bangkok Post,* March 12.

Wasi, Prawase. 2002. "An Overview of Political Reform Issues." In *Reforming Thai Politics,* edited by Duncan McCargo, 21–28. Copenhagen: Nordic Institute of Asian Studies.

Weekly Mail and Guardian. 1995. "Expensive Cure for a Sick System." June 23–29.

Weber, Max. 1978. *Economy and Society: An Outline of Interpretive Sociology.* Berkeley: University of California Press.

Wetzler, Jennryn. 2007. "Timeline on Brazil's Compulsory Licensing." Program on Information Justice and Intellectual Property, Washington College of Law.

Weyland, Kurt. 1995. "Social Movements and the State: The Politics of Health Reform in Brazil." *World Development* 23(10): 1699–1712.

——. 1996. *Democracy without Equity.* Pittsburgh: University of Pittsburgh Press.

——. 2007. *Bounded Rationality and Policy Diffusion.* Princeton, NJ: Princeton University Press.

Wibulpolprasert, Suwit. 2003. *25 Pii Khabuan Kaanpaet Chonabot Kap Phandin Thai* (25 years of the Rural Doctors' Movement in Thailand.) In Thai. Bangkok: Sangsue Publishing.

——. 2008. Presentation at High-Level Panel. International AIDS Conference. Mexico City, Mexico.

——. 2009. Senior adviser, Ministry of Public Health. Interview by author, February 18.

Wibulpolprasert, Suwit, Vichai Chokevivat, Cecilia Oh, and Inthira Yamabhai. 2011. "Government Use Licenses in Thailand: The Power of Evidence, Civil Movement, and Political Leadership." *Globalization and Health* 7(1): 32.

Wibulpolprasert, Suwit, and Paichit Pengpaibon. 2003. "Integrated Strategies to Tackle the Inequitable Distribution of Doctors in Thailand: Four Decades of Experience." *Human Resources for Health* 1(12).

Wigley, Simon, and Arzu Akkoyunlu-Wigley. 2011. "The Impact of Regime Type on Health: Does Redistribution Explain Everything?" *World Politics* 63(4): 647–77.

Wilensky, Harold. 1975. *The Welfare State and Equality: Structural and Ideological Roots of Public Expenditures.* Berkeley: University of California Press.

Wilkinson, Kate. 2014. "Is the DA's Western Cape Story a 'Good Story to Tell'? We Examine the Claims." *Africa Check,* March 28. Accessed August 21, 2016. Available at https://africacheck.org/reports/is-the-das-western-cape-story-a-g ood-story-to-tell-we-examine-the-claims.

Williams, Paul, and Ian Taylor. 2000. "Neoliberalism and the Political Economy of the 'New' South Africa." *New Political Economy* 5(1): 21–40.

Wines, Michael. 2004. "In South Africa, Democracy May Breed One-Party Rule." *New York Times,* April 14. Accessed August 21, 2016. Available at http://www.nytimes. com/2004/04/14/world/in-south-africa-democracy-may-breed-one-party-rule. html.

Winichakul, Thongchai. 2008. "Toppling Democracy." *Journal of Contemporary Asia* 38(1): 11–37.

Wisartsakul, Weeraboon. 2004. *Civil Society Movement to Revoke the Thai Patent on ddI.* Bangkok: Médecins Sans Frontières Belgium.

Wolfson, Mark. 2001. *The Fight against Tobacco: The Movement, the State, and the Public's Health.* New York: De Gruyter.

Wong, Joseph. 2004. *Healthy Democracies: Welfare Politics in Taiwan and South Korea.* Ithaca, NY: Cornell University Press.

——. 2005. "Adapting to Democracy: Societal Mobilization and Social Policy in Taiwan and South Korea." *Studies in Comparative International Development* 40(3): 88–111.

World Bank. 1993. *World Development Report 1993: Investing in Health.* New York: Oxford University Press.

World Health Organisation. 2008. *Improving Access to Medicines in Thailand: The Use of TRIPS Flexibilities.* Bangkok: NHSO.

——. 2010. *World Health Report 2010: Health Systems Financing—The Path to Universal Coverage.* Geneva: WHO.

——. 2016a. Global Health Observatory Database. Accessed August 3, 2016.

——. 2016b. National Health Accounts Database. Accessed August 3, 2016.

Worth, Katie. 2016. "'Tsunami of Disease' Slams Brazil's Health System." *Frontline,* February 24. Accessed July 29, 2016. Available at http://www.pbs.org/wgbh/ frontline/article/tsunami-of-disease-slams-brazils-health-system/.

Wutipong, Pragrom, et al. 1989. *Health Insurance Systems of Thailand.* Monograph Series No. 6. Bangkok: Mahidol University and Ministry of Public Health.

Youde, Jeremy. 2007. *AIDS, South Africa, and the Politics of Knowledge.* Burlington, VT: Ashgate.

Zille, Helen. 2015. "Premier Helen Zille's State of the Province Address 2015." Accessed August 21, 2016. Available at http://www.westerncape.gov.za/speech/ premier-helen-zilles-state-province-address-2015.

Zurcher, Sacha. 2005. "Public Participation in Community Forest Policy in Thailand." *Geografisk Tidsskrift* 105(1): 77–88.

Zwarenstein, Merrick. 1990. "Is There a Role for the Private Sector in SA Health Care?" *Critical Health* (August): 30–32.

Index

political parties (South Africa)
  Democratic Alliance, 15, 172, 180, 206
  Inkatha Freedom, 102–3
  South African Communist Party (SACP), 6,
    89–90, 103, 112–13, 116, 121, 172, 188
  National Party, 92–93, 101–2, 104, 171,
    173–74
  Economic Freedom Fighters (EFF),
    121, 172
  Congress of the People, 121, 172
  See also ANC (African National Congress)
political parties (Thailand)
  Chart Thai, 56
  Communist Party, 222n2
  Democrat Party, 46, 49, 54, 129
  Palang Mai, 37–38, 223n20
  Palang Tham Party, 55
  Thai Rak Thai, 36, 54–58, 138, 199, 223n23,
    224n22
  See also Shinawatra, Thaksin
Polokwane, 112–13, 116, 191
power-resources explanations of welfare state
    expansion, 19–20
pregnant mother-to-child transmission
    (PMTCT), 14, 132, 170–73, 180–81,
    187–89, 191–92
  See also infant mortality; maternal health
President's Emergency Plan For AIDS Relief
    (PEPFAR), 3, 190
Prince Mahidol Award Conference
    (PMAC), 201
Private Hospital Association, 60, 203
professional movements
  as distinct from identity movements,
    25–26
  durability of, 200–02
  elites and, 4–6, 8–9, 17, 19, 21, 28, 195–96,
    198–99, 211
  elites in Brazil, 73–74, 77–78, 84
  elites in Thailand, 40–41, 45–47, 62
  epistemic communities and, 26–27
  expertification, 24, 126, 152–53, 169
  health workers' unions and, 84, 94
  labor unions and, 4, 19–21
  law and, 7, 15, 148–50, 157, 164–69,
    174–184, 210–11
  Lawyers Collective, 164, 210
  left-wing parties and, 4, 19–21, 29, 157, 198
  mass movements and, 28–29, 195
  strategies of, 25
  trade unions and, 103, 107, 113
  unions and, 67–68, 97, 121, 162
  See also Rural Doctors' movement; *sanitaristas*
  See under apartheid

Program of Internalization of Health and
    Sanitary Actions (PIASS), 69, 74
protests, 4, 211
  in Brazil, 64, 70–71, 162, 165–66, 199, 204
  in South Africa, 104, 121, 180–81, 189, 191, 206
  in Thailand, 45, 47, 60–61, 143
  WTO, 136
  See also mass movements
Provisional Contribution on Financial
    Contributions Tax (CPMF), 81, 205
public health insurance
  See universal coverage; universal coverage
    program; NHI; SUS

race, 192
  See apartheid; health care: racial dynamics of
Ramphele, Mamphela, 103
Reagan, Ronald, 1–2, 93
Reconstruction and Development Programme
    (RDP), 89–90, 105
Rio de Janeiro, 67–68, 157–58, 205
robust competition, 31
Rural Doctors' movement, Thailand, 15, 18,
    35–49
  and elites, 40–41, 45–47, 62
  and international support of, 58–59
  and Ministry of Public Health and, 42–44,
    50, 55
  and opposition to, 59–62
  and Rural Doctors' Society, 36, 40–41, 55,
    128, 130
  and Thai Volunteer Service and, 38, 41–42
  and universal coverage and, 50–58
  Buasai, Supakorn, 50t2.1
  Chokewiwat, Wichai, 40, 50t2.1, 148–49,
    222n2.2, 223n19
  Chuengsatiansup, Komatra, 50t2.1
  Chunharas, Somsak, 50t2.1
  Jindawattana, Amphon, 50t2.1, 52
  Jongudomsuk, Pongpisut, 50t2.1
  Lertsuridej, Prommin, 39, 50t2.1, 55
  na Songkhla, Mongkol, 41, 57–58, 128,
    144–49, 223n24, 227n10
  Nitayarumphong, Sanguan, 35, 37, 50t2.1,
    133, 140–45
  Srivanichakorn, Supattra, 50t2.1
  Suebwonglee, Surapong, 39, 45–46, 54–58
  Tangcharoensathien, Viroj, 38, 41, 43,
    58–59, 62, 139–40, 50t2.1
  Wasi, Prawase, 41–3, 45–47, 50t2.1, 62
  Wibulpolprasert, Suwit, 38, 41, 43–44,
    50t2.1, 57–58, 145, 224n29, 227n6
  See also professional movements
Rwanda, 2

CPSIA information can be obtained
at www.ICGtesting.com
Printed in the USA
LVHW02s1825040918
589119LV00005B/282/P

9 781501 709975